TREATMENT OF ADVANCED STAGE CANCERS

Current Status and Emerging Frontiers

TREATMENT OF ADVANCED STAGE CANCERS

Current Status and Emerging Frontiers

A Symposium Organized by Ranbaxy Science Foundation and the Immunology Foundation

Editors

G.P. Talwar • O.P. Sood

Narosa Publishing House

New Delhi Chennai Mumbai Kolkata

Treatment of Advanced Stage Cancers
Current Status and Emerging Frontiers
248 pgs. | 92 figs. | 17 tbls.

Editors

G.P. Talwar
Talwar Research Foundation
E-8, Neb Valley, Neb Sarai, New Delhi

O.P. Sood
Ranbaxy Science Foundation
20, Sector 18, Udyog Vihar Industrial Area, Gurgaon

NAROSA PUBLISHING HOUSE PVT. LTD.

22, Delhi Medical Association Road, Daryaganj, New Delhi 110 002
35-36 Greams Road, Thousand Lights, Chennai 600 006
306 Shiv Centre, Sector 17, Vashi, Navi Mumbai 400 703
2F-2G Shivam Chambers, 53 Syed Amir Ali Avenue, Kolkata 700 019

www.narosa.com

ISBN 978-81-7319-932-5

Published by N.K. Mehra for Narosa Publishing House Pvt. Ltd.
22, Delhi Medical Association Road, Daryaganj, New Delhi 110 002

Printed in India

Preface

Surgery, Radiations and Chemotherapy are universally employed for treatment of cancers. Depending on the stage at which these intervention are made, the patient may experience complete remission. There are however frequent relapses and a stage arrives in most cancers that oncologists can do no more with the available armamentarium. This Symposium was intended to focus on the Advanced Stage Cancers and to take stock of emerging therapeutic modalities for treating such cancers.

As is usual in such get-togethers of scientists and clinicians , basic findings intermingle with their potential applications.

A major side effect of the available chemotherapeutic drugs is that these act not only against cancer cells but also on normal cells of the body undergoing replication. A major aim of the new therapeutics is to target *selectively* the cancer cells with none or minimal effect on normal healthy cells. Molecules such as Transglutaminase expressed in pancreatic cancers (Chapter 2) or hCG / hCGb expressed ectopically by a number of cancers at advanced stage (when they are believed to assume embryonic stage characteristics) have been identified . These can be targeted by siRNA or by antibodies of high affinity specific to the molecule. Antibodies may exercise cytotoxicity on tumour cells expressing the ligand alone or by ADCC (Antibody dependant cell toxicity). The antibodies could also be used as a vehicle to deliver drugs, toxins (Pseudomonas exotoxin) (Chapter 9) or a totally safe, anti inflammatory and anti cancerous compound, curcumin, to cancer cells resulting in their selective killing without deleterious effect on healthy cells (Chapter 8). The Symposium carries presentations on all these aspects.

Also presented is the possibility of diagnosis of cancers such as Epithelial ovarian cancer by a blood test at an early stage of the cancer improving thereby the chances of effective therapy (Chapter 23). The presence of hCG b in blood/urine in a nonpregnant female or male can again serve as an index of a possible malignancy of the type in which this molecule is expressed ectopically, its disappearance, an index of successful surgery / therapy and its reappearance in circulation, a signal of relapse.

Immune responses appear to play a cardinal role for suppressing / eliminating cells transformed to altered cancerous state. Consequently immunotherapy with antigens presented through competent dendritic cells is an active field of research and early clinical trials are already on to determine safety and efficacy. Chapters 12,14,15 provide valuable insights. Another interesting paper alludes to radiation–enhanced immunotherapy (Chapter 16) and Bhaskar Saha reviews CD40 & cancer therapy.

Leaves of Neem (Azadirachta indicus) contain a glycoprotein modulating more than one type of immune system cells against cancers. Two papers from an active team at Chitranjan National Cancer Institute (Chapters 17,18) describe their interesting studies. The possibility of blocking NFKb & APA –1 pathway by curcumin and the therapeutic action of a polyherbal tablet, Praneem in elimination of HPV 16 and regression of early cancerous changes in women with cervical dysplasia are reported in another interesting paper (Chapter 13).

Besides plants containing immunomodulating compounds, BCG (Bacillus Calmette Guerin) has been employed clinically as adjuvant in Bladder Cancer. Another non-pathogenic fast growing Mycobacterium coded as w earlier, which, has been named recently as Mycobacterium indicus pranii (MIP) shows even better properties as adjuvant. Dr. Dipankar Nandi at the Indian Institute of Science Bangalore & Dr. Om Singh at the National Institute of Immunology New Delhi find that this Mycobacteria has preventive and therapeutic action on cancers in vivo in mice. It clears of course the Bladder carcinoma also. Bakulesh Khamar summarizes these & results of other clinical trials on MIP (Mw) (Chapter 19).

The Symposium started with a Plenary Lecture by the Nobel laureate Dr. David Baltimore. This remarkable lecture was recorded and has been transcribed by Dr. Sunil Mukherjee in a form that the readers can "listen" (and not only read) his presentation. It covers the mechanisms by which immune cells recognize infections (LPS) & respond to it. How the Switch is put "on" and "off" by feedback mechanisms, Micro RNAs & their role in chronic inflammatory response & cancers are elegantly discussed. This presentation is followed by one by Kapil Mehta, wherein siRNA is used therapeutically to silence Transglutaminase expressed in pancreatic cancers. Akhil Banerjea points to the use of novel siRNA to block the carcinogenic transformation brought about by Hepatitis viruses.

It was important to project the moving front of clinical practice. Prof. S.K.Sarin presents the scenario for advanced liver cancer, followed by 2 presentations on treatment of Chronic Myeloid Leukemia. Head & Neck Cancers & metastasis are covered by Ranju Ralhan and Rakesh Kumar. Sukh Mahendre Singh draws attention to the differential role of female and male sex steroids in growth and apoptosis of a T cell lymphoma in mice. The role of sex hormones in prostate & breast cancers is of course well recognized. Subrata Sinha reviews the staging of gliomas, and Ellora Sen draws attention to the role of tumour microenvironment and inflammation in Glioblastoma progression.

This 14th Annual Symposium of Ranbaxy Science Foundation was held on 14-15 January, 2008 at the National Institute of Immunology (NII), New Delhi. It was co-sponsored by the Immunology Foundation. Ranbaxy Science Foundation is a non-profit organization dedicated to the promotion of science in the country by encouraging and rewarding excellence in medical and pharmaceutical sciences and channeling national and international knowledge and expertise. It holds Symposia and Round Table Conferences every year on relevant topics at the forefront of medical sciences and public health.

We do hope that this publication will find a unique place in the currently available scientific literature on the subject.

G.P. Talwar • O.P. Sood

Contents

1
CHAPTER

Micro RNAs and the Inflammatory Response

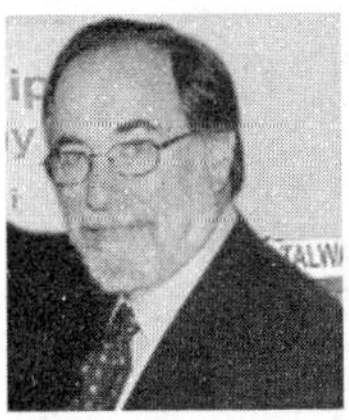

David Baltimore

President Emeritus, Robert Andrews Millikan Professor of Biology, California Institute of Technology, Pasadena, USA

Thank you very much and good morning to you all. It is an honor and a pleasure to be here to kick off this meeting and to honor the awardees, and let me add my congratulations to those of the other speakers on your great achievements and also particularly acknowledge the young people who are awarded, probably their first award in their lives, to honor both their activities and the future that they have in biomedical research. It is a pleasure for me to be in India again. I was here about a month ago. I do not recommend travel like that to anyone but when you do get here, it is always such an exciting time to be in India; the colors, the life of India, it is something I think that any visitor, when they come, responds to in a very positive and very excited way. I actually gave a talk from this podium when I was here in December and what I am telling you about now, is an entirely different part of our laboratory's work.

I originally thought I would talk about NF-kB at some length, but I would not. I use it as an introduction but really focus on microRNAs, as I think this is one of the most exciting new elements of biological control that has come along in many, many years and, although we did not discover them, we have been very excited to learn about the functions of microRNAs and how important they can be in many biological processes. I will focus on the inflammatory response as the major one. I might say that the background here is a picture taken by the Jet Propulsion Laboratory of the mountains that are behind Pasadena, California (Fig. 1.1). Caltech is somewhere down here but not particularly evident in the picture.

This story starts with NF-kB. NF-kB is a transcription factor, a factor that controls the expression of genes, which is found in the cytoplasm of almost all cells and of course, there are no genes in the

email: baltimo@caltech.edu

cytoplasm, so it is there as a reservoir, ready to respond to external stimuli and it maintains its reservoir role by being bound to an inhibitor I-kB and so it is also a dimeric transcription factor with an inhibitor bound to it. The inhibitor keeps it in the cytoplasm, keeps it from binding to DNA, makes it actually totally inert as far as we know, but it can be activated in a lot of different ways but all of them end up chewing up I-kB, getting rid of it, chewing it into pieces and liberating NF-kB to be an active molecule in a cell. This molecule then is recognized by transport proteins, then taken into the nucleus where it finds target genes, and there are many such target genes, hundreds of them, and they do a lot of things to change the nature of the cell. They actually inhibit the apoptosis leading to survival of the cell. They initiate inflammatory responses dealing with infections. They initiate growth responses and start up the proliferation of the cells and they do a lot of specialized things. If the cell happens to be a neuron, they are involved in changing the properties of nerve.

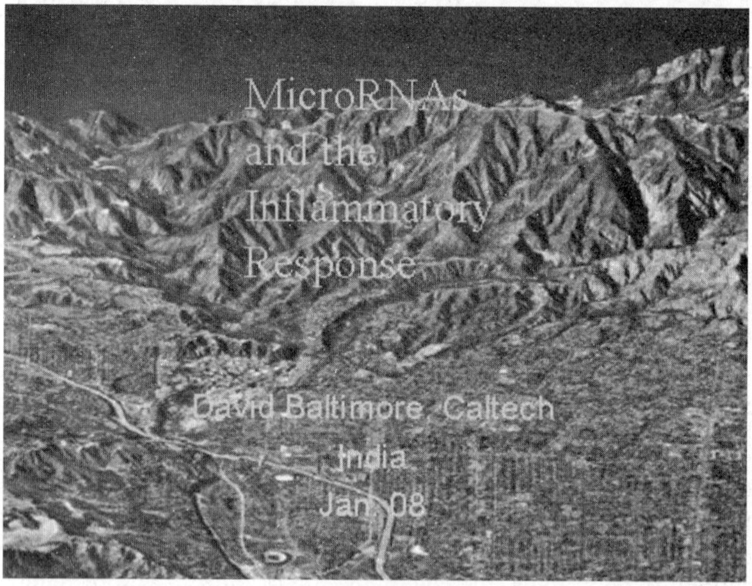

Fig. 1.1

So, what is it that leads to the activation of NF-kB? It is a whole range of stimuli. Many of them known as proinflammatory, tumor necrosis factor, IL-1 as example, some of them link to infection like lipopolysaccharide which comes from bacteria and which the body needs to recognize as an indication of infection, antigens that come from various sources and are recognized on B-cells and T-cells and activate NF-kB, and even noxious stimuli, like UV radiations and oxygen radicals activate NF-kB as well as viruses. So, this single transcription factor is activated by all sorts of noxious stimuli and the idea is to prepare the cell to be part of the body's response to invasion, allowing body to counter the invasion by immune mechanisms, in particular, innate immune mechanisms, and all of this works to the IKK complex, so each one of these little dotted lines is a signal transduction pathway (Fig. 1.2). I will show you a couple of them later, each one being different in the stimuli that I have shown here, but all of them lead to the IKK complex and that complex includes a kinase which phosphorylates IkB and signals its degradation. So, all of this comes down to the phosphorylation of two sides on IkB.

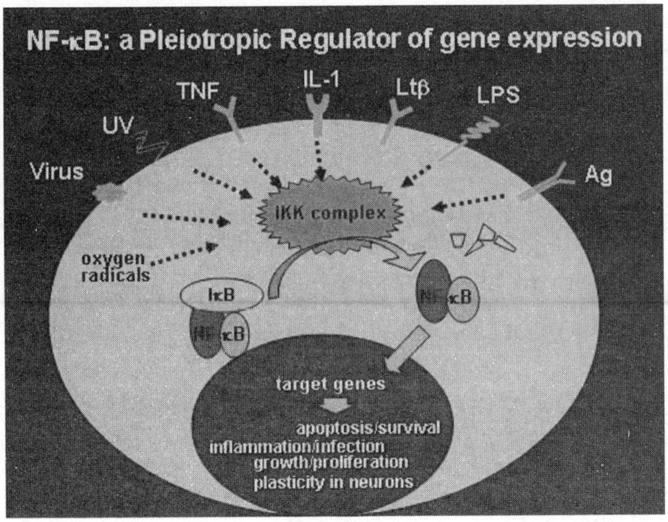

Fig. 1.2

Fig. 1.3 now shows you in much more detail what happens when either lipopolysaccharide or tumor necrosis factor binds to a cell. The lipopolysaccharide receptor called TLR4, changes its configuration, becomes the center for the formation of a complex of proteins and these proteins then send signals into the cell, leading to activation of, for instance, interferon-inducible genes, activation of a variety of elements of the transcriptional machinery. But, they particularly send signals towards the pole of the TAB and TAK complex which then sends signals to the IKK complex which is shown here, which leads, as I said, to the degradation of IkB and the release of NF-kB which is then sent to the nucleus. TNF also forms a complex using different proteins around its intracytoplasmic tail but leads to the activation of the same pathway. So, that is NF-kB and it is something we worked on now for 20 years since we discovered it in the late 1980s and it is the central mediator of the inflammatory response.

So, what is inflammation and why is NF-kB so important? Well, inflammation is really the first line of defense that we have against an infection. It is what the body uses to destroy things that are foreign, to get rid of them; macrophages, neutrophils, all sorts of cells that play roles in getting rid of foreign materials like bacteria and all of that is through NF-kB activation. So, NF-kB gets activated, but anything that causes that level of change in cellular behavior is dangerous because what it is doing is inhibiting a lot of the central functions of the cell and saying we have got to deal with infection now and that is going to be our primary interest. So, once the infection is gone, NF-kB has to go back into place and stay, so that the cell can get on with its business and so, it has to come and it has to go. And there are actually a wide range of inhibitory phenomenon that dampen NF-kB responses so that it can make a major fast response but then over time gets muted.

Why is that? Well, the rest of this slide talks about the dangers of NF-kB and the dangers of inflammation (Fig. 1.4). In many cases, responses to self-antigens occur. Right now, we have been talking about foreign materials and how the body responds to it. Even, self-antigens can activate NF-kB but this is now an inappropriate response, a dangerous response for the body. Chronic inflammation is something that you see particularly in older people quite extensively in the body for reasons that are not particularly clear; it is not clear what is driving it. Some of it maybe self antigens which you could see in the blood vessels and you could see lots of evidence that it is involved in heart disease. Chronic NF-kB activation is actually evident in many kinds but not all cancer cells and why cancer cells are displaying this chronic inflammatory condition is unclear. But, it is clear that this is part of what is driving the cancer cells and is part of actually the induction process of certain cancers, and I can go on and on.

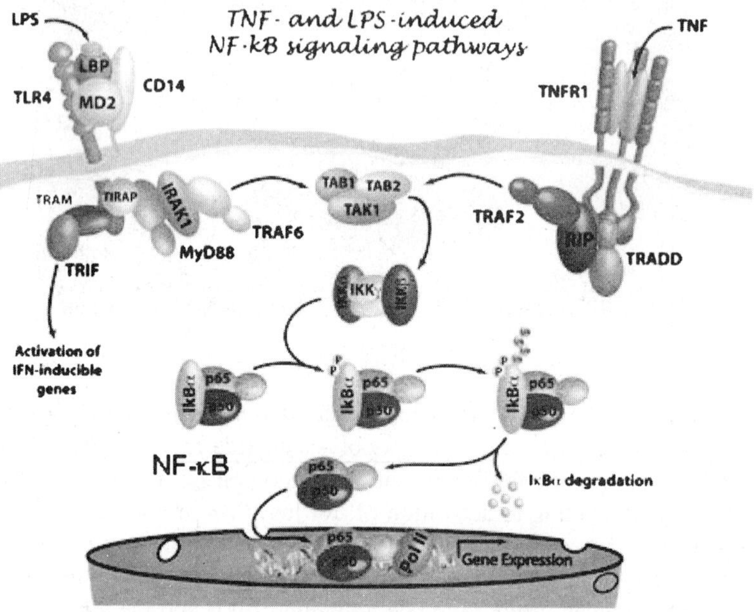

Fig. 1.3

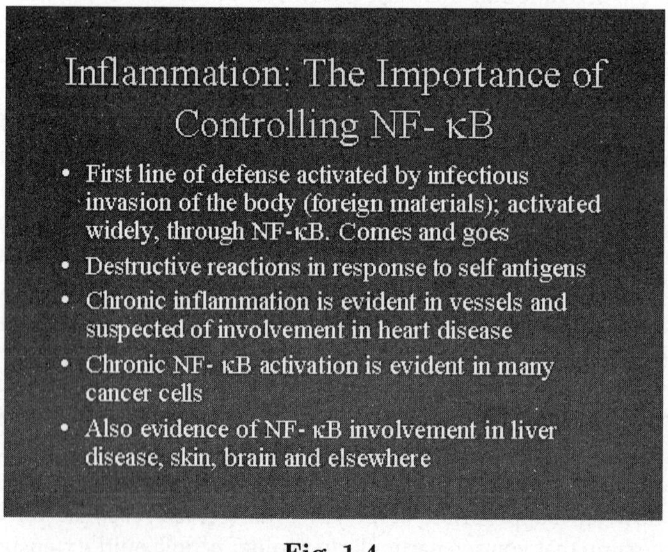

Fig. 1.4

There is evidence in liver disease and skin disease and brain disease and neurodegenerative problems and elsewhere in the body. So, this is something that has enormous potential for harm as well as potential for good.

Fig. 1.5 is a sort of colored illustration of this. When at a wound site the bacteria can get in, the wound itself as well as the bacteria sends signals through macrophages, through mast cells, and through platelet activation to the local circulation. 'Send us yourself' it says and out come neutrophils, other macrophages, and other cells to begin the process of response to inflammation and all of these cells have activated NF-kB. Also, NF-kB is a link between the innate immune system, which is much of what I have been talking about, and the adaptive immune system, which involves T-cells and B-cells and the major players here are dendritic cells and macrophages, cells that recognize the pathogen and send signals to T-cells and B-cells that activate the adaptive immune system.

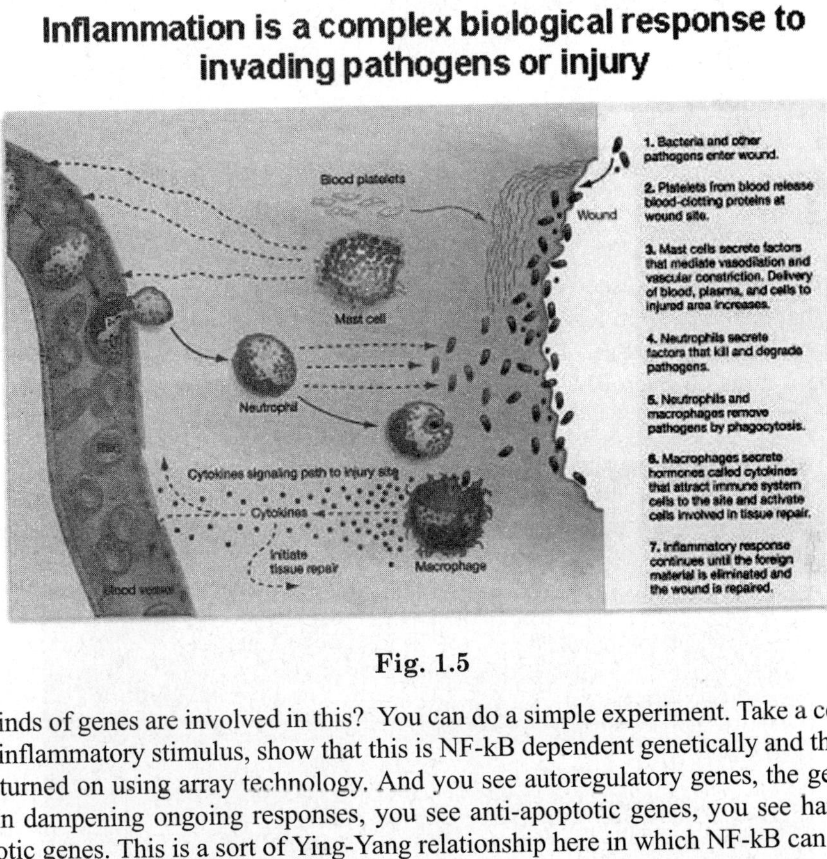

Fig. 1.5

What kinds of genes are involved in this? You can do a simple experiment. Take a cell, induce it with a proinflammatory stimulus, show that this is NF-kB dependent genetically and then ask what genes are turned on using array technology. And you see autoregulatory genes, the genes that are involved in dampening ongoing responses, you see anti-apoptotic genes, you see hardly enough pro-apoptotic genes. This is a sort of Ying-Yang relationship here in which NF-kB can both induce the apoptosis and prevent it and that obviously happens at different times you may see proinflammatory molecules, like TNF, so we may induce the cell with TNF but then it makes more TNF in a positive feedback of the inflammatory response. There will be induction of lots of chemokines which is what bring cells to the inflammatory site: IL-6, which has become an increasingly important part of protein that make the innate immune system work (Fig. 1.6). Beta interferon, proteins of the adaptive immune system, IgK, the light chain of immunoglobulin etc. are induced and lots of proteins that would mediate growth control and others (Fig. 1.7). This is all a basic introduction - the work we have been doing for 20 years.

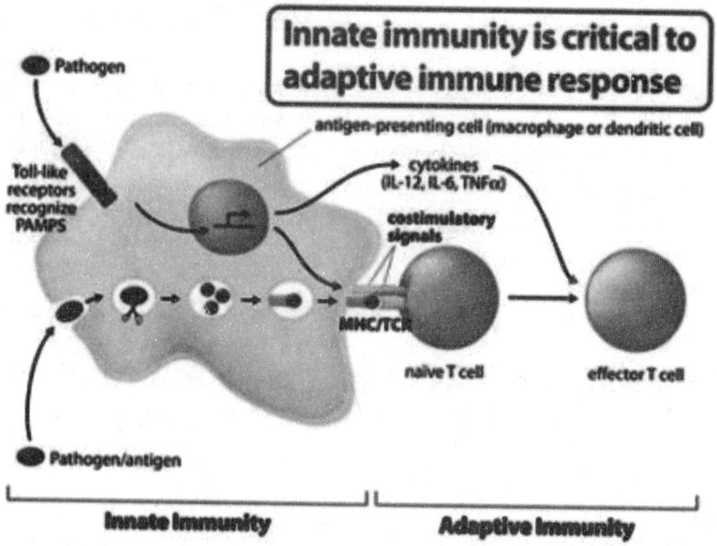

Fig. 1.6

About three years ago, we asked ourselves, might NF-kB activate microRNAs? And the reason for that was that there had been lots of evidence coming along that microRNAs play an important role in many biological processes. They are made by transcription and since this is a transcription factor, maybe it turns on microRNA genes and so Mark Boldin decided to look at this question (Fig. 1.8).

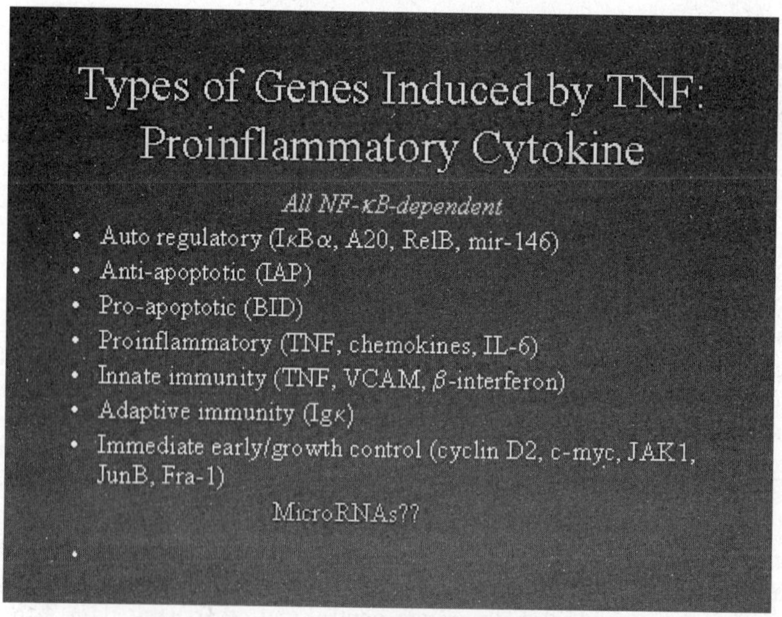

Fig. 1.7

Let me tell you a little about microRNAs because they are new and some people do not know a lot about it. MicroRNAs are derived from transcripts, which are the transcripts that look like normal gene transcripts (Fig. 1.9). They start with a cap-head and end with poly A, but in many cases there is no open reading frame that we found in that transcript, in some cases there is but in certain cases there is not. The only thing that you can find in that transcript which is conserved evolutionarily and what looks important is a little hairpin of RNA somewhere in this much larger molecule, and there is a processing system in the nucleus led by DROSHA like proteins which process out this little hairpin and gets rid of the rest of the RNA or lets it go on and do other functions in some cases. This is then exported to the cytoplasm and there it is worked upon by another nuclease called dicer. Dicer cuts off the loop leaving just a little doublestranded piece of RNA and then that is activated by helicase type of protein which chews in complicated ways one strand over the other and package a single stand of RNA what is called the RISC complex. And it is that complex which is the active form of the microRNA. That microRNA then goes searching among the messenger RNAs in the cell to find messenger RNAs that have a complementary sequence. It is only about 23 nucleotides long but it looks for complementarity over an even shorter region called the seed sequence and it finds complementarity in the 3 prime untranslated regions of messenger RNAs and that could lead to one or two consequences. Either it could lead to the degradation of the messenger RNA because at least one of the RISC protein is a nuclease or it can lead to a block in the translation of that messenger RNA by mechanisms, which are still little uncertain. So, microRNAs are 22-nucleotide long non-coding RNAs and their role is not to gene-silence (i.e. transcriptional silencing) but it is really the inhibition of translation of an existing messenger RNA: it is a post-transcriptional mechanism. MicroRNAs silence genes by a base-pairing mechanism, so this is a field there for bioinformaticists because you could look at the sequences of microRNAs, look at the sequences of messengers, and predict which messengers will be controlled by which micro-RNA.

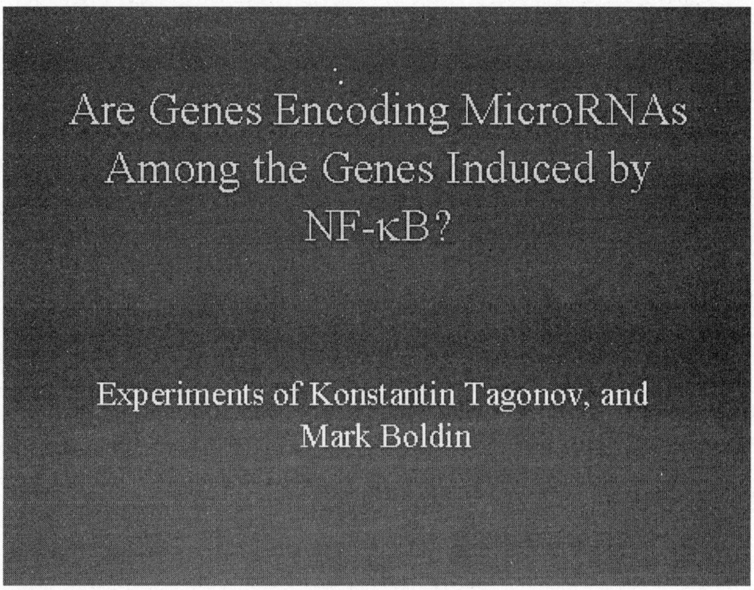

Fig. 1.8

So these computer assisted estimates predict about 1000 microRNAs in the human genome of which we really only know half, 500, the other half are guessed, and if you look at the complementarity of these to the existing complement of messenger RNAs, you would predict that many of these microRNAs attack multiple messenger RNAs, in that perhaps 30% of the protein coding capacity of the cell is controlled by microRNAs and we do not actually know if that number is right. What we know is much, much less than that, but this is what the bioinformaticists should give. And already microRNAs have been shown to be involved in differentiation. In fact, the very first microRNAs were discovered in *C. elegans*, in a worm because of the genetic set that they were involved in the control of differentiation. They are involved in organ development, cell proliferation, apoptosis, fat metabolism, insulin secretion, and lots and lots more. So, the experiment that we did was a very straightforward one. We simply took two populations of cells, one of which had been induced with lipopolysaccharide for 8 hours, the other which had not been induced at all, and we asked what was the level of microRNA expression in these two cell populations and we plotted one cell against the other and for those where there was no effect, this was a straight 45-degree line; three of the RNAs fell above that line and so were induced by the lipopolysaccharide treatment (Fig. 1.10). At the time we did this, we had an array of about 200 microRNAs. We have gone back with denser arrays, we still only see three such RNAs. So, there are three RNAs induced by this treatment. We focused on miR-146 and we focused on that because it probably has the highest degree of induction but we had no idea whether it was going to be interesting or not.

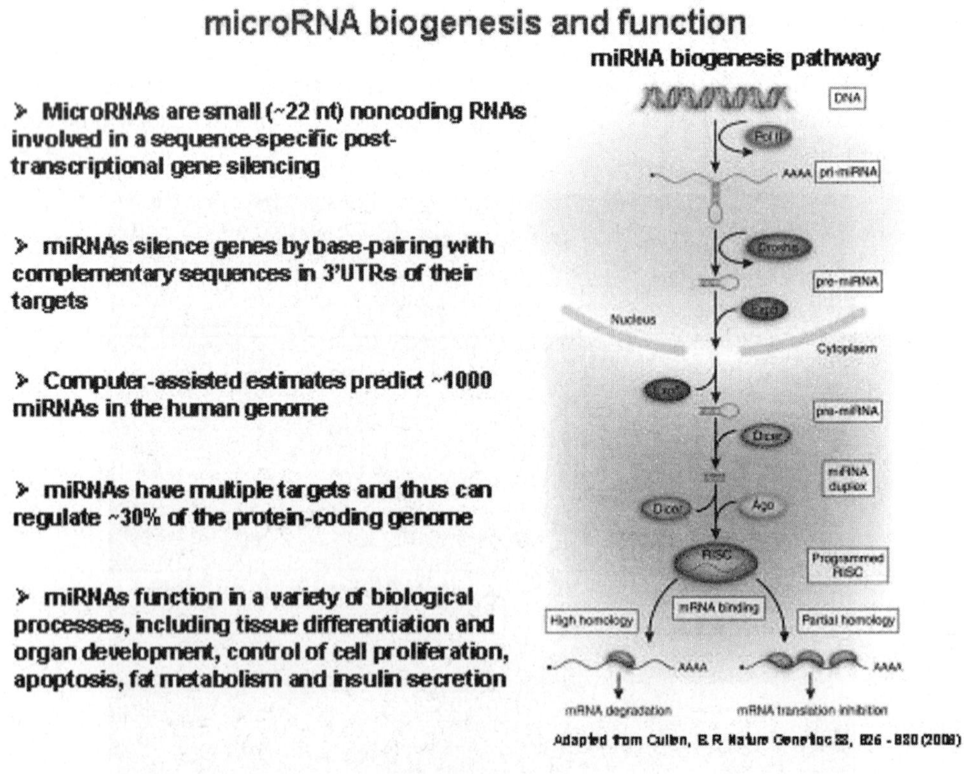

Fig. 1.9

You can see here that when induced with lipopolysaccharide in two kinds of macrophage cell lines, you will get a very obvious induction of microRNA 146 and it is about 10-fold induction by treatment with lipopolysaccharide (Fig. 1.11). And_that happens in the two cell tumors and in normal

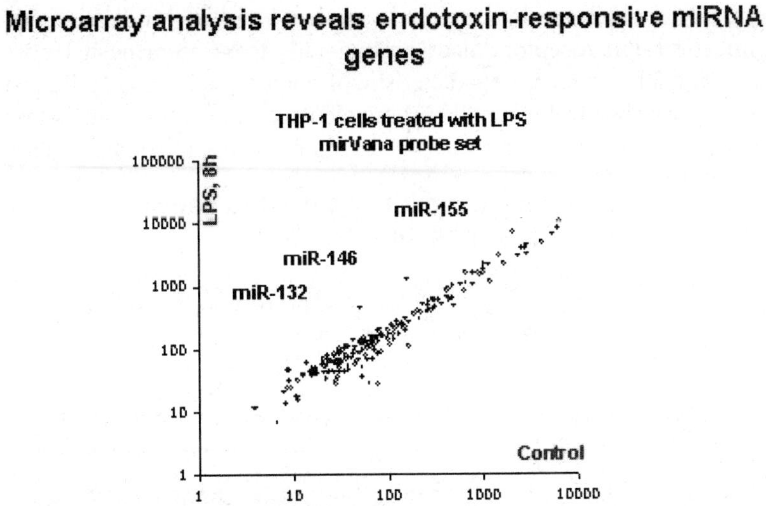

Fig. 1.10

macrophages also. You could also see the induction of the pre-microRNA and you can see the induction of the initial transcript. There are actually two RNAs of 146, called 146a and 146b. They are encoded in totally different genes in different parts of the genome but they have very, very close sequence identity and in the seed region that really searches for the complementarity, they are absolutely identical (Fig.1.12). So, they clearly have overlapping function but quite separate controls. And we know a lot about that, and it is also highly conserved in this case from fish up to humans.

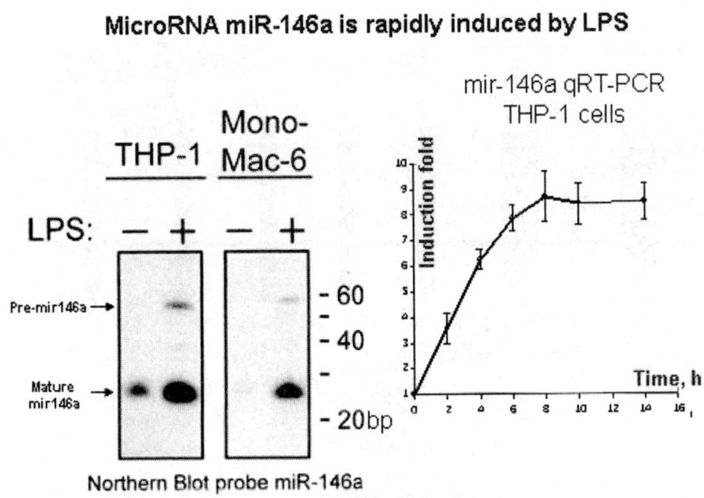

Fig. 1.11

TLR4 is the receptor for lipopolysaccharide; in fact, it is a bound protein on TLR4 called MD-2, which is the direct receptor, and structure was recently published of the bound complex. Binding of LPS leads to dimerization of TLR4, the activation of its internal cytoplasmic region, and the formation of that complex that I showed you on an earlier slide. But there are lots of other TLRs, toll-like receptors, all of which are looking for aspects of infection, indications that the body is undergoing an infection, but receptors also sense signals from gram positive organisms, CpG dinucleotide-containing DNA which is characteristic of microorganisms, flagellin, and lots of other things (Fig. 1.13). So, we asked whether all of these elements of infection, indications of infection, lead to the same microRNA induction and you can see for 146 that some do. TLR2, TLR4, and

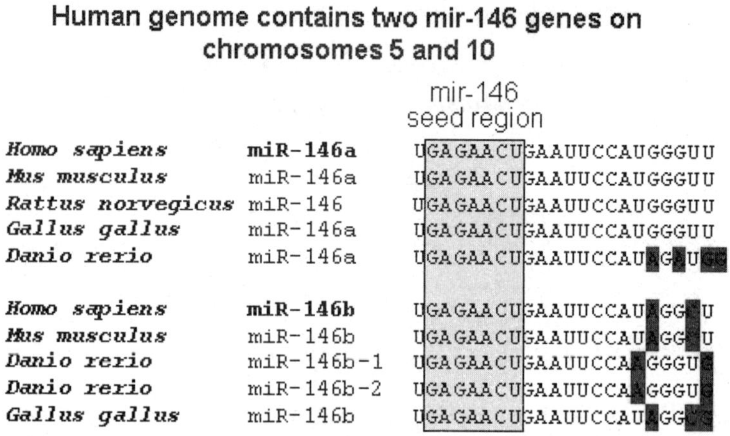

Fig. 1.12

TLR5 all cause activation of 146 transcriptions; but TLR3, TLR7 and TLR9 do not and interestingly those are intracellular toll-like receptors found in endosomes (Fig. 1.14). And so it is the surface toll-like receptors, which lead to the activation of 146. This is in the gene that contains 146

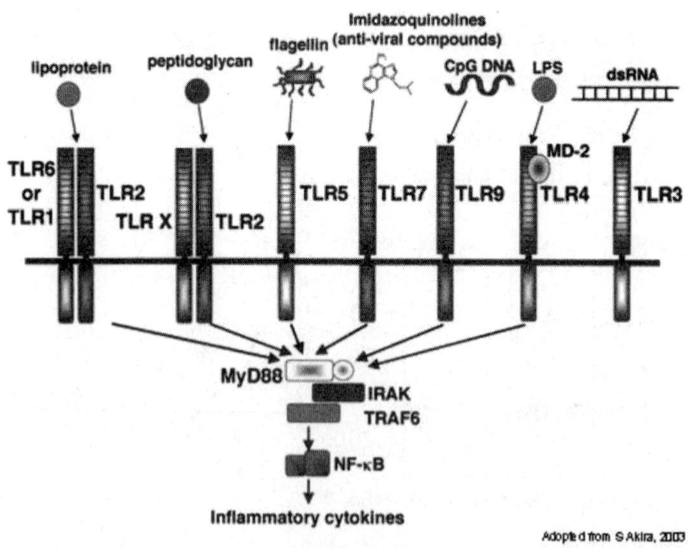

Fig. 1.13

and it is on chromosome 5 of the mousc (Fig. 1.15). It has two exons, exon 1 and 2 and this is where the microRNA is encoded, there is a huge intron here and just upstream you can see NF-kB sites and sites for the binding of IRF proteins. We wanted to ask whether we are really dealing with an NF-kB activated response. We made a reporter construct in which luciferase is being driven by this upstream region of the 146 gene. You can see that luciferase is induced very nicely about 8-fold by lipopolysaccharide and by proinflammatory cytokines IL-1 and TNF. So, then we deleted the IRF binding site and had no effect, so it is not part of the story. We deleted the NF-kB binding sites and they brought transcription down to the basal level with all of the inducers. And so quite clearly NF-kB is responsible for the induction of 146.

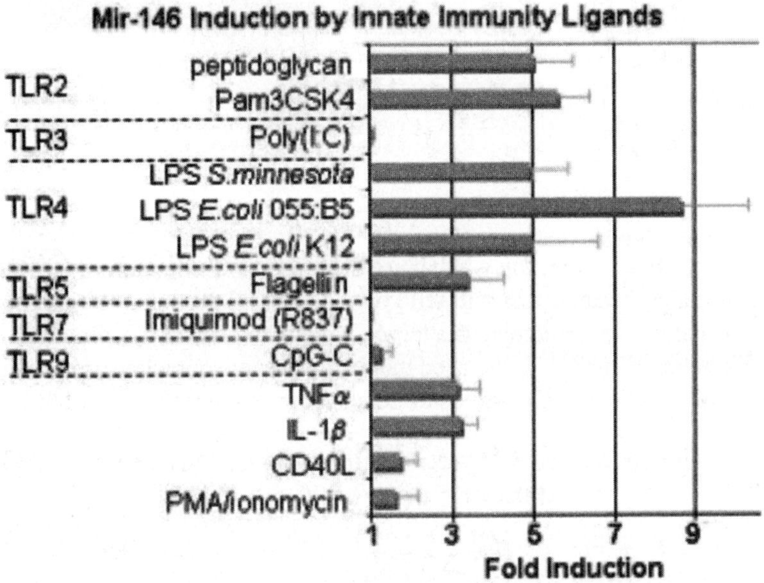

Fig. 1.14

This is actually a complex regulatory system, more complex than what we know of the answer. Because the basal level of 146 in cells, when we induce by lipopolysaccharide, goes up about 10-fold, but if we induce with lipopolysaccharide in the presence of cycloheximide, an inhibitor of protein synthesis, you get a nice induction of the pre-messenger RNA but no new induction, no increase in the amount of the matured micro-RNA (Fig. 1.16). So, there is another protein made by lipopolysaccharide activation, which is involved in the process of recognition of some sort of 146. We do not know what it is, but we do know that this is a remarkably highly regulated system. We can see that in this experiment in which we looked at, the first transcript, the precursor to miR-146 or the primary transcript for 146 that is induced by lipopolysaccharide and induced in the presence of several cyclohexamine as shown quantitatively here and that is rare because if we look at other microRNAs present, viz 132 in this experiment, which is induced probably well in cycloheximide, all the process and machinery for 132 is constitutive in cells but not for 146a.

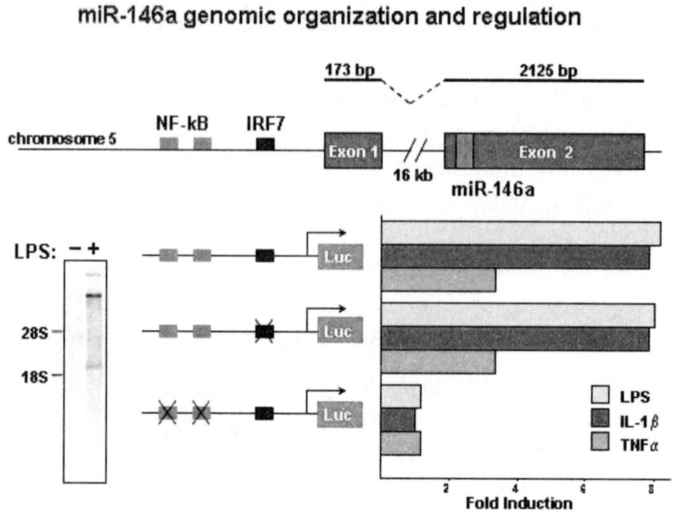

Fig. 1.15

Right now, the really key question is what are the targets? To do that, the first thing you can do is to use bioinformatics, because that will tell you what are all the candidate targets and certainly it does implicate that any given candidate is a target. And there were at this time four target prediction systems in the literature (Fig. 1. 17). We used them all, we came out with surprises- because in many cases if you do this, you will get hundreds of genes as an answer, but we got only three genes that

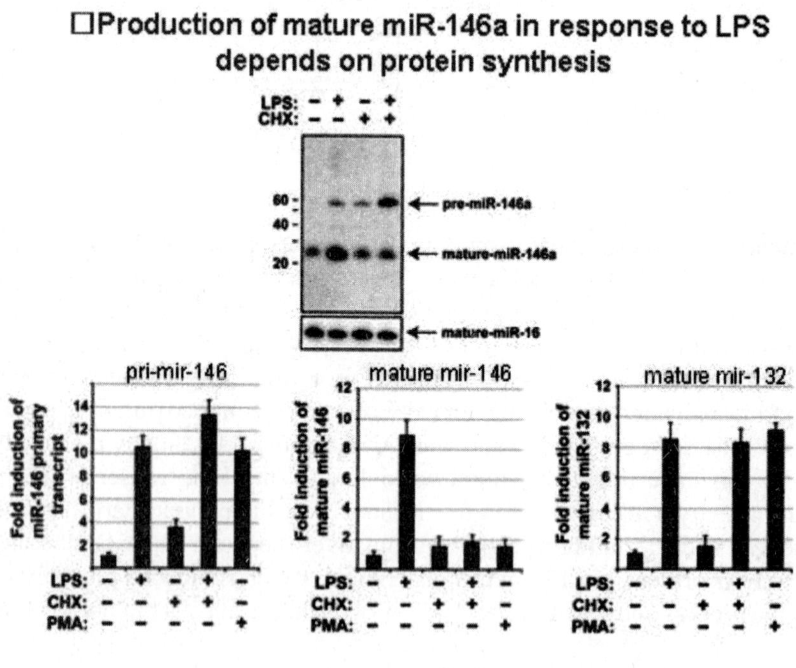

Fig. 1.16

were at the top of the list. There were lots of others for which there was a suspicion and there may yet be a story there, but there were three at the top of the list. The genes were COT/Tpl2, TRAF6, and IRAK1 (Fig. 1. 18). Now, TRAF6 and IRAK1 are proteins that are part of the complex that is activated by lipopolysaccharide, so they made sense; COT/Tpl2 is not and did not make sense. So, to test whether these really are targets of these microRNAs, we made a construct in which we have the CMV promoter driving Luciferase. We put downstream of that, the 3′ untranslated region of the three test genes (Fig. 1.18): TRAF6, which actually has two miR-146 sites, IRAK1 and COT/Tpl2. And then simply put the transfection constructs into cells and asked, if you cotransfect 146, does it inhibit the translation of Luciferase? The answer was very clearly yes, it does. So, if we are using the TRAF6-UTR, we can get a two and a half fold inhibition, which is big in this business (Fig. 1.19). While cotransfectinng 146a, if we scramble 146a or we use an irrelevant RNA like miR-21 or scramble the binding side on the UTR, then we do not get any inhibition, and so clearly this is a big and specific effect.

miRNA target prediction algorithms

TargetScanS — Lewis BP, Shih IH, Jones-Rhoades MW, Bartel DP & Burge CB
Prediction of mammalian microRNA targets
Cell 115, 787-98 (2003)

miRanda — John B, Enright AJ, Aravin A, Tuschl T, Sander C, Marks DS
Human MicroRNA targets
PLoS Biol 2, e363 (2004)

miRBase (Sequences) — Griffiths-Jones S, Grocock, RJ, van Dongen S, Bateman A & Enright AJ
miRBase: microRNA sequences, targets and gene nomenclature
Nucleic Acids Res 34, D140-4 (2006)

PicTar — Krek A, Grun D, Poy MN, Wolf R, Rosenberg L, Epstein EJ, MacMenamin P, da Piedade I, Gunsalus KC, Stoffel M, Rajewsky N
Combinatorial microRNA target predictions
Nat Genet. 2005 May;37(5):495-500

Fig. 1.17

It was the same thing too with IRAK1 but COT/Tpl2 was ineffective. So, we come down to two target genes. We do not know that they are the only two but we do know that they are two important genes.

One way to look at whether they are right or not is to make a lenti viral construct that expresses 146a or a scrambled version of it and put it into cells and ask what the consequences of continual, unregulated expressions of 146 expression in cells are. So, you can see the outcome here (Fig. 1. 20). This is the scrambled version and this is the 146, we are putting it into clones of the macrophage cell line THP-1 and you can see that we get a big increase in the amount of 146 even

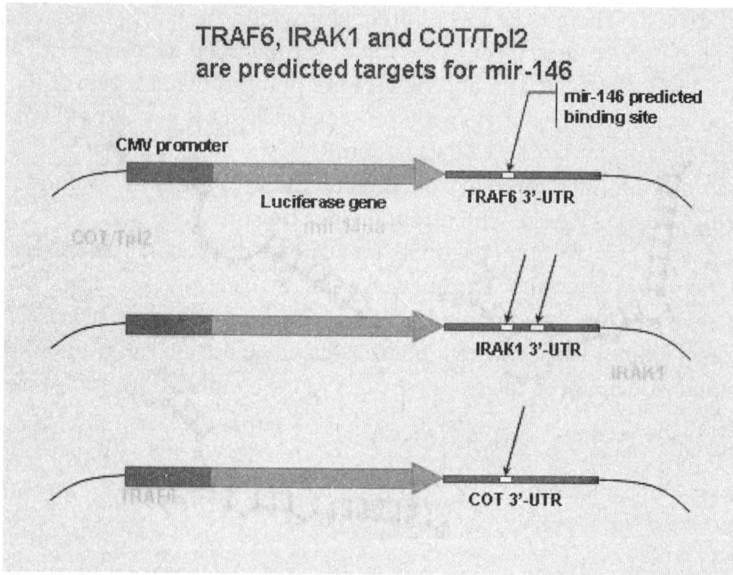

Fig. 1.18

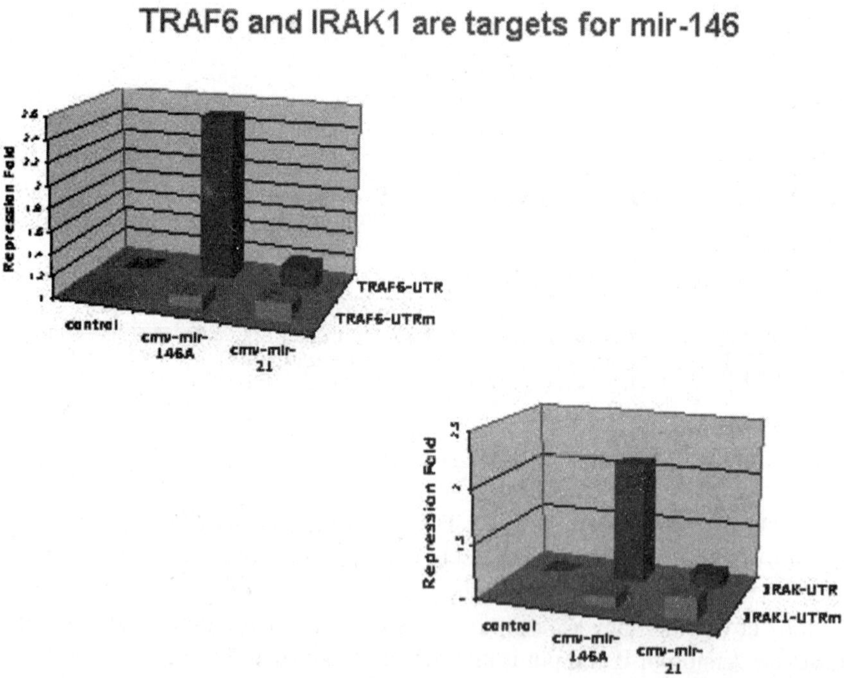

Fig. 1.19

without induction because we are expressing it from this constitutive virus construct. The level is about the same as the level you would see by induction, so it is physiologically meaningful. If we induce with lipopolysaccharide, we can actually see the two different forms because the natural form is a little smaller than the form we engineered for reasons I would not go into. The scrambled version does not give you a mature product of course. Then we asked, what is the effect on IRAK1? So, this is the normal level of IRAK1, this is the amount if we induce with lipopolysaccharide, so IRAK1 is degraded by induction with lipopolysaccharide and that degradation is found in un-induced cells if they have active 146 present and induction actually does not increase it. So, in fact, it is true that over expression of 146 does lead to the inhibition of synthesis of IRAK1; but somewhat less to TRAF6, although it inhibits the synthesis of TRAF6 also.

The consequences of that are that the cells that over express 146 are very poorly induced by lipopolysaccharide and you see that for some genes, although I am not saying that for others (Fig. 1.21). In particular, you see it in a TNF gene; you see a weaker but reproducible effect on IL-6, you see much less of an effect for IL-8. Why that specificity occurs, we do not really know. So, we can now make quite a plausible argument for the function of 146. It is feedback regulated (Fig. 1.22). It is a part of the process of dampening the NF-kB response to lipopolysaccharide. So, lipopolysaccharide is binding to the TLR4, causes the formation of this complex and leads to the activation of NF-kB. But one of the genes that NF-kB sees is the gene for 146, that then gets induced, 146 feeds back on the messenger RNAs for IRAK1 and TRAF6 and causes a down regulation of this signaling system. There are very few systems in which we know so clearly the function of a particular microRNA.

Overexpression of mir-146a downregulates IRAK1 and TRAF6 protein levels in THP-1 cells

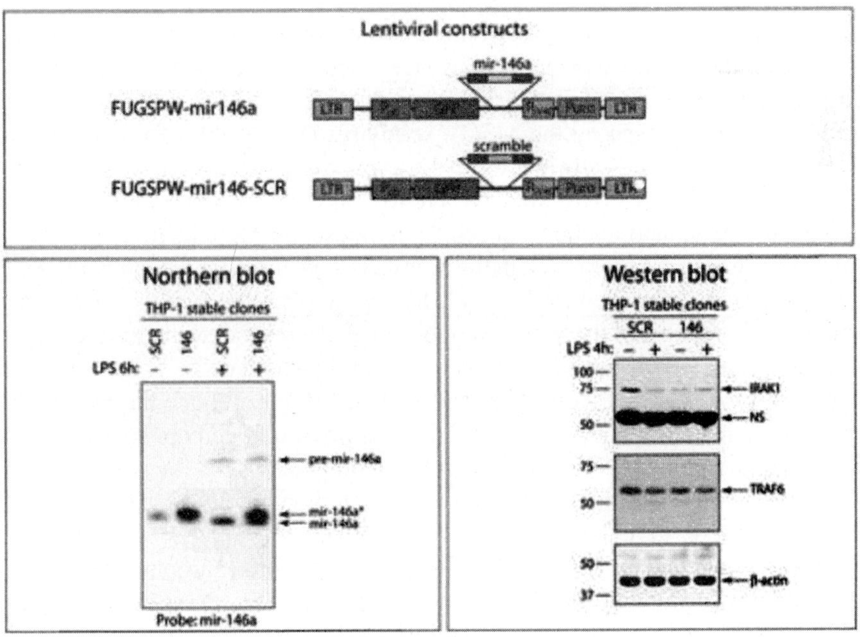

Fig. 1.20

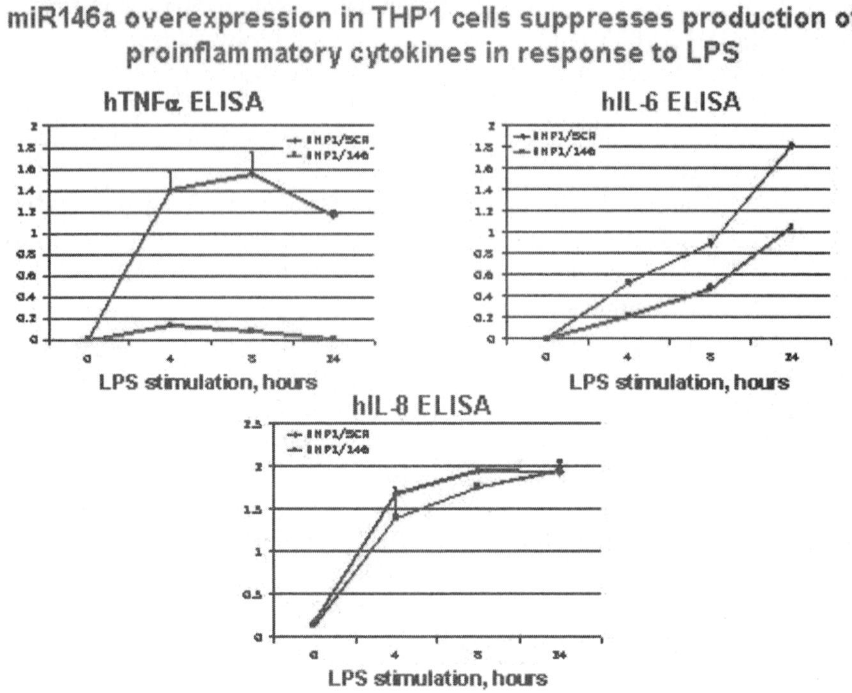

Fig. 1.21

Now, what we really want to do is to test these notions by over expressing 146 in mice. We can do that in a fairly straightforward manner and we have actually done this experiment now through a lot of different microRNAs, and for lots of other genes. What we do is, we make a little expression cassette and in this case, based on the MSCV retrovirus (Fig. 1. 23). The LTR of the retrovirus drives the expression of this cassette and we make a link cassette between GFP (Green Fluorescent Protein) and the genes of microRNA. We have a retroviral vector which contains the 146 sequences. We infect that into the hematopoietic stem cells of a mouse. So, we take these cells out, we expose them to the virus, we then put them back in the mouse, but we irradiate the mouse by lethal radiation so that the injected stem cells takeover the whole hematopoietic system of the mouse; and the mouse is now expressing, in fact, all of the normal blood cells that a mouse expresses but they all have 146 in them. It is not in the rest of the body and it is only in the blood cells. If it works quite well, you can get about a 50-fold increase in the constitutive level of 146 in bone marrow or in spleen as a consequence of reconstituting the animals with genetically modified bone marrow.

Just to be clear about this, the hematopoietic stem cell gives rise to the whole series of differentiation events: the common lymphoid progenitor, the common myeloid progenitor etc. (Fig. 1. 24). The lymphoid progenitor gives rise to T-cells, to B-cells, and of course there are many different kinds of T-cells. The myeloid progenitor gives rise to granulocytes, neutrophils, macrophages through one differentiation pathway and through another to megakaryocytes and erythrocytes, red blood cells. So, all the blood elements are made by this HSC. We put genes into it. The genes will then be expressed down here and function in these derivative cells; in particular, we are going to look at the myeloid series but not going to talk much about the lymphoid series.

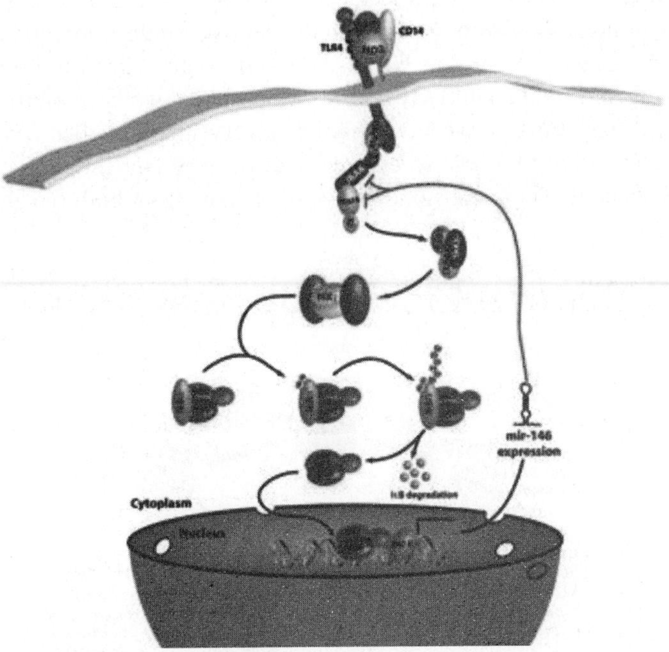

Fig. 1.22

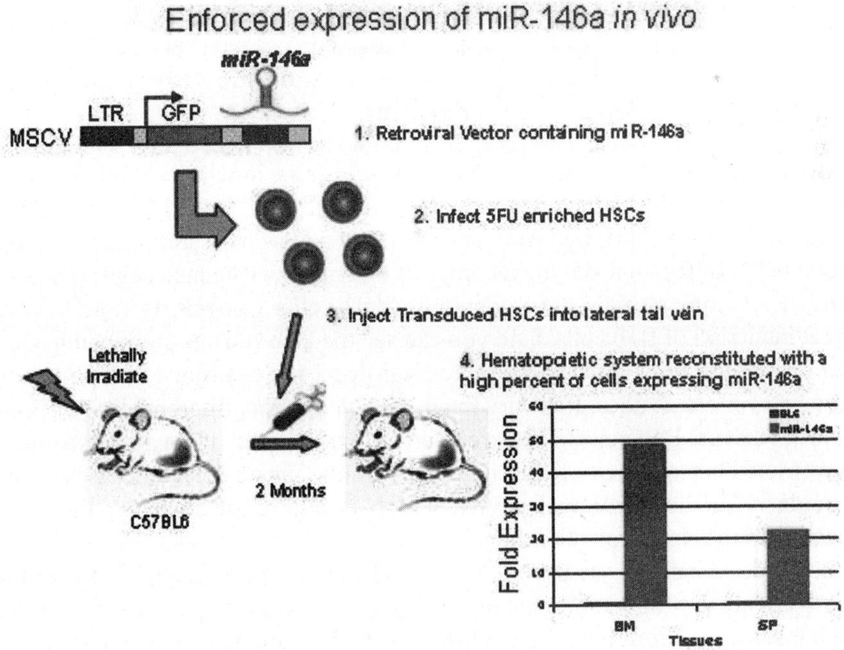

Fig. 1.23

We have also done the opposite. We knocked out the 146 gene in mice and we have done that with a targeting construct, I would not go through the details, but the consequence is that there is no 146a in bone marrow, spleen, or thymus because there is no gene for it in the mouse and we have made those mice (Fig. 1. 25). I should say before going on that we have pretty extensively characterized the overproducing animals. We have only had a very small number of the knockout animals to look at and so I would not be able to answer a lot of very interesting questions on what was happening in the knockout. There are some very clear results from both types of expression in the mouse.

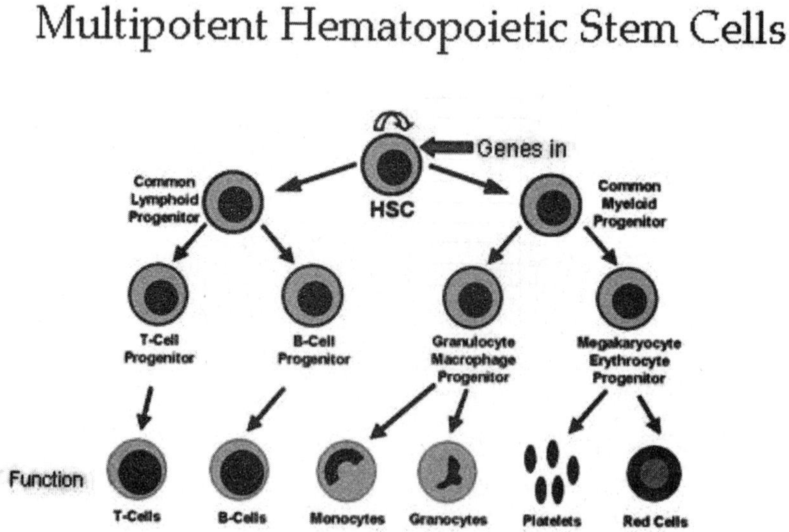

Fig. 1.24

(Fig. 1.26) So, here is a consequence of not having the gene in what are called B1b cells and the consequences that these cells, which are in this box, are affected. I would not explain why, but we are looking at CD19 and CD11b by FACS analysis. The cells which are in this box go from being 9% of the total to 2% of the total and in fact much of that may well be in background. So, we can say that 146a is critically important for the production of B1b cells. Conversely, if we over express then we see a great induction of B1b cells, here you can see the B1b cells go from being 3% up to being 15% in over expressing cells. So, it looks quite clear that 146a controls development of B1b cells, never mind whatever else it does. It is very much involved in the differentiation of B-cells to form B1b cells. Now, what are B1b cells? They are a sort of innate aspect of the adaptive immune system. They have restricted heterogeneity focused very much like innate cells on causes of infection and found particularly in the peritoneal cavity, which is where we look for them in this case. I will come back to the significance of them.

The other experiment that we have done is to look at primary macrophages in the knockout animals and asked are they now more sensitive to lipopolysaccharide, because this feedback regulation has been taken away from them by the loss of 146. And, in fact, we could see that very nicely with TNF-alpha that it is induced very highly and continuously after induction with lipopolysaccharide (Fig. 1. 27). The same thing happens with IL-6, and less evident with IL-12. So, on functional

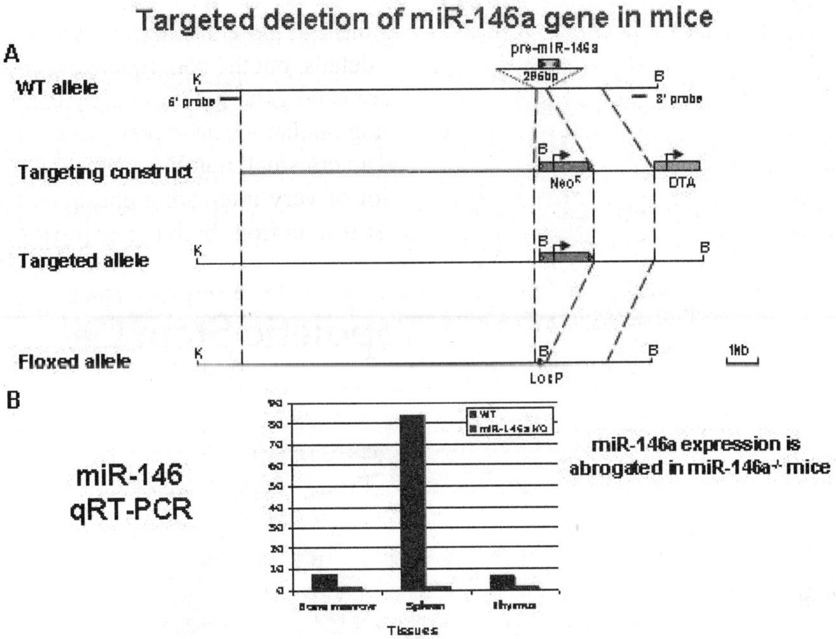

Fig. 1.25

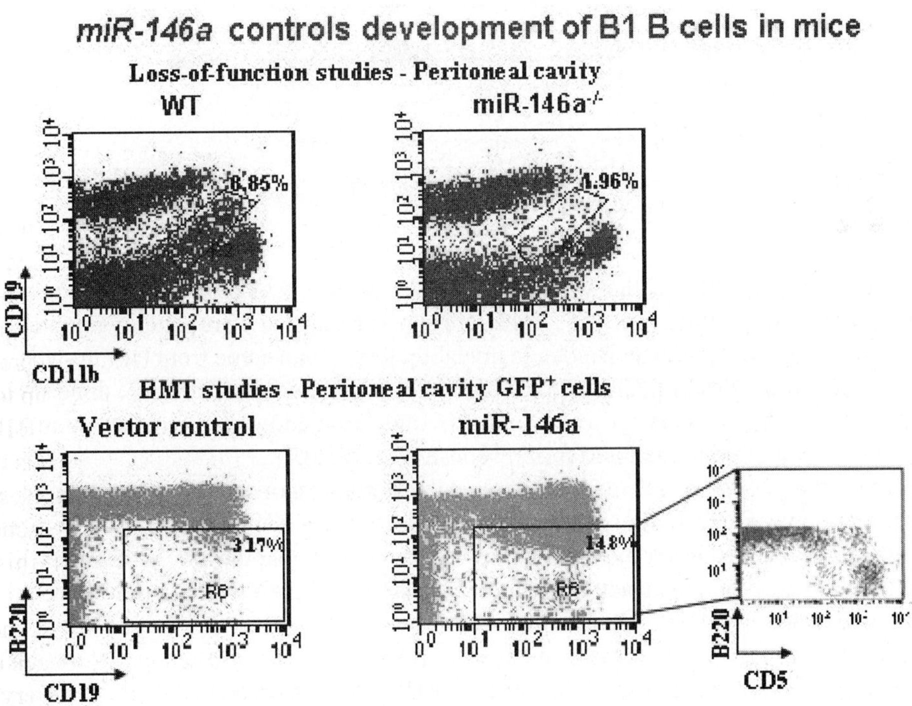

Fig. 1.26

studies, miR146 appears to be a feedback regulator of the inflammatory activation response hoping to shut down responses to the surface TLR activators. From the over expression and by knockout experiments, we confirmed that. But we have also seen that 146a contributes to modulating cell fate decisions during hematopoietic cell differentiation and it does restore the production of cells that serve in innate immune functions: B1b cells which I have shown you, gamma-delta T-cells which I have not, and then K-cells which I also have not. There are other effects and we are now trying to quantitate those and work them out in detail. So, that is one story of microRNAs that involves feedback regulation as well as differentiation control (Fig. 1. 28).

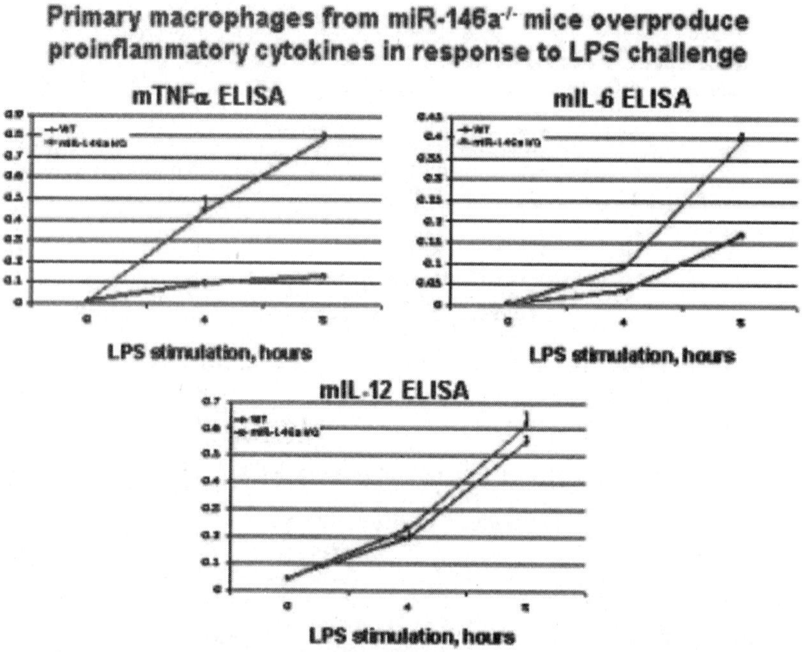

Fig. 1.27

I said there were three RNAs that were induced. We have not looked at 132 very extensively but the next story is about the third one, 155. These are experiments that were actually initiated by Ryan O'Connell working with Donovan Bolden in my laboratory. Ryan came from UCLA, where he had worked on interferon with Prof. Chang, and so he said: you know you guys have done such a great job in looking at NF-kB activation. I wonder if interferon induces microRNAs and whether microRNAs play any role in the interferon response (Fig. 1.29).

There are two ways that people possibly look at interferon responses, one is by adding interferon to cells and the other is by adding poly I: C, a doublestranded RNA analog, because partly cells respond to doublestranded RNA by making interferons thinking that they are virus infected. Poly I: C binds to TLR3 receptor, which actually is intracellular, it is shown on the surface here (Fig. 1.13) but that is wrong and I will get that slide changed.

And it works through the TRIF pathway to activate a number of transcription factors that leads to many genes being activated, but in particular the interferon production and then the interferon can bind to the interferon receptor and activate the genes that the interferon receptor activates. We can also activate the interferon receptor by just adding to cells IFN-â, and so we did both experiments. We did it in the following way: we took cells from bone marrow, differentiated them into primary macrophages. Ryan wanted to work with primary cells rather than cell lines (but I do not think there is a lot of difference), and induced them with poly I:C or with IFN-â and then did micro arrays to compare the microRNA pattern. What we saw in this case was a single RNA induced, microRNA-155 (Fig. 1.30). It was also induced by proinflammatory cytokines as I had shown you earlier, and it is induced by both the IFN-â and by poly I: C and so we say what we find looks like it is induced by interferon. It turns out that is not true and I will show you.

Mir-146 Functions

- From functional studies, Mir-146 appears to be a feedback regulator of inflammatory activation, helping to shut down responses to TLR activators
- From overexpression and knockouts, this is confirmed but have also seen that Mir-146a contributes to modulating cell fate decisions during hematopoietic cell differentiation towards production of cells that serve innate immune functions (B-1 cells, $\gamma\delta$ T cells, NK cells)

Fig. 1.28

The first clue was that poly I:C activated it better than IFN-â (Fig 1. 30). IFN-â can activate about 20-fold, poly I:C about 60-fold. That would not be true if it was all working through interferon; the rest are the controls on here.

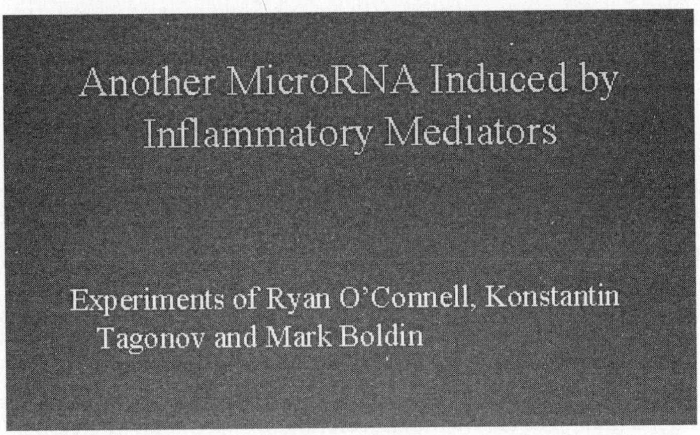

Fig. 1.29

Now, 155 has a long history and is a very interesting RNA (Fig. 1.31). It is ubiquitously expressed but generally at very low levels. It is found at its highest level in lymphoid tissue, particularly activated lymphoid tissue, and it comes from its cut out of a gene, which is called a BIC gene. BIC has a noncoding RNA like I had shown you for other primary transcripts of microRNAs, but it is a precursor of microRNA-155 but that is not how it was identified. It was identified before anybody knew anything about microRNAs by Hayward and colleagues. They identified it as the site of integration of an avian leukosis virus that causes lymphoid cancer in mice and they showed that

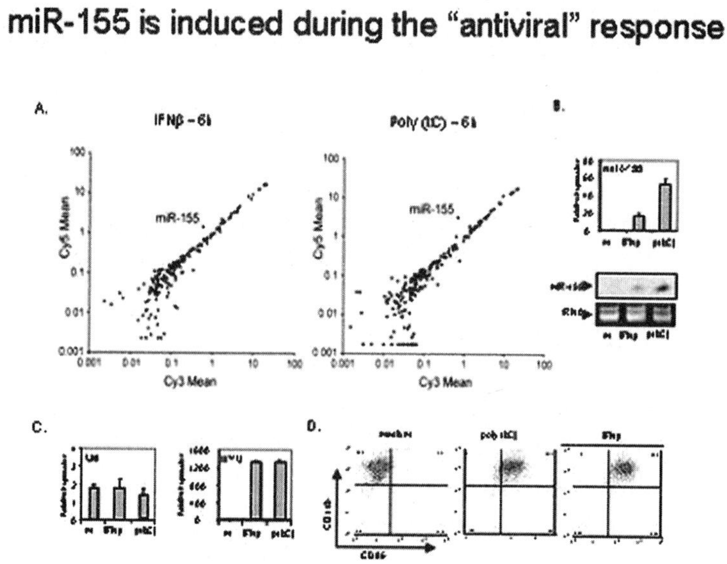

Fig. 1.30

animals that got cancer as a consequence of infection with this virus always showed or often showed integration of the virus at this BIC RNA. So, they sequenced BIC RNA and were perplexed because we did not have an open reading for them and could not feel exactly what this was telling them. That was before we understood microRNAs and so they could not see the microRNA structure. Beyond that, miR-155 has been associated with many human cancers. It is found at an elevated level in a whole variety of human malignancies, many of them are the same ones with constitutive NF-kB, suggesting that it can be induced by NF-kB. Carlo Croce did an experiment in which he expressed 155 as transgene throughout the animal but with a promoter driving it, which caused it only to be expressed in B-cells. He showed that these animals do develop B-cell lymphomas and has more recently shown, in an unpublished work, T-cell lymphoma induction by 155. So, actually 155 was the first microRNA to be shown to induce cancer.

So, this is the big noncoding transcript that has three exons, exon 1, 2, and 3. (Fig. 1.32) The 155 is found in the third exon but there is no open reading frame throughout this. You can probe the big RNA independently of its 155 content and show that it is induced by poly I:C and induced by interferon. It is induced much better and much faster by poly I:C than interferon. Again, a clue that poly I: C is not working through the induction of interferon. You see that here it has been quantitated, rapid induction by poly I:C and slower induction to a lower level by interferon.

miR-155

- Ubiquitously expressed and found at highest levels in lymphoid tissue
- BIC non-coding RNA is the precursor for miR-155 (Hayward)
- High levels of miR-155 associated with different types of human malignancies (in many cases correlated with constituitive NF-κB)
- Mice with B-cell restricted transgenic expression of miR-155 develop lymphomas (Croce)
- Normal cellular function of miR-155 not defined

Fig. 1.31

Now again, there are many TLRs and we looked at a number of those for whether they induce 155 and in this case all of them do, intracellular or extracellular, they induce 155 very nicely, and they are working through a variety of different pathways. We do not go into the pathways, but this was the killer experiment done here (Fig. 1. 33). We asked whether these would induce 155 in the absence of the interferon receptor, and in the absence of interferon receptor, interferon cannot work at all. In fact, poly I: C as well as LPS, CpG, and another activator called P3C all induce perfectly well in the absence of the interferon receptor. So, poly I: C cannot be working through interferon.

BIC and miR-155 are induced by poly (I:C) and IFNβ

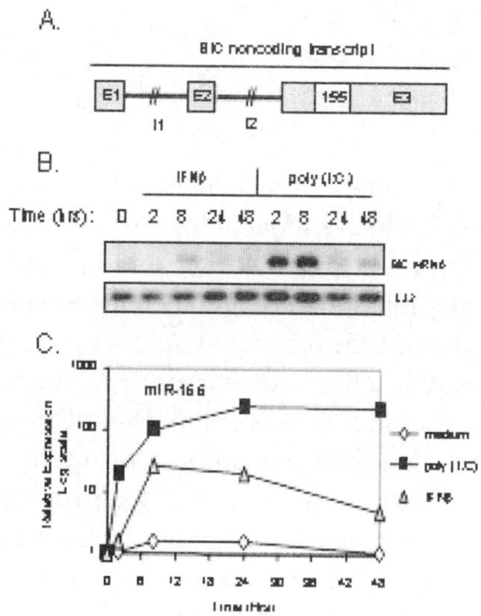

Fig. 1.32

We showed that poly I: C is working by direct TRIF activation (Fig 1.34). So, the picture that we now have is that of an activated TLR3 receptor and here it is shown appropriately in an endosome with a doublestranded RNA that leads to the direct activation of a 155 gene. The 155 gene then gets processed and searches for homologies of messenger RNAs to be inhibited. It is interferon that works indirectly. Interferon binds to the interferon receptor and to STAT proteins. They, in turn, as much as we have found out, activate the TNF gene (Fig. 1. 33). TNF gets produced. TNF crosses over and activates the TNF receptor, which then activates through the JNK kinase, the 155 gene (Fig. 1. 35). So, in fact, interferon is working indirectly and at low level; and although we started this work to look for interferon effects, the big story is TLR3 and other TLRs leading to 155 inductions.

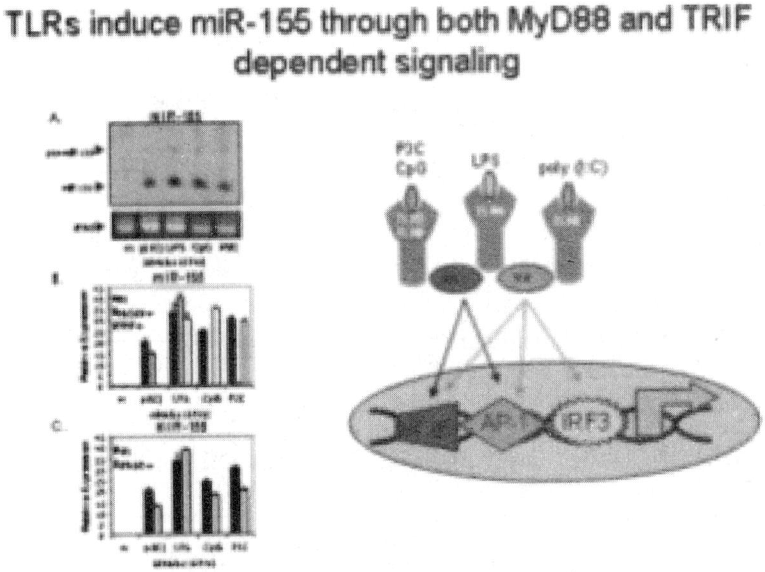

Fig. 1.33

Now, let's go through the functional consequences of 155, and here I want to show you an experiment done with normal mice which I found to be very profound (Fig. 1.36). Actually, it does not involve a discovery because you can find evidence of all of this in the literature. What we did was to inject LPS intraperitoneally into a mouse and then take out bone marrow a little while later and asked: is 155 induced and what are the other consequences of LPS treatment of the mouse? So, we looked it for 24 hours and there is a big induction of the bone marrow 155. So, this is a normal physiological response to what is in fact the sublethal dose of lipopolysaccharide and it subsides within the 72 hours. Actually, the whole cell population in the marrow turns over. I would not worry about that experiment. Now, this is a case of an animal that had been injected with buffer (PBS) at 72 hours after injection. So, this is really the normal pattern of bone marrow. What you see in it are cells, which have B220 on the surface, these are B-cells to T-cells that have B220 on their surface versus myeloid cells of various sources like macrophages and neutrophils; and you see a lot of other cells many of which are erythrocytes or pro-erythrocytes in the bone marrow. So this is the picture that you would expect from a normal bone marrow. And this is a surprising result to me that you treat an animal with lipopolysaccharide and wait 72 hours, then you see many fewer B-cells, you see

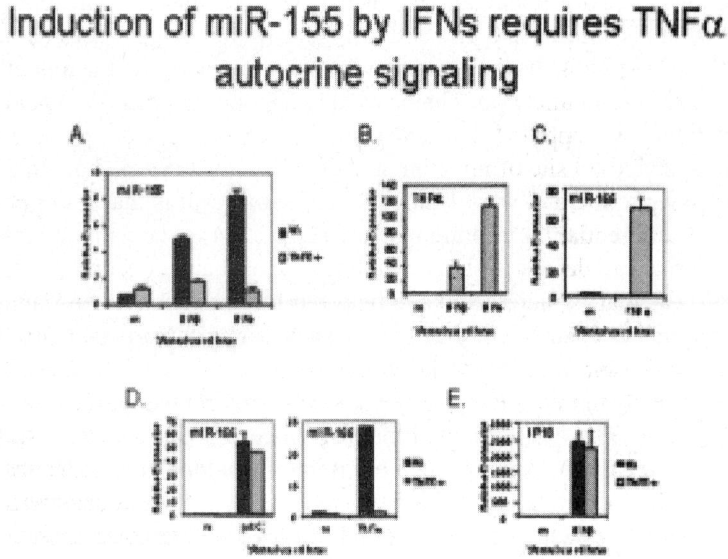

Fig. 1.34

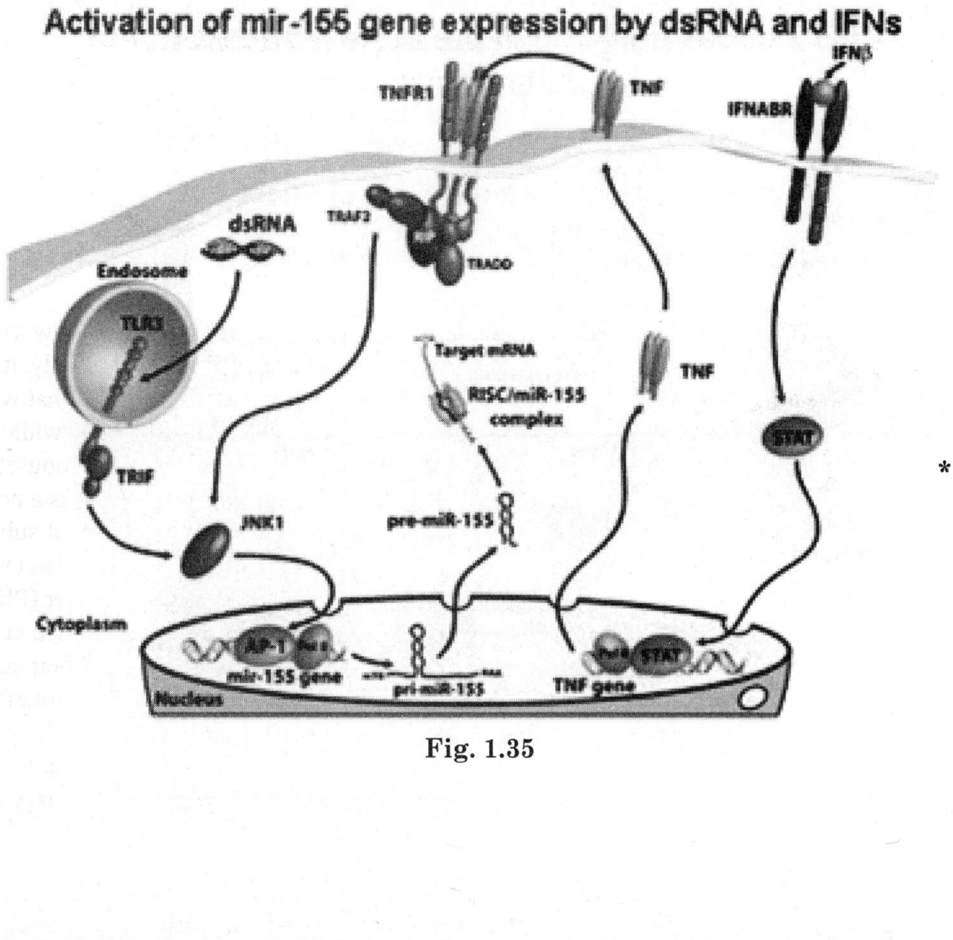

Fig. 1.35

many fewer erythrocytes, and the population in the marrow is dominated by myeloid cells. So, what is going on here? What the animal is doing is shutting down the things it does not need right away and concentrating on those cells that serve innate immune functions, as the animal thinks it is infected with a massive bacterial infection. That is what the lipopolysaccharide would indicate and so the animal is responding appropriately by increasing the outpouring from the marrow of myeloid cells which can go to supposed site of infection and get rid of the bacteria, the first line of defense. But what was surprising to me and what I think is very significant is that it implies the tree that I have showed you of differentiation in bone marrow (Fig. 1. 24) is actually a controlled series of decisions and the animal can decide to shut down one side of it and concentrate on the other side.

So, the question was that is there a linkage between the induction of 155 and this change in differentiation? So, Ryan O'Connell got together with a pathologist in my lab, Dinesh Rao and they overexpressed 155 in mice and asked what the consequences are (Fig. 1.37). Does it phenocopy the infection response- is really the question. So, we made a retroviral with Green Fluorescent Protein and now 155 in it (Fig. 1. 38). We expressed that first in cells to show that it expresses nicely, in which we got a large increase in 155. We then put it into hematopoietic stem cells, injected those back into a lithium-irradiated animal and waited two months for the hematopoietic system to reconstitute. It showed now that the hematopoietic cells have large amounts of 155 in them constitutively as well as in spleen, lymph node, bone marrow, and the thymus; and answered what are the consequences.

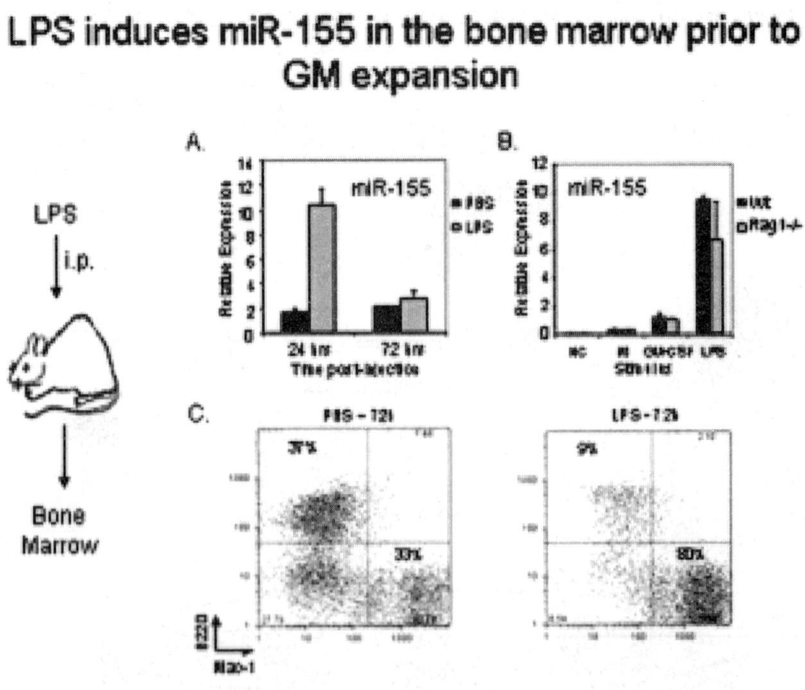

Fig. 1.36

MiR-155 causes a myeloproliferative disease in mice

Ryan O'Connell
and Dinesh Rao

Fig. 1.37

The consequences were literally very obvious (Fig. 1.39). If you take the bone out of animal, which is a controlled animal or an animal that have a scrambled RNA in it, it is red.

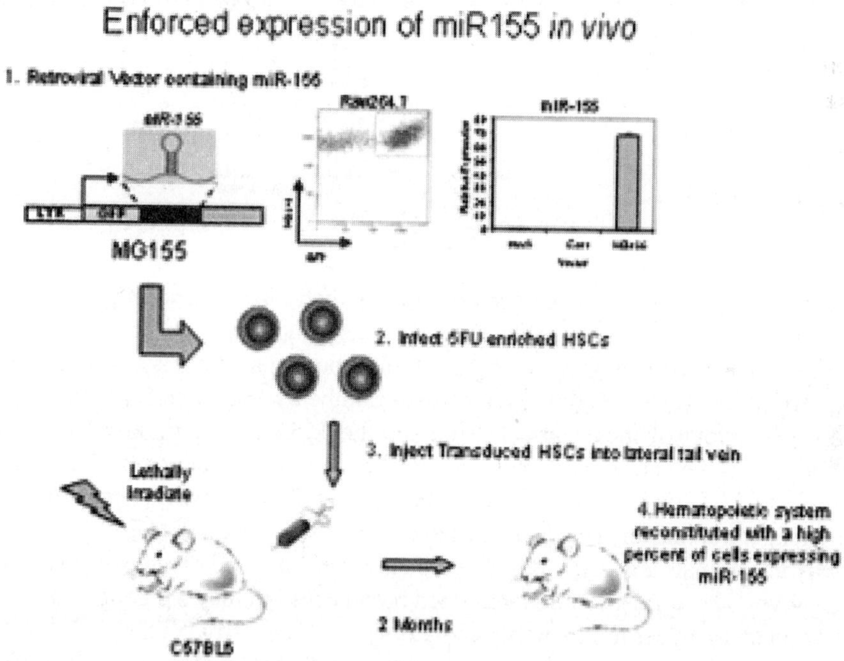

Fig. 1.38

It is red because it has got a lot of erythrocytes, pro-erythrocytes that are getting red with hemoglobin. The bone of an animal, which is over expressing 155, has no red cast to it, basically white, although it looks yellow (Fig. 1.40). If you count cells, you can see that there is a great increase in myeloid cells in the marrow, there is a great decrease in red blood cells as measured by 119, and there is a reduction in B-cells as measured by B220. So, we do get a phenocopy of the infection response; that is this response change in the pattern from here to here, is exactly what happens if you over express 155. So 155 is the causative agent in this phenomena, not just a passenger indication.

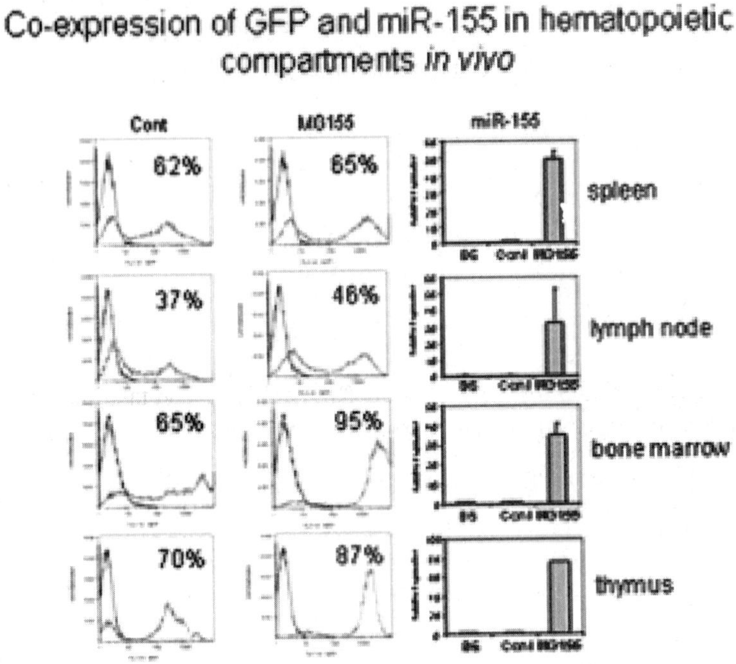

Fig. 1.39

If you like pathology, here are some very nice slides which show you normal marrow with megakaryocytes as very obvious cells, erythrocytes seen here, lymphoid cells here, and lots of myeloid cells seen (Fig. 1. 40). If we over express 155 and look at bone marrow, it is a sheet of myeloid cells, we will see very little else, although there are small numbers of other cells present (Fig. 1.41). If you take the spleens out of these animals, you see the 155 over expression has caused a huge increase in the size of the spleen, what has happened is that the production of B-cells and erythrocytes has moved to the spleen, extramedullary hematopoiesis, a consequence of the fact that the marrow is no longer making any cells, so they have to be made someway (Fig. 1.42 and 1.43). That is actually why the animals are alive. If they would not make any red blood cells in the spleen, they would not be alive. These are a sort of anemic red blood cells but they are good enough to keep the animals for as much as a year living in the laboratory.

So, then we wanted to know what are the target genes, what genes are involved in these very dramatic responses? You can do it in a lot of ways. If you do it by bioinformatics, you will get a huge number of genes back; so it is not kind of getting a nice simple picture of what we got with 146. You will get a very complicated picture. And so we made a vector that expresses 155, we put it into cells, in this case macrophages, of mouse macrophages called RAW 264.7 cells. And we took 5 clones of cells that over produce 155 and 5 clones of non-producing cells, and then we mixed

Transgenic expression of miR-155 in HSCs causes myeloid dysplasia and proliferation in the bone marrow

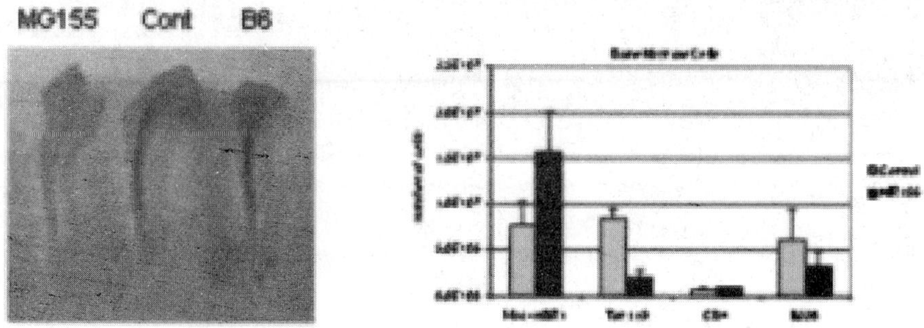

Fig. 1.40

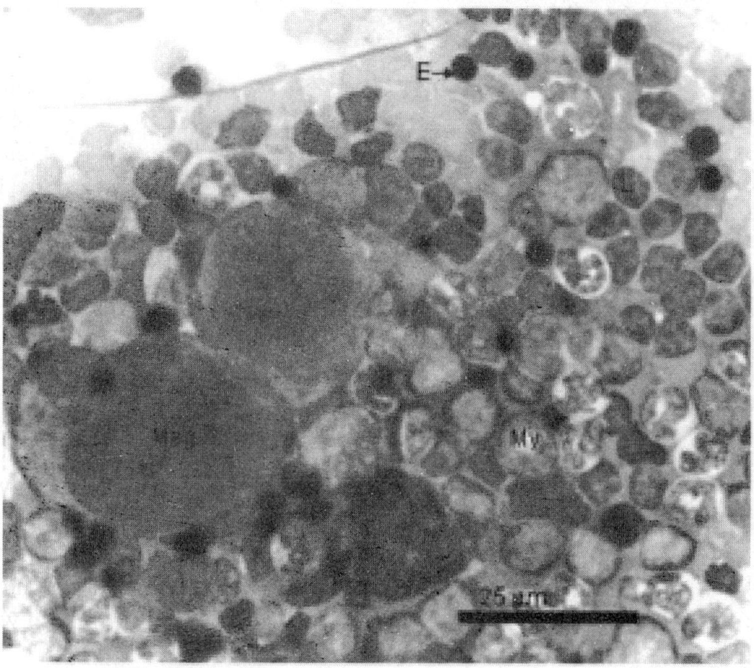

MIG bone marrow smear, Wright-stained. Meg, Megakaryocyte; My, myeloid/ granulocytic lineage; E, erythroid lineage; L, lymphoid lineage

Fig. 1.41

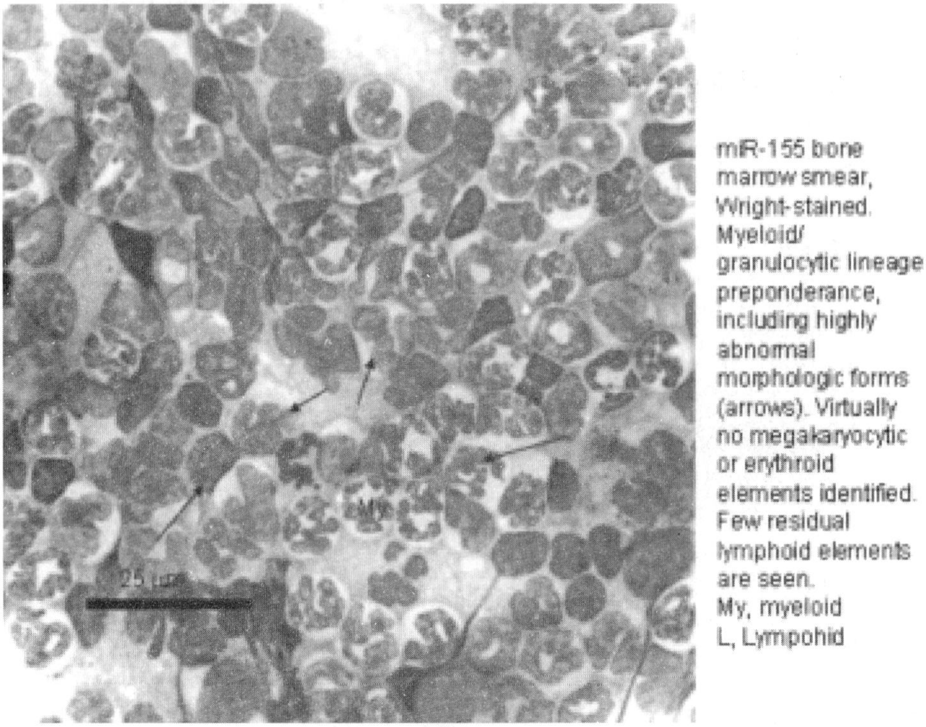

Fig. 1.42

them. The reason for doing that is just to get rid of the clonal effect and we looked at micro arrays. What you see is that certain genes are heavily down regulated in these cells as a consequence of the expression of 155 (Fig. 1.44). The genes have become specialized. As you go through the literature,

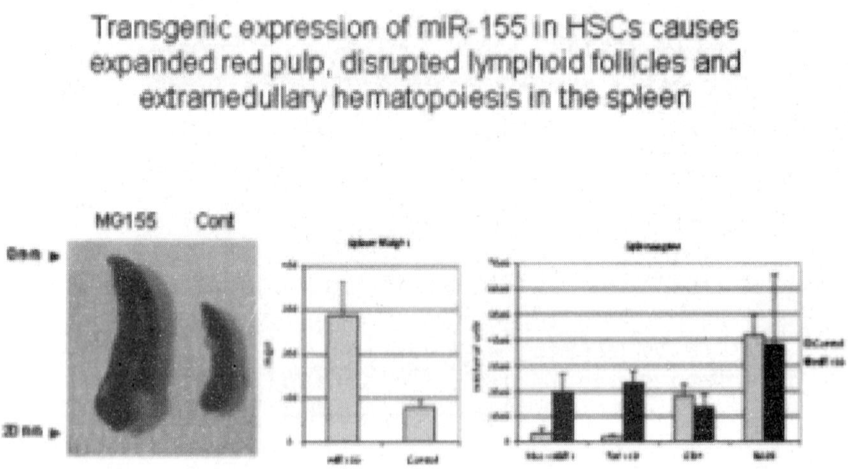

Fig. 1.43

you discover that many of these are genes that have been identified as causing myeloid malignancies through loss of functions. These are genes, whose expression when reduced, cause myeloid leukemia and this has to deal with how myeloid cells differentiate. They ordinarily require all these proteins to differentiate and if those are not there, they do not differentiate and become immature cells that lead to cancer- not true of all of the genes but it is true of many of them. I would not go into the details about the individual ones.

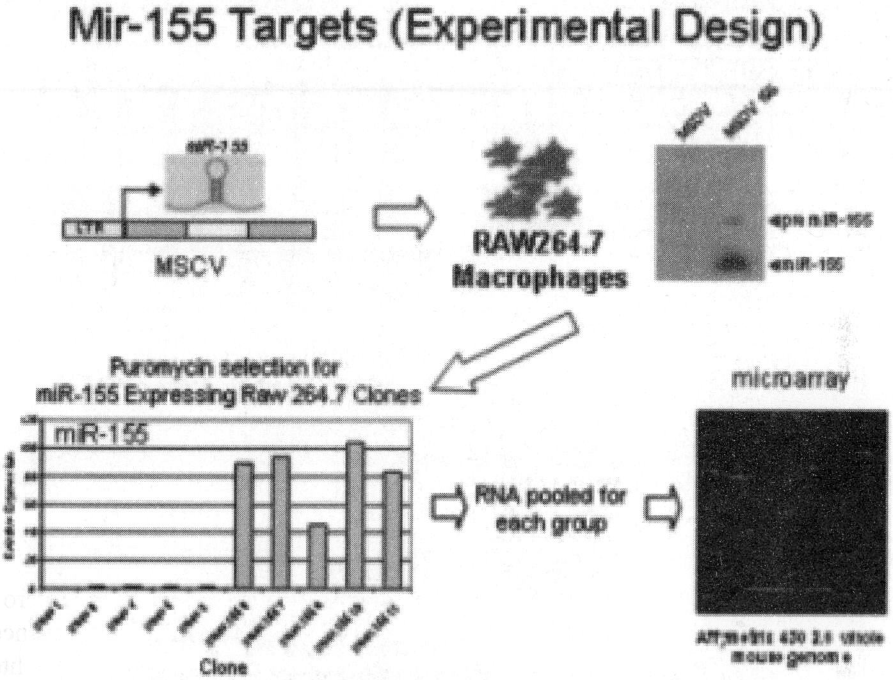

Fig. 1.44

We have also shown using reporter assays with the appropriate 3 prime external regions that all of these genes are sensitive to 155 (Fig. 1.45 and Fig. 1.46). And then we looked in human acute myeloid leukemia and we find that many cases of acute myeloid leukemia have increased levels of 155 expression (Fig. 1.47). I would not go into the details of that, but it suggests that this could be involved in human myeloid cancer as well as in their important normal functions.

So, the summary for 155 is that like 146, it is induced by proinflammatory stimuli, actually induced via a wider range of stimuli than 146, but unlike 146 we do not see any indication to place a feedback really (Fig. 1.48). It was shown in published papers of a year or two ago that it has multiple effects on the lymphoid lineage, suggesting that it may play important roles in lymphoid development. We are looking now at myeloid development. As I showed you, uncontrolled expression of miR-155 leads to myeloid proliferation and it does control myeloid related genes. And, so I think the idea that there is a link between unregulated NF-kB expression and cancer involving 155 might be worthwhile to test although it might take a lot longer to really prove that.

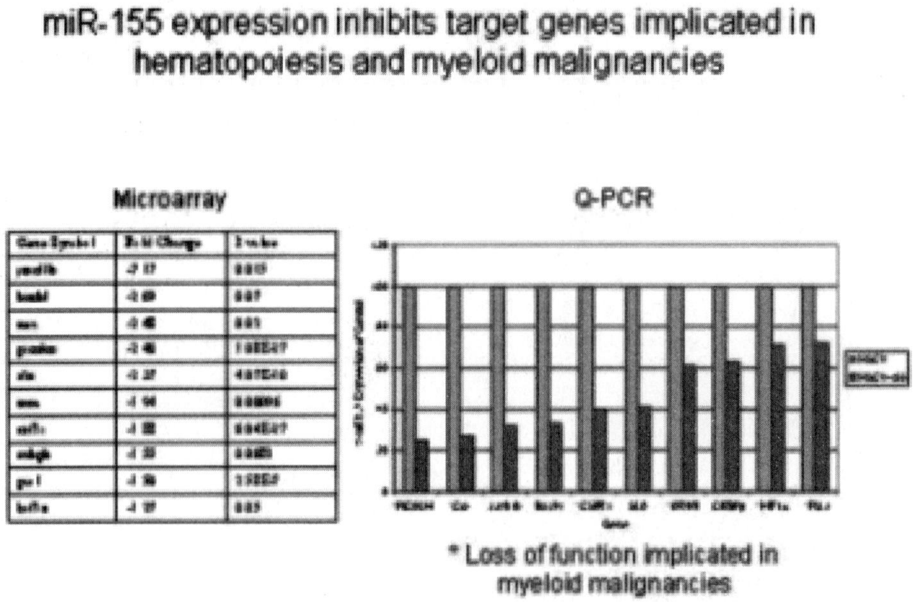

Fig. 1.45

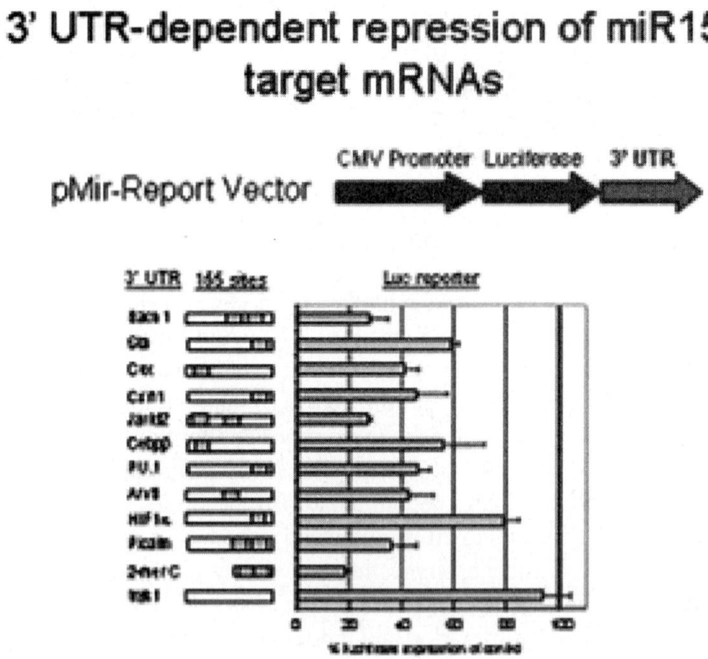

Fig. 1.46

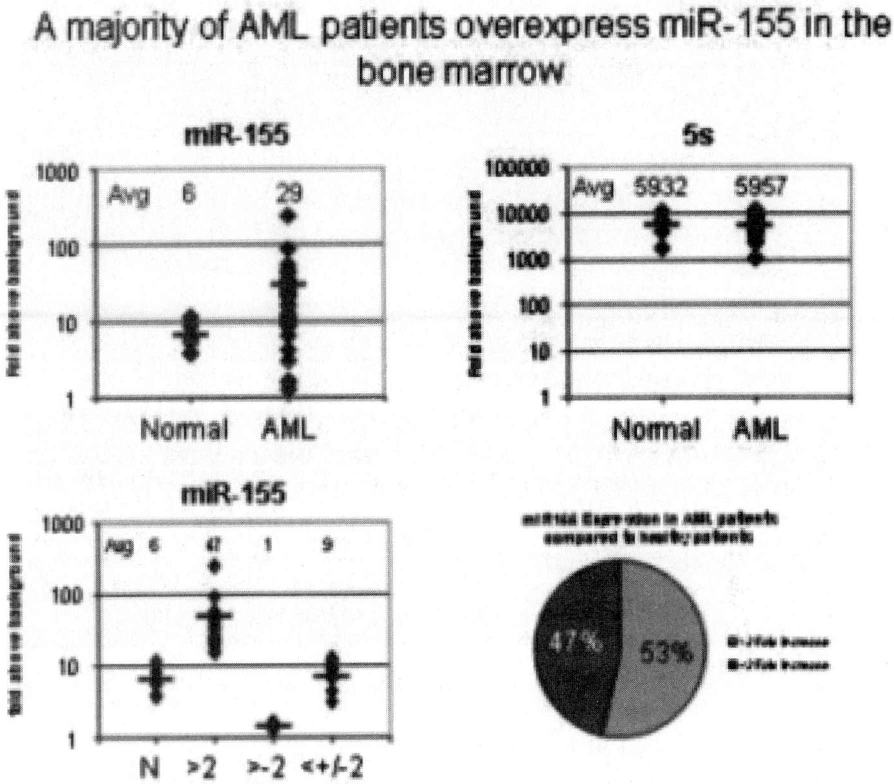

Fig. 1.47

Let me finish by just a sort of speculative look at what we learned about microRNAs from this work and from certain other in the literature (Fig. 1. 48). We know that there are very different kinds of decisions in cells, which are controlled by microRNAs: developmental decisions and feedback regulatory pathways that I have told you about. But when you look at them in detail, at the behavior of cells that over-express 146 or 155, you will get a surprising generality; which is that those choice points in hematopoiesis may be controlled in general by microRNAs, which should be 146 and 155. The 146 is involved in the decision of whether to make B1b cells or conventional B2b cells. It is also involved in other decisions way down the tree of lymphoid cells. I have shown you that 155 is involved in the decision of whether to make myeloid cells or to make erythrocytes or B cells, and over expression of it causes a shift to myeloids. Another microRNA, I forgot its number, has been shown in unpublished work or maybe recently published work to effect the decision about whether to make platelets or erythrocytes way down in the decision tree of myeloid lineage. And, in fact, in 2004, Lodish and Bartel showed that mir181 could increase the B cell output of HSCs from 32% to 80%, a huge effect. So you get this picture that microRNAs are regulators of genes involved in choice points during hematopoiesis and that this may be a clue to their important rolc in cancer; and with that, I thank you very much for your attention.

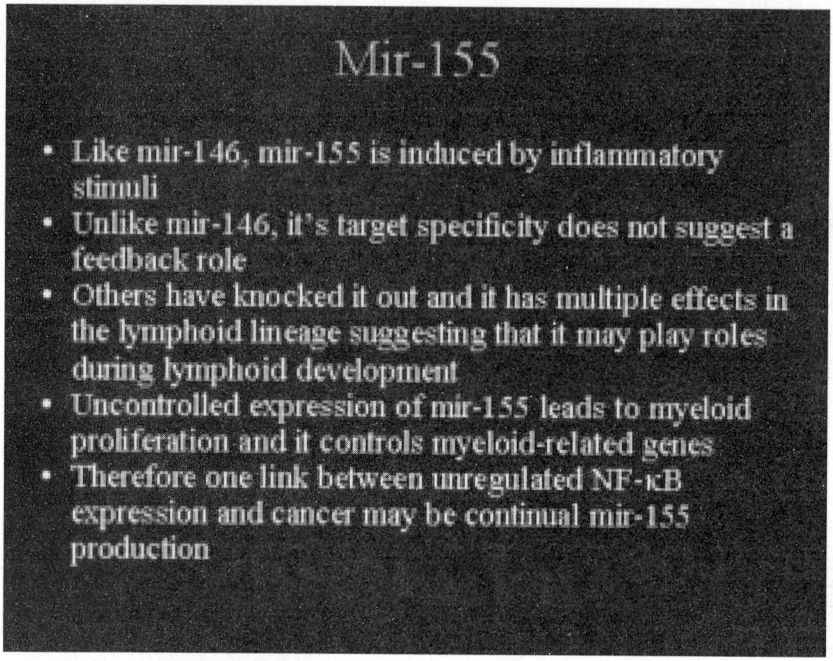

Fig. 1.48

(The organizers are grateful to Dr. Sunil Mukherjee of the International Centre for Genetic Engineering & Biotechnology for putting together this manuscript from a recorded version of the opening plenary lecture given by Dr. David Baltimore.)

2

CHAPTER

Therapeutic Significance of Increased Tissue Transglutaminase Expression in Pancreatic Cancer

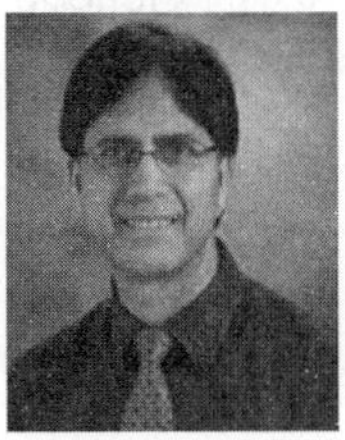

Kapil Mehta

Department of Experimental Therapeutics, The University of Texas, M. D. Anderson Cancer Center, Houston, TX 77030, USA

ABSTRACT

Pancreatic ductal adenocarcinoma (PDAC) is a serious health problem worldwide. Approximately, 33000 new patients are diagnosed annually with PDAC and about the same number die of the disease. Difficulty in early diagnosis, rapid metastasis and profound resistance to drugs are major factors that contribute to dismal survival rates in these patients. Therefore, understanding the molecular pathways and proteins that contribute to the development of intrinsic resistance and invasive behavior of PDAC cells are likely to yield immediate clinical benefits by offering new and novel therapeutic targets against PDAC. We recently found that: a) the majority of PDAC tumors and cell lines express elevated levels of tissue transglutaminase (TG2), a unique multifunctional protein implicated in such diverse functions as cell adhesion, matrix-stabilization, wound healing, apoptosis and invasion; b) TG2 by forming stable complexes with certain beta- members of the

email: kmehta@mdanderson.org

integrin family of proteins can promote constitutive activation of focal adhesion kinase (FAK), PI3K/Akt and NF-kB cell survival pathways; c) inhibition of TG2 by small interfering RNA (siRNA) inhibited the invasiveness and induced autophagic death in PDAC cells; whereas, ectopic expression of TG2 promoted cell survival and invasive functions in PDAC cells. These results clearly suggest that aberrant expression of TG2 in cancer cells plays a pivotal role in conferring chemoresistance and metastatic phenotypes. Indeed, in a preclinical mouse model, target-specific ablation of TG2 significantly retarded tumor growth and inhibited local dissemination of orthotopically growing tumors.

INTRODUCTION

Pancreatic cancer (pancreatic ductal adenocarcinma; PDAC) represents one of the most aggressive neoplastic diseases. Although, gemcitabine (Gemzar™) remains the drug of choice for treating PDAC patients but either alone or in combination with other anicancer modalites, this drug has minimal impact on patient survival. Moreover, most patients with PDAC exhibit marked resistance to other conventional chemotherapies which leaves surgical resection the only curative therapy for PDAC. Unfortunately, the disease is so aggressive that only 10-20% patients qualify for surgery at the time of diagnosis (1). These dismal figures clearly suggest the need for identifying new therapeutic targets for effective control and treatment of PDAC.

In this respect our recent observations that irrespective of the source or type, cancer cells selected for resistance to chemotherapeutic drugs or isolated from metastatic sites express elevated levels of the multifunctional protein, tissue transglutaminase (TG2) (2-5). Importantly, increased expression of TG2 is associated with an increased resistance of cancer cells to apoptosis. Indeed, a common feature among aggressive forms of cancer cells is that they exhibit profound resistance to apoptosis (6, 7), the property that enables tumor cells not only to grow and survive successfully in foreign tissue microenvironments (i.e., metastasize) but could also confer protection against chemotherapeutic drugs (8).

TG2 PROMOTES DRUG RESISTANCE AND METASTATIC PHENOTYPE

The realization that majority of anticancer drugs kill tumor cells by activating common apoptotic pathways raises an interesting possibility that dysregulation of intrinsic apoptotic pathways may be a key determinant in the development of chemoresistance in tumor cells. Indeed, several alterations that confer resistance to apoptosis in cancer cells have been identified. For example, activation of pro-survival signal transduction pathways, such as those mediated by Ras, PI3K/Akt, and NF-kB are frequently observed during advance stages of cancer (6-8).

Several recent reports have supported the conviction that increased expression of TG2 promotes cell-survival functions by preventing apoptosis (9-13). Many cancer cell types selected for resistance to chemotherapeutic drugs or isolated from metastatic sites exhibit elevated levels of TG2 expression (2-5). Importantly, downregulation of endogenous TG2 by siRNA, antisense or ribozyme approach reversed the drug-resistance phenotype in breast cancer (3, 11) and lung cancer cells (12). Conversely, treatment of cancer cells with the growth factor, epidermal growth factor (EGF) upregulated the expression of TG2 and protected cells from doxorubicin-induced apoptosis (13). Similar to drug-resistance, the development of metastatic phenotype in breast cancer (5, 14), malignant melanoma (4) and ovarian cancer (15) cells, is associated with increased levels of TG2 expression. These observations were indirectly supported by Jiang et al. (16) who in an attempt to identify metastasis-associated proteins by proteomic analysis, identified TG2 as one of the 11 proteins that were selectively amplified in metastatic human lung carcinoma.

Notably, downregulation of TG2 by siRNA resulted in increased propensity of cancer cells to undergo apoptosis and inhibited their invasiveness (3, 14, 17). Similarly, retinoic acid-induced TG2 expression was associated with increased migration and invasion of the neuroblastoma SH-SY5 cells. More recently, Satpathy et al. (15) extended these observations *in vivo* and demonstrated that increased expression of TG2 in ovarian cancer cells enhanced their adhesion to fibronectin and directional cell migration. Accordingly, ovarian cancer cells with knockdown TG2 showed diminished tumor dissemination on peritoneal surface and mesentery in an intraperitoneal ovarian xenograft mouse model. Thus, aberrant expression of TG2 in cancer cells could contribute to the development of drug resistance and metastatic phenotypes by promoting cell survival and invasive functions. These observations clearly suggest that aberrant expression of TG2 in cancer cells promotes cell survival and invasive functions.

TG2 IN PANCREATIC CANCER

Recently, we reported that the majority of PDAC tumors and cell lines have high basal levels of TG2 expression (18). Figure 1 demonstrates the extent of TG2 in selected pancreatic cancer samples and cell lines. Ten of the 12 PDAC cell lines that we tested showed high basal levels of TG2. The two well-differentiated PDAC cell lines (BxPC-3 and HPAF II) contained low but detectable levels of TG2 whereas, normal immortalized pancreatic epithelial cells (HPV E6E7) completely lacked the expression.

We also examined the expression of TG2 in patients' samples using tissue microarray containing 65 PDAC samples and 9 normal pancreatic tissue samples. We found high basal levels of TG2 expression in 51 of the 65 (78%) tumor samples (Fig.2.1). However, only one of the nine (11%) normal pancreatic tissue samples showed weak cytoplasmic staining for TG2. Thus, TG2 expression was significantly higher in PDAC tumor samples than in normal ducts ($P < 0.0001$). We observed no staining in sections treated with control isotypic IgG instead of an anti-TG2 antibody. High TG2 expression in tumor samples was significantly associated with nodal metastasis, lymphovascular invasion, and clinical stage. In an independent study by Iacobuzio-Donahue *et al.* (19) analysis of >33000 genes using three different technologies, revealed TG2 as one of the most differentially expressed genes in PDAC tumors.

Importantly, the level of TG2 expression in PDAC cells directly correlated with their resistance to gemcitabine, the most commonly used drug for treatment of pancreatic cancer (18). Thus, high-TG2 expressing Panc-28 cells showed minimal sensitivity to gemcitabine (IC_{50}=10 μM) when compared with TG2-deficient BxPC3 cells (IC_{50}= 0.1 μM). Similar to PDAC, the development of drug-resistance in breast and lung cancer cells has been associated with elevated levels of TG2 expression. Downregulation of endogenous TG2 by antisense or siRNA approach resulted in the reversal of drug-resistance in these cells. These results were recently confirmed by Kim *et al.* (11) who reported that inhibition of TG2 expression in drug-resistant MCF-7 breast cancer cells is associated with inhibition of the transcription factor NF-kB activation and reversal of drug resistance. These results clearly suggest that aberrant expression of TG2 in PDAC cells contributes to their intrinsic resistance to chemotherapeutic drugs.

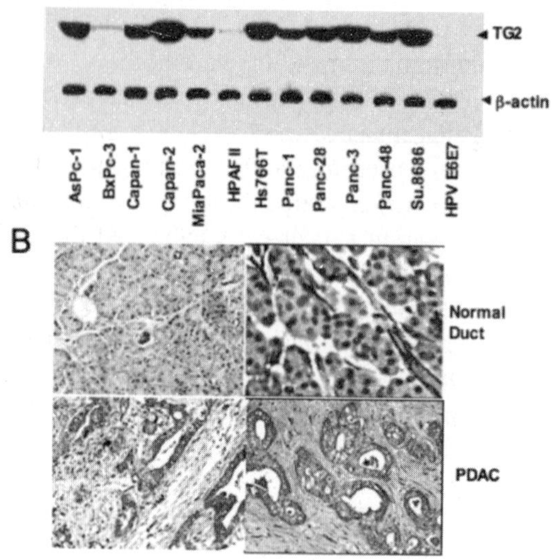

Fig. 2.1 High basal expression of TG2 is observed in PDAC tumors and cell lines. *A,* The 10 poorly-differentiated PDAC cell lines show high basal expression of TG2; the 2 well-differentiated (BxPC3 and HPAF-II) PDAC cell lines show low TG2; whereas, infinite normal pancreatic epithelial (E6E7) cells totally lack the expression. *B,* Representative tissue samples showing no TG2 staining and faint TG2 staining of endothelial cells in a normal pancreatic ductal epithelium samples (upper panel) and strong TG2 staining in a PDAC tumor sample (lower panel) (adopted from reference #18).

Moreover, overexpression of TG2 in PDAC cells is associated with increased invasiveness through the Matrigel- transwell inserts. Thus, high-TG2 expressing Panc-28 cells showed significantly more invasion than the low-TG2 expressing BxPC-3 cells (Fig. 2.2). To elucidate the role of TG2 in invasive functions, we downregulated the expression of endogenous TG2 in Panc-28 cells by siRNA approach.

We identified two TG2 sequences that are potential target sites for siRNA and do not share homology with any known sequences in the database except the human TG2 (14). Using commercially synthesized siRNA (siRNA1 and siRNA2) we transfected Panc-28 cells. As a control, cells were also transfected with scrambled siRNA (control siRNA) in which the sequence was scrambled but the nucleotide composition was the same as that in the siRNA2. Forty-eight hours later, cells were harvested and subjected to Western blot analysis and the enzymatic activity was determined. The siRNAs but not the scrambled siRNA, inhibited TG2 expression by 70-80% when compared with sham-transfected (transfection reagent alone) or untreated control; the amount of ?-actin (loading control) was identical in all samples (Fig. 2.2C). Consistent with the notion that TG2 expression promotes cell invasion, the ability of Panc-28 cells to invade through the Matrigel-transwell membrane was dramatically decreased in TG2 knockdown Panc-28 cells (Fig. 2A/B; lower panel). These results confirmed that TG2 expression by siRNA is feasible and that endogenous TG2 promotes invasive phenotype in PDAC cells. In an inverse experiment, the infection of low-TG2 expressing BxPC-3 cells with TG2-adenoviral construct (Fig. 2A/B, upper panel), rendered the cells highly invasive when compared with non-infected or 'adenovirus-alone' infected control cells.

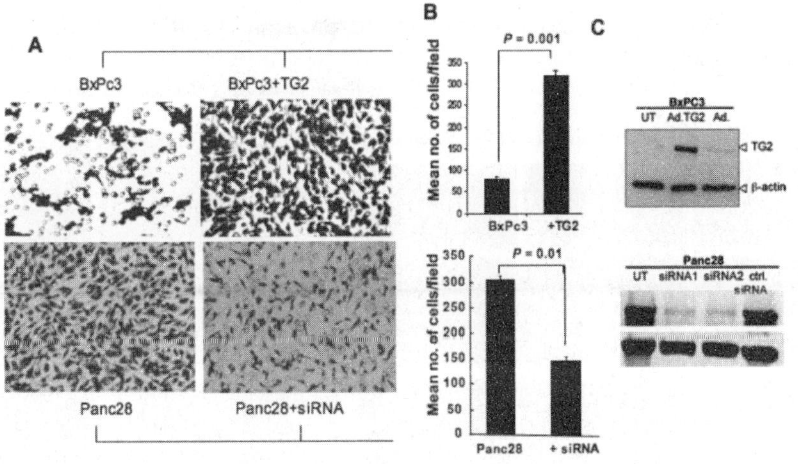

Fig. 2.2 TG2 overexpression promotes invasion of PDAC cells. *A,* Invasion of untreated and TG2-infected BxPC-3 (upper panel) cells and untreated or TG2-siRNA-transfected Panc-28 cells (lower panel) through the Matrigel-Transwell inserts after 48 h incubation. *B,* Mean number of TG2-infected (+TG2) and vector alone-infected BxPC-3 cells (upper panel) and TG2 siRNA (+siRNA)-transfected or control siRNA-transfected Panc-28 cells in 10 random microscopic fields was calculated and plotted. *C.* TG2 expression in BxPC-3 cells before and after TG2 infection (upper panel) and in Panc-28 cells before and after siRNA-transfection (Adopted from reference #18).

DOWNREGULATION OF TG2 INDUCES AUTOPHAGIC DEATH

An important observation we made during siRNA transfection of PDAC cells was that downregulation of endogenous TG2 was associated with onset of autophagic cell death (type II programmed cell death). Thus, transfection of Panc-28 cells with TG2 siRNA (but not control-siRNA) was associated with massive accumulation of autophagic vacuoles as revealed by phase-contrast microscopy (Figure 2.3A, left column). The vacuoles were highly acidic in nature as determined by acridine orange staining (Figure 2.3A, middle column) and were accompanied by accumulation of microtubule-associated light chain (LC3) protein (Figure 2.3A, right column), the hallmarks of autophagy. In control siRNA treated cells none of these changes were evident. We further analyzed the autophagy in TG2 downregulated Panc-28 cells by transmission electron microscopy (TEM). Results in Figure 3B clearly demonstrated formation of autophagosomes containing cellular organelles in TG2 siRNA treated cells. Prolonged inhibition of TG2 by siRNA resulted in severe damage and irreversible death of PDAC cells.

TG2 AS THERAPEUTIC TARGET FOR PDAC

Based on our observations discussed in the preceding section, we speculated that inhibition of TG2 could be a promising therapeutic target for reversing intrinsic resistance of PDAC to chemotherapeutic drugs. Using DOPC liposomes as the delivery system, we showed that TG2 siRNA could effectively downregulate TG2 expression in tumors and inhibit their growth and metastatic spread (Fig. 2.4; ref. 20). Notably, downregulation of TG2 expression by siRNA-DOPC rendered PDAC cells sensitive to gemcitabine.

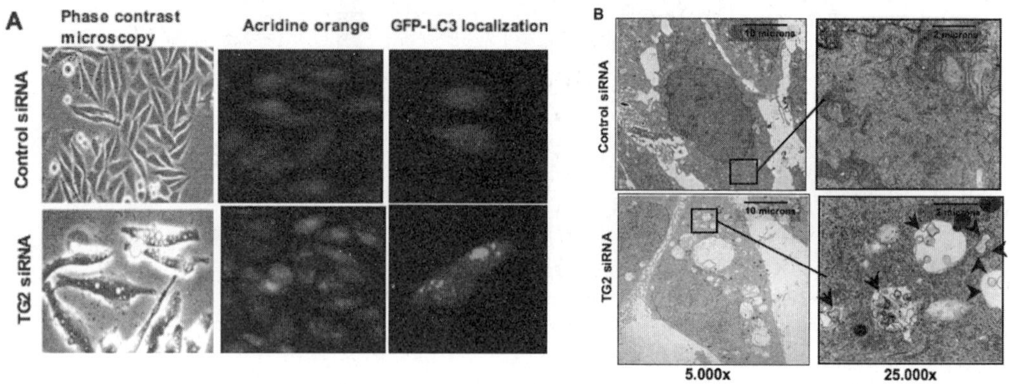

Fig. 2.3 Downregulation of TG2 induces autophagic death in PADC cells. *A*. Detection of autophago-lysosomes. Panc-28 cells were treated with either control siRNA or TG2 siRNA for 72 h. *Left panel*, morphologic changes seen under the phase-contrast microscope; *Middle panel*, acridine orange staining of the acidic vesicular organelles under the fluorescent microscope; *Right panel*, localization of LC3 at autophagosomes in Panc28 cells co-transfected with GFP-LC3 plasmid. *B*. Electron micrographs showing ultrastructural changes induced in Panc-28 cells in response to TG2 downregulation by siRNA (96 h). Numerous autophagic vacuoles (indicated by arrows) were evident in TG2 siRNA treated cells. (Adopted from reference #17).

To determine potential mechanisms underlying the antitumor effect of TG2 siRNA-DOPC, we examined its effect on several biological end-points, including cell proliferation (Ki-67), angiogenesis (CD31), and apoptosis (TUNEL). More than 90% reduction in Ki-67 expression was evident ($p < 0.001$) in tumors obtained from mice given TG2 siRNA-DOPC alone or in combination with gemcitabine. Tumors obtained from mice given gemcitabine alone or control siRNA-DOPC consistently showed high levels of Ki-67 staining (20). We also evaluated the blood vessel density in tumors obtained from mice treated with control siRNA-DOPC, gemcitabine, TG2- siRNA-DOPC or combination of gemcitabine plus TG2-siRNA-DOPC. The results obtained revealed a significant decrease in the mean blood vessel density in tumors recovered from mice that received TG2 siRNA-DOPC or gemcitabine alone. Densitometric analysis showed a significant difference in the mean microvascular density ($P < 0.0013$) in the mice that received TG2 siRNA-DOPC plus gemcitabine as gemcitabine can affect the neovascularization process in a paracrine manner by affecting VEGF levels rather than due to downregulation of TG2 in endothelial cells. Finally, we evaluated apoptosis in orthotopic tumors using TUNEL assay. PDAC tumors treated with gemcitabine alone or in combination with TG2 siRNA-DOPC showed significant increases in the numbers of apoptotic cells. No differences in the apoptotic index in TG2 siRNA-DOPC-treated tumors were evident, and the extent of apoptosis in this group was similar to that in the control siRNA-DOPC group.

The mechanism by which TG2 contributes to the development of chemoresistance and metastatic phenotypes remains unknown. A recent report by Akimov *et al.* (21) suggested that TG2

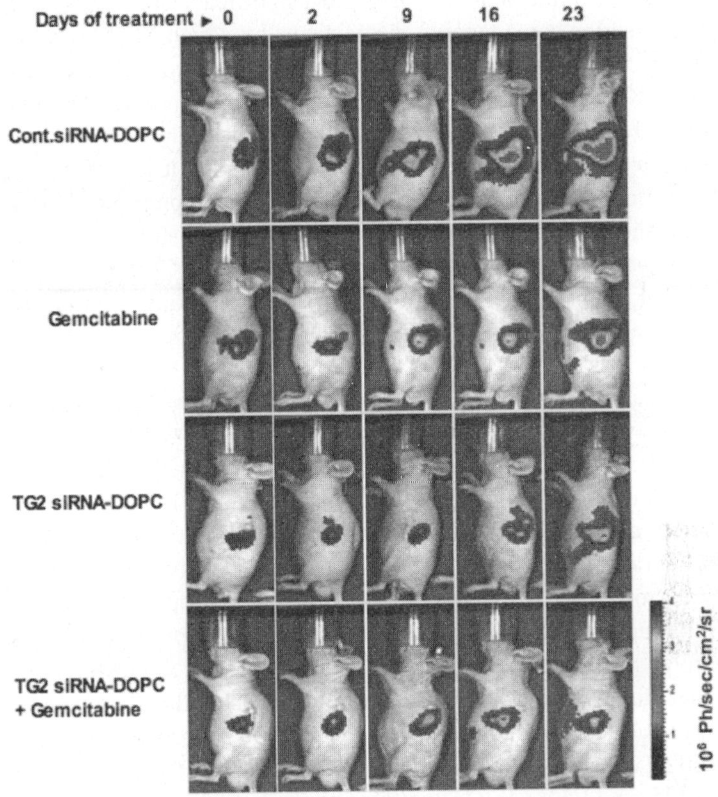

Fig. 2.4 TG2 targeted therapy of PDAC tumors in nude mice. Human pancreatic (Panc-28) cells stably tranduced with *luciferase* gene, were orthotopically implanted in the pancreases of nude mice. After 2 weeks of tumor cell implantation mice were randomly divided into 4 groups and treated with either control siRNA-DOPC, gemcitabine alone, TG2-siRNA DOPC alone or combination of gemcitabine plus TG2-siRNA-DOPC. The IVIS images of representative mice in each treatment group taken at the indicated days of treatment are shown. Mice were imaged in the ventral view using the LivingImage Software program (adopted from reference # 20).

could interact and form stable complexes with b1 and b3 integrins. This finding led to the delineation of significance of increased TG2 expression in cancer cells. Our own studies revealed that in addition to b1-integrin, compared to the mice that received control siRNA-DOPC. Taken together, these results suggested that downregulation of TG2 expression in combination with gemcitabine can result in decreased VEGF expression and decreased mean blood vessel density. Thus, treatment with TG2 siRNA-DOPC plus TG2 could bind to and form stable complex with ?b4 and ?b5 integrin in breast cancer, malignant melanoma , and pancreatic cancer cells. TG2 is known to associate with integrins primarily in the extracellular domains of integrins and to promote their interaction with the extracellular matrix (ECM) ligands, such as fibronectin, collagen, and vitronectin. Therefore, it is possible that TG2 contributes to the aggressive behavior of PDAC by constitutively activating integrin-mediated cell survival signaling pathways.

Work in our laboratory to understand the biological significance of increased TG2 expression in PDAC cells led us to describe some tenable mechanisms by which TG2 expression could result in constitutive activation of FAK, Akt, and NF-kB (18, 22). Thus, TG2 expression activated and autophosphorylated FAK (pY397), and downregulation of TG2 expression inhibited this activation. Moreover, TG2-induced activation of FAK results in activation of the PI3K/Akt cell survival signaling pathway (23). More recent studies provided some interesting leads and suggested that expression of TG2 in PDAC cells is inversely correlated with PTEN expression (Verma A *et al.,* unpublished). TG2 inhibited the phosphorylation of PTEN at serine-380 and promoted its degradation via the ubiquitin/proteasome pathway. Thus, TG2 plays a dual role in the FAK/PI3K/Akt signaling pathway by: promoting direct phosphorylation of FAK and inhibiting its upstream phosphatase, PTEN, resulting in constitutive activation of the PI3K/Akt pathway.

Moreover, TG2 expression results in constitutive activation of NF-kB (11, 22). Under normal conditions, the inflammation-induced NF-kB activation is transient, which is critical for the controlled growth and survival of normal cells. Thus, TG2-mediated constitutive activation of NF-kB in cancer cells may be critical to conferring chemoresistance and metastatic phenotypes. Indeed, our recent data support such contention and suggested that downregulation of TG2 expression by siRNA in drug-resistant breast cancer and PDAC cells results in inhibition of NF-kB and increases their sensitivity to chemotherapeutic drugs (3, 12, 24). Kim *et al.* (11) have observed a similar correlation between TG2 expression, drug resistance, and NF-kB activation in breast cancer cells. Taken together, these results suggest that TG2 plays an important role in promoting cell survival signaling and thus confers protection to PDAC cells against drug-induced cell death.

In conclusion, our studies have provided the proof of concept that therapeutic delivery of gene-specific siRNA to PDAC tumors can be achieved using DOPC liposomes. Two recent reports documented a similar effect of DOPC liposomal delivery of siRNA to silence the expression of the oncoprotein EphA2 (25) and FAK (26). Using this approach, both studies documented encouraging responses to the treatment of ovarian tumors in mice. Thus, the significance of the results of this study can be rapidly translated into the clinical setting for treatment of aggressive forms of cancer, including PDAC.

REFERENCES

1. Maheshwari V, Moser AJ. Current management of locally advanced pancreatic cancer. Nat Clin Pract Gastroenterol Hepatol 2005;2:356–64.
2. Mehta K, Fok JY, Mangala LS. Tissue transglutaminase: from biological glue to cell survival cues. Front Biosci 2006;11:173-85.
3. Herman JF, Mangala LS, Mehta K. Implications of increased tissue transglutaminase (TG2) expression in drug-resistant breast cancer (MCF-7) cells. Oncogene 2006;25:3049-58
4. Fok J, Ekmekcioglu S, Mehta K. Implications of tissue transglutaminase expression in malignant melanoma. Mol Cancer Therp, 2006;5:1493-503.
5. Mehta K, Fok J, Miller FR, Koul D, Sahin AA. Prognostic significance of tissue transglutaminase in drug resistant and metastatic breast cancer. Clin Cancer Res 2004;10:8068-76.
6. Igney FH, Krammer PH (2002) Death and anti-death: tumor resistance to apoptosis, *Nature Rev* **2**: 277-288.

7. Fesik, S. W. (2005) Promoting apoptosis as a strategy for cancer drug discovery. Nat. Rev Cancer. **5:** 876-885

8. Krebel RS, Kobayashi H, Graham CH (1994) Intrinsic or acquired drug resistance and metastasis: Are they linked phenotypes? *J Cell Biochem* **56**:37-47.

9. Milakovic T, Tucholski J, McCoy E, Johnson JVW (2004) Intracellular localization and activity state of tissue transglutaminase differentially impacts cell death. *J Biol Chem* **279**:8715-8722.

10. Boehm JE, Singh U, Combs C, Antonyak MA, Cerione RA (2002) Tissue transglutaminase protects against apoptosis by modifying the tumor suppressor protein p110 Rb. *J Biol Chem* **277**:20127-20130.

11. Kim DS, Park SS, Nam BH, Kim IH, Kim SY (2006) Reversal of drug resistance in breast cancer cells by transglutaminase 2 inhibition and nuclear factor-kB inactivation. *Cancer Res* **66**:10936-10943.

12. Han JA, Park SC (1999) Reduction of transglutaminase-2 expression is associated with an induction of drug sensitivity in the PC-14 human lung cancer cell line. *J Cancer Res Clin Oncol* **125**: 89-95.

13. Antonyak MA, Miller AM, Jansen JM, et al. (2004). Augmentation of tissue transglutaminase expression and activation by epidermal growth factor inhibit doxorubicin-induced apoptosis in human breast cancer cells. *J Biol Chem* **279**, 41461-41467.

14. Mangala LS, Fok JY, Zorrilla-Calancha IR, Verma A, Mehta K. Tissue transglutaminase expression promotes cell attachment, invasion and survival in breast cancer cells. Oncogene. 2007; 26: 2459-70.

15. Satpathy M, Cao L, Pincheira R, *et al.* Enhanced peritoneal ovarian tumor dissemination by tissue transglutaminase. Cancer Res 2007;67:7194-202.

16. Jiang W, Ying Y, Lu J. Identification of metastasis- associated proteins by proteomic analysis and functional exploration of interleukin-18 in metastasis. Proteomics 2003;3:724-37.

17. Akar U, Ozpolat B, Mehta K, Fok J, Kondo Y, Lopez-Berestein G. Tissue transglutaminase inhibits autophagy in pancreatic cancer cells. Mol Cancer Res. 2007;5:241-49.

18. Verma A, Wang H, Manavathi B, et al. Increased expression of tissue transglutaminase in pancreatic ductal adenocarcinoma and its implications in drug resistance and metastasis. Cancer Res 2006;66:10525-33.

19. Iacobuzio-Donahue CA, Ashfaq R, Maitra A et al. Highly expressed genes in pancreatic ductal adenocarcinomas: a comprehensive characterization and comparison of the transcription profiles obtained from three major technologies. Cancer Res. 2003;63:8614-22.

20. Verma A, Guha S, Diagaradjane P, Kunnumakkara AB, Sanguino AM, Lopez-Berestein G, Sood AK, Aggarwal BB, Krishnan S, Gelovani JG, Mehta K. Therapeutic significance of elevated tissue transglutaminase expression in pancreatic cancer. Clin Cancer Res (In press), 2008.

21. Akimov SS, Krylov D, Fleischman LF, and Belkin AM. Tissue transglutaminase is an integrin-binding adhesion coreceptor for fibronectin. J Cell Biol 2000;148:825-38.

22. Mann AP, Verma A, Sethi G, et al. Overexpression of tissue transglutaminase leads to constitutive activation of nuclear factor- {kappa} B in cancer cells: delineation of a novel pathway. Cancer Res 2006;66:8788-95.

23. Verma A, Mehta K. Tissue transglutaminase-mediated chemoresistance in cancer cells. Drug Resist Updates 2007;10:144-51.

24. Verma A, Mehta K. Transglutaminase-mediated activation of nuclear transcription factor-kB in cancer cells: a new therapeutic opportunity. Curr Cancer Drug Targets 2007;7:559-65.
25. Landen CN, Jr., Chavez-Reyes A, Bucana C, et al. Therapeutic EphA2 gene targeting *in vivo* using neutral liposomal small interfering RNA delivery. Cancer Res 2005;65:6910-18.
26. Halder J, Aprana AK, Landen CN, et al. Focal adhesion kinase targeting using in vivo short interfering RNA delivery in neutral liposomes for ovarian carcinoma therapy. Clin Cancer Res. 2006;12:4916-24.

3

CHAPTER

Novel Si-RNA-Ribozyme Constructs Against HIV-1 and X Gene of Hepatitis B Virus

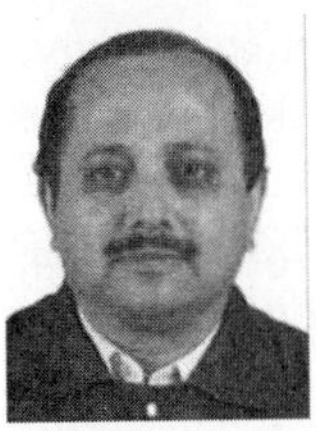

Nidhi Gupta, Aalia S. Bano, Yogeshwar Sharma, Vikas Sood and Akhil C. Banerjea

National Institute of Immunology, Division of Virology, New Delhi

INTRODUCTION

Catalytic nucleic acids made up of either RNA (ribozyme) or DNA (the DNA-enzymes or DNAzymes) are promising therapeutic molecules that possess the ability to interfere with the expression of any target gene in a sequence-specific manner (1-5). There are several kinds of ribozymes but the hammerhead motif containing ribozymes are exploited more extensively followed by hairpin motif containing ribozyme besides others. Lately, short catalytic DNA molecules, called DNA-enzymes or DNAzymes (Dzs) have gained lots of importance. Prominent among them are the 10-23 and 8-17 motif containing DNA-enzymes that have attracted the most attention and currently being exploited for gene therapy (5, 6 -8). The emergence of evolutionary conserved small interfering RNA (siRNA) technology in its ability to silence a target gene in more potent and sequence-specific manner have led to very important discoveries ranging from probing the cellular functions of the genes (functional genomics), targeted drug discovery to its possible use in a therapeutic setting. One of the major features about an effective siRNA is that only few molecules per cell are able to knock down the gene expression as compared to catalytic RNA/DNA or antisense

(RNA or DNA) which usually require more amounts that often leads to toxicity problems. Although siRNA provides very promising approach to knock down the gene expression, occasionally off target effects and non-specific stimulation of the innate immune system mediated by specific sequences of siRNAs have been reported. Besides, significant progress has to be made for effective and safe delivery for human applications. Since the recognition of siRNAs as a powerful tool to silence the expression of any target gene, it has rapidly become the preferred means to interfere with the replication of several pathogens including variety of viruses (9 -10). We shall briefly review the results achieved in our laboratory at National Institute of Immunology, New Delhi along with few others using this approach taking the example of two viruses of great public health importance for India and worldwide, namely, HIV-1 and hepatitis B.

Catalytic RNA, DNA and siRNAs Against X Gene of Hepatitis B Virus

The X gene of hepatitis B (HBx) is strongly associated with hepatocellular carcinoma and may involve other tumor specific genes as well. It alone can activate several heterologous (cellular and viral) promoters including the HIV-1 LTR promoter. We recently showed that HBx protein potently activates both LTR-B and LTR-C driven reporter gene (11). Interestingly, the LTR-C mediated activation was significantly more than LTR-B and we additionally showed that both HIV-1 Tat and HBx protein can act synergistically in activating the HIV-1 LTR promoter. The fact that LTR-C promoter is activated by X protein more potently suggests that HIV-1 subtype-C (the major subtype that is causing the epidemic in India) replication may be accelerated. Several investigators have attempted to use nucleic acid based approaches against the HBx gene and they include ribozymes (12), DNA-enzymes) (13) and siRNAs (14). While impressive intracellular inhibition of HBx gene was obtained, different antiviral approaches (like Ribozymes, aptamers or siRNAs) need to be combined to make the antiviral approach more efficacious. We combined the earlier known hammerhead ribozyme (Rz-170) (12) with the small hairpin RNAi using a known cleavable linker (we subsequently intend to engineer a 10-23 DNA-enzyme cleavage site in place of the cleavable linker). A T7 RNA polymerase based construct was used to generate such an RNA construct as described earlier (15, 16) as showed in figure 1. The selectively disabled mutants (figure 1, panel B) were engineered to determine if the antiviral efficacy could be modulated with these mutants. These RNAs (wild-type and mutant versions) were introduced into mammalian cells along with the target gene expressing construct and monitored for downregulation of X RNA by RT-PCR techniques. Wild-type construct interfered very strongly, and as expected, the selectively disabled versions were less effective and siRNA component was the major contributor for inhibition of expression (figure 2, panels A and B). Not only the RNA levels were severely reduced, the wild type construct completely knocked down the intracellular levels of X protein by western blot analysis (figure 3, compare lanes 3 and 2). A prominent X protein specific band (16.5Kda) can be seen when the target encoding DNA was transfected (lane 2). Thus, we provide proof of concept that the inhibitory properties of Rz and siRNAs can be harnessed using the same construct and using selectively disabled constructs, it is possible to modulate this activity. These constructs are ready to be placed under a powerful pol III (CMV) or pol II (U6) promoter which can be placed in viral vectors, the most preferred being the lentivirus based vectors, for gene therapeutic approaches as used by one of us earlier (17, 18).

Fig: 3.1(A) 110 nt long chimeric construct having siRNA and Rz-170 linked by an intracellular cleavable spacer, designed against X-gene of Hepatitis B virus. This construct has a T7 promoter sequence at the 3' end for the hybridization of T7 oligo required for in vitro transcription by T7 polymerase. (B) The Chimeric transcript after in vitro transcription.

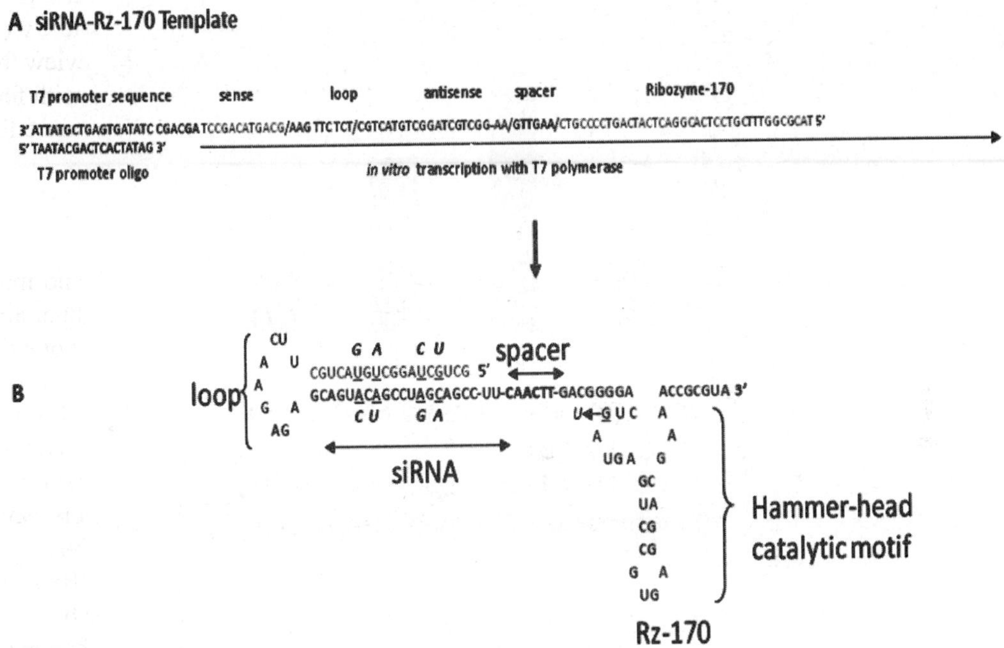

Fig. 3.1

Fig: 3.2 (A) Total RNA was isolated using trizol from HEK-293 cells transfected with HBx encoding plasmid and wt-siRNA-wtRz170, mt-siRNA-wtRz170 and wt-siRNA-mtRz170. After 48 hrs of transfection, the cells were subjected to RT-PCR to check the level of expression of HBx transcript along with the control RNA (huGAPDH). (B) Quantiatative estimation of the target RNA.

Fig: 3.3 Western blot was performed to study the level of HBx expression 48 hrs after transfection of HEK-293 cells with wt-siRNA-wtRz-170.

Inhibition of HIV-1 Gene Expression By Hammerhead Ribozymes and DNA-Enzymes

Both Ribozymes containing hammerhead and DNA-enzyme possessing 10-23 catalytic motifs have been described by us and others targeting different regions of either virus genes, namely TAT/Rev, Gag, Nef and HIV-1 coreceptors (for review reference # 5) etc. A multitarget ribozyme has been designed against TAT/Rev and also HIV-1 envelope (19 -20). While most studies utilized mono- (21) or a bi-specific ribozymes (22, 23) or DNA-enzymes, remarkably 9 ribozymes targeted against HIV-1 envelope RNA in tandem were placed together which was found to be very effective against HIV-1 as no escape variants were observed. Very recently we showed that both ribozyme and Dz when used in combination, are capable of cleaving HIV-1 target RNA more effectively under in

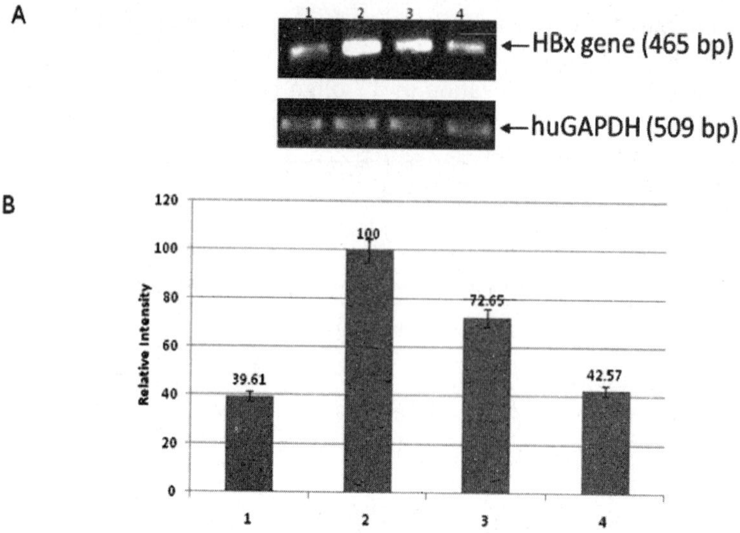

Lane1:HBx+ wt-siRNA-wtRz-170(1μg each)
Lane2:HBx(1μg)
Lane3:HBx+mt-siRNA-wtRz-170(1μg each)
Lane4:HBx+wt-siRNA-mtRz-170(1μg each)

Fig. 3.2

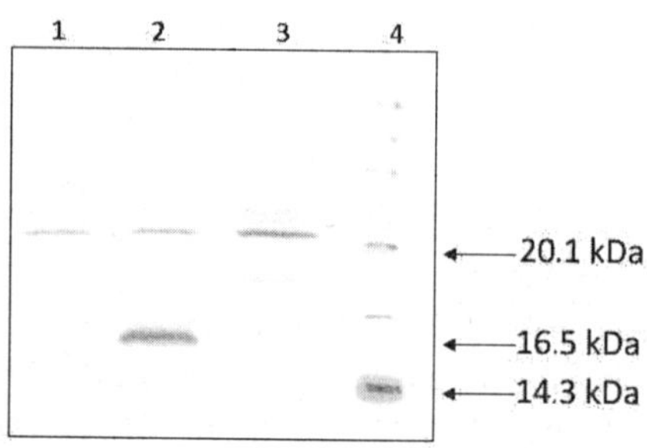

Lane1: control cells
Lane2: HBx(1μg)
Lane3: HBx+wt-siRNA-wtRz-170(1μg each)
Lane4: Rainbow marker 756

Fig. 3.3

vitro conditions and also in a synergistic manner intracellularly (24). HIV-1 infection is established by HIV-1 co-receptor CCR5 using virus (R5 tropic) and in advanced stages it is usually seen that that the virus is using another corecptor-CXCR4 present on the CD4+ve T lymphocytes. Individuals who possess a remarkable mutation (Δ32 mutant of CCR5) exhibit strong resistance to HIV-1 infection. This mutation is quite common in people with European descent but extremely rare among Asians and Africans as supported by our studies (25, 26). The fact that individuals who are homozygous for Δ32 CCR5 mutation are physically normal and R5 tropic virus needs it to initiate a successful infection, provides a unique opportunity to target this gene as an antiviral approach. We (21, 27) and others (28) therefore designed several Rzs and Dzs against the HIV-1 co-receptors (CCR5 and CXCR4).

Si-RNA Construct + Specific Antisense DNA Molecules Potently Knock Down Intracellular HIV-1 Tat/Rev RNA

Lately, we made an siRNA (small hairpin structure) construct against HIV-1 Tat/Rev (position 8369 to 8386 from pNL4-3 HIV-1 DNA – obtained from NIH, MD, USA) region using the T7RNA polymerase based system as described earlier. An antisense DNA molecule was synthesized immediately downstream of siRNA target sequence as shown by arrow (figure 3.4 panel A). The strategy has been described by one of the authors in some detail before (29 -30). Briefly, Si RNA (small hairpin loop) is synthesized using T7 promoter derived transcripts using T7 RNA polymerase construct as described earlier (15, 16). We then made a disabled version of this construct by creating

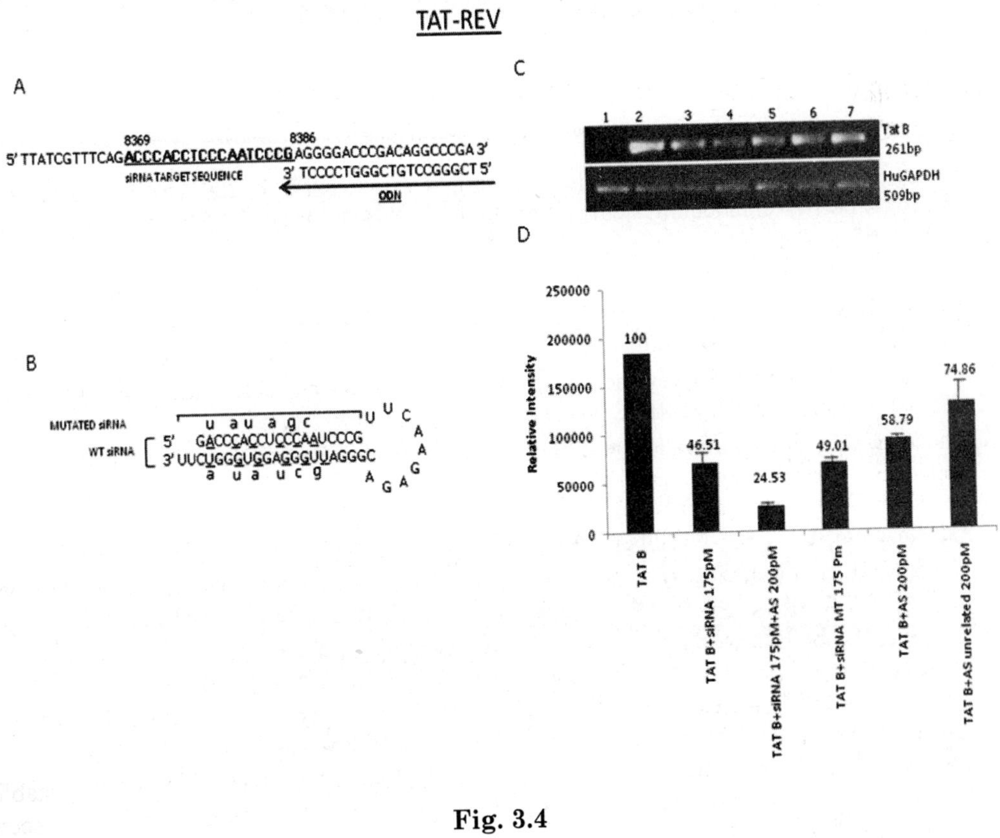

Fig. 3.4

six point mutations in the stem region (figure 3.4, panel B as shown by small case letters). When wild-type construct was co-transfected into a mammalian cell along with the target gene expressing expression vector, a potent reduction was observed (panel C and D). Remarkably, the level of target RNA was further reduced in the presence of antisense molecules. Unrelated antisense failed to interfere with the intracellular expression. This is the first report where target RNA levels could be modulated by the unique combination siRNA and antisense DNA molecule.

Fig. 3.4 (A) The target sequence (8369-8386) against which siRNA was designed and 20 mer antisense ODN was designed downstream to the siRNA target sequence. B) Wild type siRNA oligo with 3' two nucleotide overhangs was synthesized by sigma Aldrich and the mutant siRNA was synthesized having 6 point mutations in the stem region of the siRNA. (C) Total RNA was isolated using trizol, 48 hrs after transfection of HEK-293 cells with Tat pcDNA, siRNA and antisense ODN and subjected to RT-PCR to check the level of expression of Tat transcript. (D) Quantitative estimation of the target RNA indicating a fourfold reduction of Tat expression on addition of siRNA and antisense.

In summary, the novel siRNA-Ribozyme constructs possess the ability to knock down target gene expression either on their own or more potently when combined with either hammerhead ribozyme or specific antisense DNA molecules.

Acknowledgement: This work was supported by grants from Department of Biotechnology, Government of India to NII, ND and to the corresponding author (ACB).

REFERENCES

1. Akkina, R., Banerjea, A., Bai, J., Anderson, J., Li, M. J. & Rossi, J. J. (2003) Si-RNAs, ribozymes, and RNA decoys in modeling stem cell based gene therapy for HIV/AIDS. Anticancer Res. 23, 1997-2005.
2. Joyce, G. F. (2004) Directed evolution of nucleic acid enzymes. Annu. Rev. Biochem. 73, 791-836.
3. Santoro, S. W., and Joyce, G.F. (1997) A general purpose RNA-cleaving DNA enzyme. Proc. Natl. Acad. Sci. USA 94, 4262-4266.
4. Silverman, S. K. (2005) Survey and Sumary. In vitro selection, characterization, and application of deoxyribozymes that cleave RNA. Nucleic Acids Res. 33, 6151-6163.
5. Banerjea AC, Chakraborti S, Unwalla H, Goila R, Shrbani S, Dash BC et al. Potential therapeutic application of DNA enzymes and siRNAs against viral and cellular genes. In synthetic nucleic acids as inhibitors of gene expression: mechanisms, applications, and therapeutic implications. Ed. Khachigian, L. M., CRC Press, Florida, USA, 2004; pp115-134.
6. Unwalla, H., and Banerjea, A. C. (2001) Novel mono- and Di-DNA-enzymes targeted to cleave TAT or TAT-Rev RNA inhibit HIV-1 gene expression. Antiviral Res. 51, 127-139.
7. Unwalla, H., and Banerjea, A. C. (2001a) Inhibition of HIV-1 gene expression by novel macrophage-tropic –DNA-enzymes targeted to cleave HIV-1 TAT/Rev RNA. Biochemical J. 357, 97-105.
8. Dash, B. C., and Banerjea, A. C. (2004) Sequence specific cleavage activities of DNAenzymes targeted against HIV-1 Gag and Nef regions. Oligonucleotides 14, 41-47.
9. Lee, N. S, Taikoh, D., Bauer, G., Li, H., Li, M-J., Ehsani, A., Salvaterra, P., and Rossi, J. (2002) Expression of small interfering RNAs targeted against HIV-1 rev transcripts in human cells. Nat. Biotechnol. 20, 500-505.
10. Yu, J. Y., DeRuiter, S. L., and Turner D, L. (2002) RNA interference by expression of shortinterfering RNAs and hairpin RNAs in mammalian cells. Proc. Natl. Acad. Sci. USA 99, 6047-6052.
11. Nidhi Gupta, Vikas Sood, Aalia Bano and Akhil C. Banerjea (2007). X protein of hepatitis B virus potently activates HIV-1 subtype C LTR promoter: implications for faster spread of HIV-1 subtype C. AIDS 21, 1491-1492.

12. Goila, R., and Banerjea, A. C. (2004). Sequence specific cleavage of hepatitis X RNA in cis and trans by novel monotarget and multitarget hammerhead motif-containing ribozymes. Oligonucleotides 14, 249-262.

13. Goila, R., and Banerjea, A. C. (2001) Inhibition of hepatitis B virus X gene expression by novel DNAenzymes. Biochemical J. 353, 701-708.

14. Hung, L., and Kumar, V. (2004). Specific inhibition of gene expression and transactivation functions of hepatitis B virus X protein and c-myc by small interfering RNAs. FEBS Lett. 560, 210-214.

15. Anderson J, Banerjea A and Akkina R. (2003). Bispecific short hairpin siRNA constructs targeted to CD4, CXCR4 and CCR5 confer HIV-1 resistance. Oligonucleotides 13, 303-312.

16. Bispecific Akkina R, Banerjea A, Bai J, Anderson J, Li M, Rossi J. (2003). Si-RNAs, ribozymes, and RNA decoys in modeling stem cell based gene therapy for HIV/AIDS. Anticancer Research 23, 1997-2006.

17. Banerjea A, Li M, Bauer G, Remling L, Lee NS, Rossi J and Akkina R. (2003). Inhibition of HIV-1 by lentiviral vector-transduced siRNAs in T lymphocytes differentiated in SCID-humice and CD34+ progenitor cell-derived macrophages. Molecular Therapy, 8, 62-71.

18. Banerjea, A., Li, M-J., Remling, L., Rossi, J and Akkina, R. (2004). Lentiviral transduction of Tar decoy and CCR5 ribozyme into CD34+ progenitor cells and derivation of HIV-1 resistant T cells and macrophages. AIDS Research & Therapy, On line 17th December, Biomed Central.

19. Unwalla, H., Chakraborti, S., Sood, V., Gupta, N. and Banerjea, A.C. (2006). Potent inhibition of HIV-1 gene expression and TAT mediated apoptosis in human T cells by novel mono- & multitarget anti-TAT/Rev/Env ribozymes and a general purpose RNA-cleaving DNAenzyme. Antiviral Research 72, 134-144.

20. Chen, C-J., Banerjea, A.C., Harmison, G.G., Haglund, K., and Schubert, M.(1992). Multitarget-ribozyme directed to cleave at up to nine highly conserved HIV-1 env RNA regions inhibits HIV-1 replication - potential effectiveness against most presently sequenced HIV-1 isolates. Nucleic Acids Research, 20, 4581-4589.

21. Goila, R., and Banerjea, A. C. (1998). Sequence specific cleavage of the HIV-1 coreceptor- CCR5 gene by a hammer-head ribozyme and a DNA-enzyme: Inhibition of the coreceptor function by DNA-enzyme. FEBS Letters 436, 233-238

22. Shahi, S., Shanmugasundaram, G. K., Banerjea, A. C. (2001). Ribozymes that cleave reovirus genome segment S1 also protects cells from pathogenesis caused by reovirus infection. Proc. Natl. Acad. Sci. USA, 98, 4101-4106.

23. Shahi S and Banerjea, AC. (2002). Multitarget ribozyme against the S1 genome segment of reovirus possesses novel cleavage activities and is more efficacious than its constituent monoribozymes. Antiviral Research 55, 129-140.

24. Sood, V., Unwalla, H., Gupta, N., Chakraborti, S., and Banerjea, A.C. (2007). Potent knock down of HIV-1 replication by targeting HIV-1 Tat/Rev RNA sequences synergistically with catalytic RNA and DNA. AIDS 21, 31-40.

25. Husain – Gene Husain, S., Goila, R., Shahi, S., Banerjea, A. C. (1998). First report of a healthy Indian heterozygous for . 32 mutant of HIV-1 coreceptor- CCR5 gene. Gene, 207, 141-147.

26. Husain, S., Goila, R., Shahi, S., Banerjea, A. C. (1998). Inheritance pattern of mutant human immunodeficiency virus type 1 coreceptor gene in an Indian family. J. Human Virology, 1, 187-192.

27. Basu, S., Sriram, S., Goila, R., and Banerjea, A. C. (2000). Targeted cleavage of HIV-1 coreceptor – CXCR-4 by RNA cleaving DNA-enzyme: Inhibition of coreceptor function. Antiviral Research, 46,125-134.

28. Quin, X.F., An, DS., Chen, IS, Baltimore, D. (2003). Inhibiting HIV-1 infection in human T cells by lentiviral-mediated delivery of small interfering RNA against CCR5. Proc. Natl. Acad. Sci. USA, 100, 183-188.

29. Sood, V., Gupta, N., and Banerjea, A.C. (2007). DNA-enzyme mediated cleavage of HIV-1 Gag RNA is significantly augmented by antisense-DNA molecules targeted to hybridize close to the cleavage site. Oligonucleotides 17, 113-121.

30. Gupta N, Bano, AS., Sharma, Y., Sood, V., Banerjea, AC. (2007). Potent intracellular knock down of hepatitis B virus X RNA by catalytic hammerhead ribozymes or DNA-enzymes with antisense DNA-oligonucleotides or 10-23 DNA-enzymes that powerfully augment in vitro sequence specific cleavage activities. The Open Biotechnology Journal, 1, 81-92.

4

CHAPTER

Newer Treatment Options for Advanced Liver Cancer

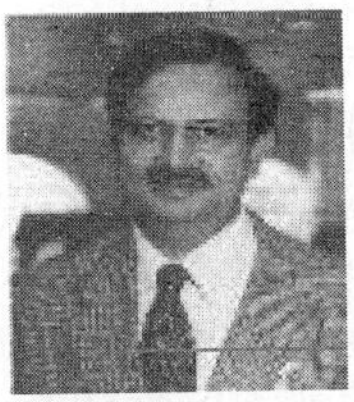

S.K. Sarin[1]* and Kaushal Madan[2]

[1]Department of Gastroenterology, G B Pant Hospital
[2]Department of Hepatology, Institute of Liver and Biliary Sciences, New Delhi

INTRODUCTION

Hepatocellular carcinoma (HCC) is the 5th most common form of cancer in the world and 3rd most common cause of cancer related deaths.[1]

The management of HCC differs from other forms of solid organ malignancies because of the following reasons. HCC is probably the only cancer which arises in an underlying organ whose functional status is already compromised. So, the prognosis of the patients with HCC depends not only on the extent of the tumor, but also on the functional status of the underlying cirrhotic liver. In addition, the management of HCC involves treatment of the tumor, treatment of complications of cirrhosis and treatment of the etiology of cirrhosis (eg HBV, or HCV). For this reason, the definition of advanced liver cancer includes not only the spread of the tumor beyond curative stages but also the presence of poor liver function which does not allow the application of a potentially curative therapy even if the tumor is limited in its extent. For this So reason any patient with multiple liver tumors, with vascular involvement (especially portal vein and its branches), or with child's class C or poor performance status scores, is said to be having advanced HCC.[2]

When the tumor itself becomes advanced, the problem of managing such patients gets compounded. The expected median survival of patients with advanced liver cancer has been reported to be less than 10-12 months. The Unfortunately, fact is that in most parts of the world the majority of HCCs are detected in an advanced stage.[3] Systemic chemotherapy with the conventional chemo-

*email: shivsarin@gmail.com

therapeutic agents have shown very poor results in HCC which has grown beyond the limits of cure. These studies have used drugs like doxorubicin, cisplatinum, gemcitabine and paclitaxel. These drugs not only do not produce a good response, but also lead to significant adverse effects. It has been demonstrated that hepatocellular carcinoma tumor cells express multidrug resistant (MDR1) gene which may be one of the reason for the poor response.[4,5] The management of such cases require coordinated efforts by hepatologists, endoscopists, interventional radiologists, oncologists, and surgeons. In the recent years a number of newer treatment modalities and drugs have been reported to have significant effect on the survival of HCC patients. In the forthcoming paragraphs we will try to elaborate the newer developments in the management of patients with advanced liver cancer.

Newer Therapeutic Options for Advanced HCC

Intra-hepatic Arterial Therapies

The typical prototype of intra-arterial therapies is the trans-arterial chemoembolization (TACE). The principale of intra-arterial therapies is based on the fact that liver has a dual blood supply (75% derived from portal vein and 25% derived from hepatic artery). When the HCC forms, it gets its blood supply from neo-vessels derived from the hepatic artery or its branches. As the tumor grows, the portal venous supply becomes less and less and the tumor progressively acquires more and more blood supply from the hepatic artery. In the later stages, almost the entire blood supply of an HCC is derived from hepatic artery or its branches. On the other hand the major blood supply to the rest of the liver continues to be from the portal vein. So, selective infusion of drugs or chemotherapeutic agents in to the branch of the hepatic artery which is supplying the HCC, leads to concentration of the drug within the tumor without affecting the rest of the liver. This branch can then be embolized with gel foam or metallic coils leading to ischemic necrosis of the tumor (some thing which is done in trans-arterial chemoembolization [TACE]). However, in the advanced stages of HCC, when the portal vein is also blocked or invaded by the tumor, the only source of blood supply to the rest of the liver is the hepatic artery. Blocking the hepatic artery in such cases can result in ischemic necrosis of the rest of the liver, leading to liver failure. So in advanced HCC when the portal vein is also invaded we have to resort to other forms of intra-arterial therapies such as continuous intra-arterial chemotherapy infusions or intra-arterial radioembolization.

Trans-arterial infusion chemotherapy

In this form of therapy, continuous infusion of a chemotherapeutic drug is given in to a branch of hepatic artery via an indwelling catheter left in situ in the branch of hepatic artery. The drug is administered through a port implanted subcutaneously in the thigh and connected to the indwelling catheter. In this form of therapy, the hepatic artery is not embolized and therefore there is no risk of ischemic liver failure even if the portal vein is blocked. This is usually administered along with subcutaneous injections of either standard or pegylated interferons, since chemotherapy alone has not been found to be effective in HCC patients as has been discussed earlier. The effectiveness of this strategy was first described in 1993.[6] The addition of interferon leads to induction of p53 gene leading to accelerated apoptosis of cancer cells.[7] Obi et al, evaluated 116 patients with HCC and portal vein invasion, who received standard interferon 5Million IU on days 1, 3 5 of every week, along with intra-arterial infusion of 5 fluororacil (5-FU) from day 1 to 5 of 1st and 2nd week of each 4 week cycle. 16% patients could achieve a complete response as defined by complete disappearance of the lesion as well as the portal vein tumor, maintained for at least 4 weeks. The 1 and 2 year survival rates were 34% and 18% respectively and these were significantly higher than retrospective controls (5915% and 5% respectively).[8] There have been other reports as well, mainly from Japan, of the use of intra-arterial infusion chemotherapy with interferon in advanced HCC patients with results showing an improvement in survival.[9,10] Infusion chemotherapy in to the hepatic artery along with subcutaneous interferon thus remains a useful option for patients with portal vein tumor thrombus, since these patients are not candidates for any form of curative therapy. Larger randomized trials in future may give this therapy its appropriate place in the treatment algorithm for HCC.

Radioembolization

Another novel method of taking care of patients with locally advanced HCC is by intra-hepatic arterial instillation of radio-nuclides such as ^{90}Yttrium, ^{188}Rhenium and ^{166}Holmium-Chittosan complex. This has the advantage of delivering a locally concentrated dose of radiation to the tumor without causing much systemic side effects of radio-therapy. In essence, it is a form of liver directed brachytherapy.

^{90}Yttrium is incorporated in to glass microspheres or microbeads called TheraSphere (MDS Nordion, Ottawa, Canada). A recent study reported the use of ^{90}Yttrium theraspheres in 108 patients with advanced HCC, 34% of whom had portal vein thrombosis. The partial response rate using the EASL criteria was 70% and there were no cases of radiation induced gastroenteritits or pneumonitis.[11] In another study using intra-arterial ^{188}Rhenium labeled iodized oil in 93 patients with advanced HCC, complete response was demonstrated in 8%, partial response in 26% and stabilization of the disease in 35%. The 1, 2 and 3 year survival rates in those who achieved some objective tumor response were 90%, 58% and 30% respectively.

While ^{90}Yttrium is available commercially, the use of other radio-isotopes is in the experimental stages only and the high costs of Yttrium prohibits its routine use. However intra-arterial infusion brachytherapy does hold promise for the treatment of inoperable locally advanced HCC.

Newer Systemic Therapies

Vitamin K therapy

How vitamin K produces its anti tumor effect is still a subject of research and many mechanisms have been proposed including, induction of oxidative stress, tyrosine kinase inhibition, induction of cell cycle arrest and apoptosis.[12,13]

A few human trials have used vitamin K1 for HCC. Vitamin K1 40 mg per day given orally to 30 patients with HCC, resulted in partial tumor response in 7 patients and disease stabilization in 6.[14] In addition, the des gamma carboxy-prothromin levels normalized. In another study, 40 patients received oral vitamin K1 and all patients had 20% tumor response and 5 patients lived longer than 1 year on treatment.[15]

We recently conducted a randomized controlled trial in 42 consecutive patients with advanced HCC, comparing high dose infusion of vitamin K3 (n=23) [iv infusion of 50mg on day 1 followed by 50mg increments everyday up to 6 days, followed by 20mg intramuscularly twice a day for next two weeks] with placebo (n=19). One patient (4.3%) had complete response and 3 (13%) had partial response. Those who had an objective response had a significantly longer survival (22.5 ± 12.2 months) as compared to those who did not achieve any objective response (6.1 ± 4.6 months); $p=0.002$. One patient had complete resolution of the portal vein tumor thrombus.[16] However this response may not be sufficient and future studies employing more patients need to be carried out before vitamin K therapy can become a standard therapy for patients with advanced HCC.

Thalidomide

Thalidomide is an anti-angiogenic drug and a number of small studies have used thalidomide either alone or in combination with other chemotherapeutic agents to demonstrate significant anti-tumor effect against advanced HCC.[17]The advantage is the oral intake and the dose limiting adverse events include sedation, neurotoxicity and gastro-intestinal toxicity. But despite the initial enthusiasm, most of these studies have demonstrated only modest tumor response rates, ranging from 0 to 6.5% (table1).[18,19,20,21]

Physical Methods

High frequency focused ultrasound (HIFU)

Recently a new and innovative method for managing patients with large unresectable HCCs has been introduced. It makes use of the principal of high frequency ultrasonic beams generating heat energy at the focal points causing tumor necrosis. The advantage of this method is the non-invasive nature of the procedure which allows ablation of large tumor areas of any shape. The image guidance is done by real time B mode ultrasonography. It was first approved for HCC in China in 1999.[22] Since then a number of reports demonstrating the usefulness of HIFU have appeared in the literature.[23,24,25] Li et al, compared 151 patients treated with HIFU with 30 controls. The over all response rate was significantly higher in the HIFU group (88.8%) than in the controls (16.7%); $p<0.01$. In the HIFU group, complete and partial response rates were achieved in 28.5% and 60.3% respectively, compared to 0% and 16.7% respectively in the placebo group. The 1 and 2 year survival rates were 50% and 30.9% in the HIFU group compared with 3.4% and 0% respectively in the placebo group.[26]

HIFU thus appears to be an effective modality for therapy of advanced liver cancer but presently its wide spread use is limited by its cost and availability.

Molecular Therapies

The molecular therapies are based on the use of small molecules which are multikinase inhibitors and block either the cell surface receptors like vascular endothelial growth factor receptor (VEGFR), platelet derived growth factor receptor (PGDFR), epidermal growth factor receptor (EGFR) or down stream signaling kinases such as Raf kinase, mitogen activated kinase (MAK), extracellular signal regulated kinase (ERK). In addition monoclonal antibodies directed against the above mentioned receptors can be used to block the singnaling pathways regulated by these receptors. The blockage of signal transduction of these pathways leads to blockage of processes involved in tumor growth, tumor progression, metastasis and angiogenesis. The prototype drug which has been most successfully tested is sorafenib. Other drugs in this category are sunitinib, geftinib, erlotinib, capecitabine, bevacizumab (monoclonal antibodies against VEGFR) and cetuximab (monoclonal antibodies against EGFR).

Sorafenib

Sorafenib (Nexavar, Bayer pharmaceuticals, West Haven, Conn) is an oral multikinase inhibitor that exerts an anti-angiogenic effect by blocking the VEGFR-2 and PDGFR-â as well as by inhibiting tumor cell proliferation by targeting the Raf/MAK/ERK signaling pathways.[27] In phase II trial of Sorafenib, it was administered in a dosage of 400 mg BD in 4 weeks cycle to 137 patients with inoperable HCC. 3 patients (2.2%) achieved a complete response, 8 (5.8%) had a minor response and 46 (33.6%) had stable disease for at least 16 weeks. The median over all survival was 9.2 months.[28] Subsequently, a large phase 3 placebo controlled trial was conducted, in which 299 patients received sorafenib and 303 received placebo. The over all survival was significantly higher in the sorafenib group (46.3 weeks) as compared to placebo (34.4 weeks); p=0.0005. Similarly the time to progression was significantly more in the sorafenib treated patients (24 weeks), than in the placebo group (12.3 weeks); p=0.000007. The adverse events included, fatigue, diarrhea and hand & foot syndrome.[29]

Sunitinib

Sunitinib again is another small molecule, which is a multikinase inhibitor. Two phase 2 studies have evaluated the efficacy and safety of this drug in patients with inoperable HCC. It was tried at a dose of 37.5 mg daily or 50mg daily in a 4 weeks on and 2 weeks off schedule. One patient in each trial had a partial response and about 37% had a stable disease. The adverse events were significant and included, thrombocytopenia, neutropenia, CNS symptoms, asthenia and hemorrhage.[30,31]

Other small molecules and monoclonal antibody drugs are undergoing phase 2 and 3 trials and the results will be available in near future. However the preliminary results of the use of these agents in advanced HCC (published as proceedings) do suggest moderate effect on survival.[32] There is no doubt that these molecular based therapies are going to be the most important drugs if not the first line for the future management of inoperable HCC.

Tumor vaccine

It is known that body's immune system can remove a large number of tumor cells as part of the innate defenses by recognizing the antigens on the tumor cells as foreign. If the body's immune system can be boosted to fight against the cells/tissues expressing tumor antigens, it can form an interesting systemic therapeutic approach for HCC patients. This forms the basis for development of tumor vaccines. Dendritic cells are the most important antigen presenting cells and dendritic cells specifically modulated to react against autologous HCC tissue antigens can be used to induce immune reaction against liver cancer cells. Lee et al, used dendritic cell vaccination intravenously in 31 patients with advanced HCC. 12.9% patients had a partial response and 54.8% had a stable disease.[33] Another form of tumor vaccine is a DNA vaccine expressing alpha-fetoprotein (AFP) gene, which leads to specific T-cell responses against the AFP expressing cells.[34]

In conclusion, the newer therapeutic modalities (outlined above) which have become available for the management of advanced HCC are definitely going to improve the dismal prognosis of this disease. The results up till now have demonstrated improvement in overall survival but whether this can be improved further or whether it is associated with improvement in the quality of life of these patients is yet to be seen. The future is going to see these treatments being offered either singly or in combination, with molecular targeted therapies being integral parts of the regimen.

Table 4.1 Response rate to thalidomide based systemic therapy for HCC

Series	Agent used	N	Response(%)
Wang, 2004[18]	Thalidomide	99	6.1
Hsu, 2003[19]	Thalidomide	68	6.3
Zhu, 2005[20]	Thalidomide+epirubicin	19	0
Schwartz, 2005[21]	Thalidomide + IFN	70	5.5

REFERENCES

1. Parkin DM, Bray DF, Ferlay J, Pisani P. Estimating the world cancer burden gobocan 2000. Int J Cancer 2001; 94: 153-56.
2. Bruix J, Sherman M, Llover JM, Beaugrand M, Lencioni R, Burroughs AK, et al. Clinical management of hepatocellular carcinoma. Conclusions of the Barcelona-2000 EASL conference. J Hepatology 2001; 35: 421-30.
3. Llovet JM, Burroughs A, Bruix J. Hepatocellular carcinoma. Lancet 2003; 362: 1907-1917.
4. Kato A, Miyazaki M, Ambiru S, Yoshitomi H, Ito H, Nakagawa K,e t al. Multidrug resistance gene (MDR1) expression as a useful prognostic factor in patients wi th humna hepatocellular carcinoma after surgical resection. J Surg Oncol 2001; 78: 110-5.
5. Li G, Chen X, Wang Q, Xu Z, Zhang W, Ye L. The roles of four multi-drug resistance proteins in hepatocellular carcinoma multidrug resistance. J Huazhong Univ Sci Technolog Med Sci. 2007; 27: 173-5.
6. Patt YZ, Yoffe B, Charnsangarej C, et al. Low serum alpha-feto protein levels in patients with hepatocellular carcinoma as a predictor of response to 5FU and interferon alpha 2b. Cncer 1993; 72: 2574-82.
7. Hagiwara S, Kudo M, Nakatani T, Sakaguchi Y, Nagashima M, Fukuta N, et al. Combination therapy with PEG-IFN á and 5-FU inhibits Hep-G2 tumor cell growth in nude mice by apoptosis of p53. British Journal of Cancer 2007; 97: 1532-37.
8. Obi S, Yoshida H, Toune R, Unuma T, Kanda M, Sato S, et al. Combination ther apy of intra-arterial 5-fluorouracil and systemic interferon alpha for advanced hepatocellular carcinoma with portal venous invasion. Cancer 2006; 106: 1990-7.
9. Urabe T, Kaneko S, Matsuhita E, Unoura M, Kobayashi K. Clinical pilot study of intrahepatic arterial chemotherapy with methotrexate, 5-fluorouracil, cisplatin and subcutaneous interferon alpha 2b for patients with locally advanced hepatocellular carcinoma. Oncology 1998; 55: 39-47.
10. Nagano H, Miyamoto A, Wada H, Ota H, Marubashi S, Takeda Y, et al. Interferon-alpha and 5-fluorouracil therapy after palliative hepatic resection in patients with advanced hepatocellular carcinoma, portal venous tumor thrombus in the major trunk, and multiple nodules. Cancer 2007; 110: 2493-501.
11. Kulik KM, Carr BI, Mulcahy MF, Lewandowski RJ, Atassi B, Ryu RK, et al. Safety and efficacy of 90Y radiotherapy for hepatocellular carcinoma with and without portal vein thrombosis. Hepatology 2008; 47: 71-81.
12. Gant TW, Rao DN, Mason RP, Cohen GM. Redox cycling and sulphydryl arylation; their relative importance in the mechanism of quinine cytotoxicity to isolated hepatocytes. Chem boil Interact 1988; 65: 157-73.

13. Cole MD, McMahon SB. The Myc oncoprotein: a critical evaluationof trasnacativation and target gene regulation. Oncogene 1999; 18: 2916-24.

14. Carr BI, Wang Z, Virji MA, Piper M. Vitamin K (VK) inhiits hepatoma cell growth invitro and in patients [Meeting abstract]. Proc. AACR 1996; 37: A1485.

15. Carr BI. Suppression of DCP/PIVKA-2 and alpha-fetopro tein levels in human hepatocellular carcinoma (HCC) by high doses of vitamin K1 (VK1). Hepatology 1996; 22: 348A.

16. Sarin SK, Kuamr M, Garg S, Hisar S, Pandey C, Sharma BC. High dose vitamin K3 infusion in advanced hepatocellular carcinoma. J Gastroenterol Hepatol 2006; 21: 1478-1482.

17. Ouek R, Lim ST, Ong S. Hepatocellular carcinoma-pathological complete reseponse to oral capecitabine, megestrol and thalidomide. Acta oncol 2006; 45: 95-7

18. Wang TE, Kao CR, Lin SC, Chang WH, Chu CH, Lin J, et al. Salvage therapy for hepatocellular carcinoma with thaliodmide. World J Gastroenterol 2004; 10: 649-53.

19. Hsu C, Chen CN, Chen LT, Wu CY, Yang PM, Lai MY, et al. Low-dose thalidomide treatment for advanced hepatocellular carcinoma. Oncology 2003; 65: 242-9.

20. Zhu AX, Fuchs CS, Clark JW, Mizukansky A, Taylor K, et al. A Phase II study of epirubicin and thalidomide in unresectable or metastatic hepatocellular carcinoma. The Oncologist 2005; 10: 392-98.

21. Schwartz JD, Sung M, Schwartz M, Lehrer D, Mandeli J, Liebes L, et al. Thalidomide in advanced hepatocellular carcinoma with optional low-dose interferon-alpha 2A upon progression. Oncologist 2005; 10: 718-27.

22. Wu F, Chen WZ, Bai J. A preliminary study of high intensity focused ultrasound inthe trea tment of hepatocellular carcinoma. Chin J Ultrasound. 1999; 8: 213-16.

23. Kennedy JE, Wu F, ter Haar GR, Gleeson FV, et al. High-intensity focused ultrasound for the treatment of liver tumors. Ultrasoincs 2004; 42: 931-5.

24. Li CX, Xu GL, Jiang ZY, et al. Analysis of clinical effect of high-intensity focused ultrasound on liver caner. World J Gastroenterol 2004; 10: 2201-4.

25. Wu F, Wang ZB, Chen WZ, et al. Advanced hepatocellular carcinoma: treatment with high intensity focused ultrasound ablation combined with transcatheter arterial embolization. Radiology 2005; 235: 659-67.

26. Li YY, Sha WH, Zhou YJ, Nie YQ. Short and long term efficacy of high intensity focused ultrasound therapy for advanced hepatocellular carcinoma. J Gastroenterol Hepatol 2007; 22: 2148-54.

27. Wilhelm SM, Carter C, Tang L, et al. BAY43-9006 exhibits broad spectrum anti-tumor activity and targets the RAF/MEK/ERK pathway and receptor tyrosine kinases involved in tumor progression and angiogenesis. Cancer Res 2004; 64: 7099-7109.

28. Abou-Alfa GK, Schwartz L, Ricci S, et al. Phase II study of sorafenib in patients with advanced hepatocellular carcinoma. J Clin Oncol 2006; 24: 4293-4300.

29. Llovet J, Ricci S, Mazaferro V, et al. Sorafenib improves survival in advanced hepatocellular carcinoma (HCC): results of a phase III randomized placebo controlled trial (SHARP trial). J Clin Oncol (Meeting Abstracts). 2007; 25 (18S). Abstract LBA1.

30. Zhu AX, Sahani DV, di Tomaso E, et al. A phase II study of sunitinib in patients with advanced hepatocellular carcinoma. J Clin Oncol (Meeting Abstracts). 2007; 25 (18S). Abstract 4637.

31. Faivre SJ, Raymond E, Douillard JBE, et al. Assessment of safety and drug-induced tumor necrosis with sunitinib in patients with unresectable hepatocellular carcinoma (HCC). J Clin Oncol (Meeting Abstracts). 2007; 25 (18S). Abstract 3546.

32. Zhu AX. Development of sorafenib and othe molecularly targeted agents in hepatocellular carcinoma. Cancer 2008; 112: 250-59.

33. Lee WC, Wang HC, Hung CF, Huang PF, Lia CR, Chen MF. Vaccination of advanced hepatocellular carcinoma patients with tumor lysate-pulsed dindritic cells: a clinical trial. J Immunother 2005; 28: 496-504.

34. Lan YH, Li YG, Liang ZW, Chen M, Peng ML, Tang L, et al. A DNA vaccine against chimeric AFP anhanced by HSP 70 suppresses growth of hepatocellular carcinoma. Cancer Immunol Immunother 2007; 56: 1009-16.

5

CHAPTER

Tyrosine Kinase Inhibitors in Chronic Myeloid Leukemia

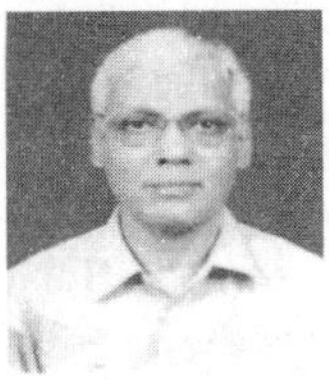

Tapan K. Saikia

Head, Department of Medical Oncology, Prince Aly Khan Hospital, Nesbit Road, Mazagaon Mumbai 400010

INTRODUCTION

It all started in 1959-60 with the discovery by Nowell and Hungerford of a minute chromosome in patients with chronic myeloid leukemia (CML (1). This came to be known as Philadelphia chromosome (Ph). Later seminal works by Janet Rowley led to identification of t(9;22)(q11;q34) (2). In subsequent years research in the molecular arena identified BCR-ABL oncogene, which is the product of Ph 22q, encodes a chimeric BCR-ABL protein of 210-kD in CML, (and 185-kD in Ph+ acute lymphoblastic leukemia) that has constitutively activated ABL tyrosine kinase activity (3-5). Protein kinases are a large family of homologous proteins comprising two major subfamilies, the protein serine/threonine kinases and protein tyrosine kinases (PTKs); subsequent work in the field had implicated their role in development of cancers (6). These kinases, being a component of the signal transduction pathways, play a central role in diverse biological processes such as cell growth, metabolism, differentiation, and apoptosis. Ever since it became apparent that the Bcr-Abl kinase could be the functional target in CML, scientists became interested in developing therapeutic molecules targeting this disease causing pathology (7-10). Daley et al have demonstrated that expression of p210 mBcr-Abl induces a myeloproliferative disease in mice that resembles CML, thus confirming the ability of this chimeric protein to be etiological factor (11).The search culminated in development of the tyrosine kinase inhibitor (TKI) imatinib mesylate (4-[(4-methyl-

email: tapan.saikia@gmail.com

1-piperazinyl)methyl]-N-[-methyl-3-[[4-(3-pyrimidinyl]amino]phenyl]benzamide methanesulfonate; also known as STI571, (trade name Gleevec or Glivec, Novartis Pharma), screened from a large number of such organic compounds (7-10). The drug has been tested in a number of preclinical models and was found to be inhibitor of autophosphorylation of v-Abl, PDGF receptor, and Kit receptor in a submicromolar concentration (9, 10). The field has been expanding exponentially at the present time in an attempt to discover more potent TKIs and other targeted agents (12).

Prior to the advent of the TKIs, the effective modalities of treatment of CML that could target BCR-ABL included low-dose cytarabine, interferon-alpha, and high-dose cytotoxic therapy + allogeneic hematopoietic stem cell transplantation (HSCT). Till date allogeneic HSCT remains the only curative treatment for CML, although long-term follow up shows drug therapy, particularly imatinib mesylate to be superior to transplantation in terms of safety and overall survival (13).

Tyrosine Kinase Inhibitors

First generation BCR-ABL inhibitor (Imatinib Mesylate)

STI571 (formerly known as CGP57148B, now known as imatinib mesylate), a specific inhibitor of the BCR-ABL tyrosine kinase, a synthetic compound, was the first of its kind to be brought into clinical trial after the molecule was found to be effective in preclinical models (14). It acts through competitive inhibition at the ATP-binding site of the enzyme, which leads to inhibition of tyrosine phosphorylation of proteins involved in BCR-ABL signal transduction. It shows high degree of specificity for BCR-ABL, the receptor for platelet-derived growth factor (PDGFR), and c-kit tyrosine kinases. It causes arrest of growth or apoptosis in hematopoietic cells that express BCR-ABL but does not affect normal cells. The investigators postulated that continuous inhibition of the Bcr-Abl will be required for an optimal clinical benefit and this was the case (14). In studies they could rescue the Bcr-Abl expressing cells if the drug could be washed out within 16 hours of initial exposure. The drug is orally bio-available with a half life if 14-16 hours, suggesting a clinical efficacy with once daily dose.

A phase 1 study showed its safety and significant antileukemic activity in interferon failure chronic phase CML (CML-CP) patients (table 5.1) (15). At 300 mg daily and above almost all patients achieved a complete hematologic response and major cytogenetic response in s third to half of the patients. The hematologic and non-hematologic toxicity profiles were mild in majority with grade 3 & 4 in a minority of cases.

Table 5.1 Hematologic and Cytogenetic Responses to Imatinib: Phase 1 Study

Dose (mg/day)	Patients	CHR (%)	MCyR/CCyR (%)	mCyR (%)
200 or 250	16	56	NA	NA
300 – 1000	54	98	see below	
300 – 350	13	–	38	15
400	6	–	50	33
500	6	–	17	17
600	8	–	50	50
750	6	–	33	0
800	8	–	12	25
1000	7	–	14	14

83 patients & 54 patients respectively evaluated for hematologic & cytogenetic responses; CHR-complete hematologic response; MCyR – major cytogenetic response; CCyR – complete cytogenetic response; mCyR – minor cytogenetic response; NA – not available

It also was found to be effective in a fraction of patients in blast crisis (CML-BC) as well as in Ph+ acute lymphoblastic leukemia (Ph+ ALL) (Table 5.2) (16).

Table 5.2 Responses in CML-BC & Ph+ ALL to Imatinib: Phase 1 Study (300 – 1000 mg)

Disease	No. patients	CHR (%)	Marrow (≤5% blasts)
CML-MBC	38	4(11)	8(21)
CML-LBC or Ph+ALL	20	4(20)	7(35)

This opened up vistas for a number of phase 2 studies and establishing its effectiveness in all phases of CML as well as in certain other tumors where c-kit and PDGFR play crucial roles in pathogenesis of the diseases. The phase 3 IRIS trial initiated in 2000 (June 2000- January 2001) comparing imatinib with interferon alpha + low-dose cytarabine in 1106 patients (553 patients each arm with a cross-over design) has confirmed the role of the molecule in newly diagnosed CML patients as the standard of care (Table 5.3) (17).

Table 5.3 Long-term Outcome in IRIS Trial

Response	at 12 months (%)	at 60 months (%)	Best Response (%)
CHR	96	98	97
CCyR	69	87	82
EFS	-	83	-
OS	-	89	-
Progression to AP/BC	-	7	-

The 5-yr outcome data has shown overall survival (OS) of 89%, event-free survival (EFS) of 83% and an estimated 7% patients progressing to advanced phase disease of accelerated phase or blast crisis (17). The study has also proved that achieving a complete cytogenetic response by 12 months and a major molecular response by 18 months is crucial for prolonged progression-free survival (17, 18). Very significantly it has been able to reduce the progression of the disease with the passage of time (Table 5.4). The safety profile is usually excellent with grade 3/4 hematologic and non-hematologic reported in a small proportion of patients (Table 5.5). Currently recommended daily dose of imatinib is 400 mg. Some clinical studies have explored higher doses of 600 mg – 800 mg daily. However, at present time, many clinicians are showing concern about some bothersome long-term toxicity. The cardiac toxicity noted in animal experiments has not been a clinical concern in most of the patients followed over a long period of time.

Table 5.4 Progression of disease or Treatment Failure in the IRIS Trial

Year	Failure (%)	AP/BC (%)
Yr 1	3.3	2.5
Yr 2	7.5	2.8
Yr 3	4.8	1.6
Yr 4	1.5	1.6
Yr 5	0.9	0.6

Table 5.5 Grade 3 & 4 Adverse Events on Imatinib as First-line Therapy (IRIS Trial)

Events	Total Events (%)	yr-1&2	yr-3&4	>yr-4
Neutropenia	17	14	3	1
Thrombocytopenia	9	8	1	<1
Anemia	4	3	1	<1
Raised liver enzymes	5	5	<1	0
Other events	17	14	4	2

Despite its excellent clinical profile, it has now become clear that while receiving imatinib both primary and secondary resistance develop in a significant number of patients (19-26). Although only a small number of patients with early chronic phase disease develop resistance to imatinib, it is much higher in patients with late chronic phase, accelerated phase and blastic phase disease. This resistance is usually caused by point mutations in the kinase domain of the BCR-ABL enzyme that reduce sensitivity towards imatinib. There are also other BCR-ABL-independent mechanisms of imatinib resistance. Such resistance might arise through low-to-undetectable background level of BCR-ABL mutations (less than 1% of tumor cells) that exist before imatinib treatment (12). During treatment with the drug further mutations are acquired and leads to re-emergence of the tyrosine kinase activity. A detailed account of imatinib resistance is being described in another chapter of this book. This has led to intense research for development of next generation TKIs. A number of those have been found to have significant activity in vitro and in vivo. Clinical studies have shown significant activity of dasatinib (sprycel) and nilotinib (tasigna) in imatinib resistant and intolerant patients of all phases. Some others are being investigated in clinical trials – INNO 406, SKI 606, and Aurora kinase inhibitors like MK 0457, etc (12).

Second Generation BCR-ABL Inhibitors

Structural biology studies have been helpful in developing new drugs to overcome resistance acquired by the BCR-ABL protein (14). Such drugs target the integrity and/or stability of the protein as well as signaling pathways downstream of BCR-ABL. Classes of these new inhibitors include selective ABL inhibitors, ABL and Src-family kinase inhibitors, Aurora kinase inhibitors, and non-ATP competitive inhibitors of BCR-ABL.

Selective ABL inhibitors

Nilotinib. AMN – 107 (nilotinib; Novartis, tasigna). This selective inhibitor of ABL kinase is about 30-fold more potent than imatinib (28-30). The drug appears to be much more selective in inhibition of ABL kinase. It does not have ability to inhibit Src-family kinases. In vitro, it could inhibit 32 of 33 mutant BCR-ABL forms resistant to imatinib (31). The mutation T315I has been found to confer absolute resistance to this molecule. It is well tolerated orally and a phase 1 study in imatinib-resistant CML-CP patients exploring the doses of 50 mg – 1200 mg daily, significant responses were noted (Table 5.6) (32). Following a phase 2 study, the recommended dose is 400 mg twice daily (33). The plasma half-life is 15-24 hours. Common side-effects are cytopenia, bilirubinemia, fluid retention, etc.

Table 5.6 Hematologic and Cytogenetic Responses to Nilotinib in CML-CP

	Patients with response		
Response	**IM-resistant =194**	**IM-intolerant =86**	**All patients =280**
CHR	92 (68)	45 (90)	137 (74)
Cytogenetic response			
Major	94 (48)	40 (47)	134 (48)
Complete	58 (30)	30 (35)	88 (31)
Partial	36 (19)	10 (12)	46 (16)
Minor	16 (8)	6 (7)	22 (8)
Minimal	25 (13)	14 (16)	39 (14)

ABL and Src-family inhibitors

The Src family of tyrosine kinases plays important roles in physiological conditions by modulating multiple intracellular signal transduction pathways involved in cell growth, differentiation, migration and survival. BCR-ABL activates Src kinases both through phosphorylation and direct binding. Thus, targeting of BCR-ABL and Src kinases simultaneously may overcome drug resistance in CML.

Dasatinib. BMS- 354825 (dasatinib; Bristol-Myers-Squibb, sprycel) is a dual inhibitor of BCR-ABL and Src-famliy kinases (34, 35). It is almost 300-fold more potent than imatinib and orally active. This inhibition of Src-family kinases is probably responsible for its ability to bind to the active conformation of the ABL kinase domain whereas imatinib appears to bind catalytically inactive conformation of the kinase. Dasatinib could directly inhibit 21 of 22 mutant forms of BCR-ABL resistant to imatinib (36). Like nilotinib it has also been found to be unable to override T315I mutation. It has a plasma half-life of 3-4 hours and because of this a twice daily dosing schedule was developed and approved (70 mg twice daily) (Table 5.7) (37, 38). However, a recent four-arm randomized trial has shown that a 100 mg once daily dose is optimally active and safe (39). The twice daily dose could be responsible for some of the clinically side-effects. Based on this, an approval for 100 mg daily has come through for imatinib-resistant patients. Cytopenia were common in multiply pre-treated cases and fluid retention occurred with development of pleural effusion, pericardial effusion, and pulmonary edema in some patients. The mechanism for fluid retention might be due to the inhibition of PDGFRb or through an autoimmune mechanism. Clinical trials are on evaluating the feasibility of using dasatinib as a first line therapy in CML.

Table 5.7 Hemtologic and Cytogenetic Response to Dasatinib in CML-CP

		At 8 months follow-up	
	Total	**Imatinib-resistant**	**Imatinib-intolerant**
number	186	127	59
CHR, n (%)	168 (90)	111 (87)	57 (97)
Cytogenetic, n (%)			
Major	97 (52)	50 (39)	47 (90)
Complete	73 (39)	35 (28)	38 (64)
Partial	24 (13)	15 (12)	9 (15)
Minor	7 (4)	6 (5)	1 (2)
Minimal	16 (9)	15 (12)	1 (2)

Bosutinib SKI – 606 (bosutinib; Wyeth) is also dual Src kinase and BCR-ABL inhibitor (40). An orally active compound and has shown clinical efficacy in phase 1/2 studies in all phases of CML and Ph+ ALL (41). However, it does not inhibit KIT or PDGFR. It showed in vitro activity against all imatinib-resistant mutants except T315I, as is the case in nilotinib and dasatinib. Further studies are on and it also may find approval for clinical use in near future.

INNO-406 Earlier known as NS-187 (Innovive), is a potent BCR-ABL and LYN dual kinase inhibitor. It is structurally related to imatinib and nilotinib and is about 20-fold more potent than imatinib (42). As it is an inhibitor of LYN kinase alone, not the all members of the Src-family, the side-effects could possibly be lower. Clinical trials are on studying its clinical efficacy in CML.

Non-ATP-competitive Inhibitors of BCR-ABL

An alternative approach is being explored to develop molecules that inhibit the kinase activity either by a non-ATP competitive allosteric mechanism or by preventing the binding substrates to the kinase. Such an approach might side track the resistant mutants and bind to different sites. One such molecule is ONO12380 that interacts with the substrate-binding sites of these kinases (43). Clinical trials are to begin with this agent.

Aurora kinase inhibitors

The Aurora family of serine/threonine kinases is essential for mitotic progression; Aurora A has a crucial role in mitotic spindle formation and centrosome maturation (44). Inhibition of this kinase disrupts cell cycle progression. Aurora B is a chromosomal passenger protein essential for chromosomal congression and cytokinesis.

MK-0457. MK-0457 (Known earlier as VX-680; Merck) can inhibit all three Aurora kinases as well FLT3 (44). It also has moderate inhibiting potential of ABL and JAK2. Clinical study has shown its effectiveness in CML patients and acute lymphocytic leukemia with T315I mutation (45).

CONCLUSION

Improvement in the field of structural biology has been crucial in development of targeted molecules for control of CML activity in humans. Currently, there are multiple protein kinase structures in the Protein Data Bank. The availability of this structural information from multiple members of the protein kinase family allows us to realize how small changes in the primary structure, even those remote from the ATP-binding site, can be exploited to develop selective kinase inhibitors. Imatinib mesylate has been the first of its kind (9, 17). Subsequent years, especially with the pressure exerted by development of kinase domain mutations in some of the patients receiving imatinib have led the scientists to develop more potent compounds like dasatnib, nilotinib, bosutinib, Aorura kinase inhibitors and many such small-molecules (12). It is hoped that in near future clues would be found to eliminate diseases like CML through combination targeted agents or another molecule that might have potential to eradicate leukemia stem cells (46)

REFERENCES

1. Nowell PC, Hungerford DA (1960). *A minute chromosome in human chronic granulocytic leukemia.* Science 132:1497-1501.
2. Rowley JD (1973). *A new consistent chromosomal abnormality in chronic myelogenous leukemia identified by quinacrine fluorescence and Giemsa staining.* Nature 43:290-293.
3. Bartram CR et al (1983). *Translocation of c-abl oncogene correlates with the presence of a Philadelphia chromosome in chronic myelocytic leukemia.* Nature 306:277-280.
4. Groffen J, et al (1984). *Philadelphia chromosomal breakpoints are clustered within a limited region, bcr, on chromosome 22.* Cell 36:93-99.
5. Lugo TG, Pendergast AM, Muller AJ, Witte ON (1990). *Tyrosine kinase activity and transformation potency of bcr-abl oncogene products.* Science 247:1079-1082.
6. Kolibaba KS and Druker BJ (1997). *Protein tyrosine kinases and cancer.* Biophys. Acta 1333:F217-F248.
7. Buchdunger E, et al (1996). *Inhibition of the Abl protein-tyrosine kinase in vitro and in-vivo by a 2-phenylaminopyrimidine derivative.* Cancer Res 56:100-1-4.
8. Zimmermann J, et al (1996). *Phenylamino-pyrimidine (PAP) derivatives: a new class of potent and selective inhibitors of protein kinase C (PKC).* Arch. Pharm. (Weinheim) 329:371-376.
9. Druker BJ, et al (1996). *Effects of a selective inhibitor of the ABL tyrosine kinase on the growth of BCR-ABL positive cells.* Nat Med 2:561-566.
10. Deininger MW, Goldman JM, Lydon N and Melo JV !1997). *The tyrosine kinase inhibitor CGP57148B selectively inhibits the growth of BCR-ABL-positive cells.* Blood 90:3691-3698.
11. Daley GQ, van Etten RA, Baltimore D (1990). *Induction of chronic myelogenous leukemia in mice by the p210 BCR/ABL gene of the Philadelphia chromosome.* Science 247:824-830.
12. Weisberg E, et al (2007). *Second generation inhibitors of BCR-ABL for treatment of imatinib-resistant chronic myeloid leukemia.* Nature Review 7:345-356.
13. Hehlmann, R, et al (2007). *Drug treatment is superior to allografting as first-line therapy in chronic myeloid leukemia.* Blood 109:4686-4692.
14. Druker BJ and Lydon NB (2000). *Lessons learned from the development of an Abl tyrosine kinase inhibitor for chronic myelogenous leukemia.* J Clin Invest 105:3-7.
15. Druker BJ, Talpaz M, Resta DJ, et al (2001). *Efficacy and safety of a specific inhibitor of the BCR-ABL tyrosine kinase in chronic myeloid leukemia.* N Engl J Med 344:1031-1037.

16. Druker BJ, Sawyers CL, Kantarjian H, et al (2001). *Activity of a specific inhibitor of the BCR-ABL tyrosine kinase in the blast crisis of chronic myeloid leukemia and acute lymphoblastic leukemia with the Philadelphia chromosome.* N Engl J Med 344:1038-1042.
17. Druker B, et al (2006). *Five-year follow-up of patients receiving imatinib for chronic myeloid leukemia.* N Engl J Med 355:2408-2417.
18. Hughes T, et al (2006). *Monitoring CML patients responding to treatment with tyrosine kinase inhibitors – review and recommendations for harmonizing current methodology for detecting BCR-ABL transcripts and kinase domain mutations and for expressing results.* Blood 108:28-37.
19. Weisberg E & Griffin JD (2000). *Mechanism of resistance to the ABL tyrosine kinase inhibitor STI571 in BCR-ABL-transformed Hematopoietic cell lines.* Blood 95:3498-3505.
20. Mahon FX, et al (2000). *Selection and characterization of BCR-ABL positive cell lines with differential sensitivity to the tyrosine kinase inhibitor STI571: diverse mechanisms of resistance.* Blood 96:1070-1079.
21. le Coutre P, et al (2000). *Induction of resistance to the abelson inhibitor STI571in human leukemic cells through gene amplification.* Blood 95:1758-1766.
22. Gorre ME, et al (2001). *Clinical resistance to STI-571 cancer therapy caused by BCR-ABL gene mutation or amplification.* Science 293:876-880.
23. Schindler T, et al (2000). *Structural mechanism for STI-571 inhibition of Abelson tyrosine kinase.* Science 289:1938-1942.
24. Shah NP, et al (2002). *Multiple BCR-ABL kinase domain mutations confer polyclonal resistance to the tyrosine kinase inhibitor imatinib (STI571) in chronic phase and blast crisis chronic myeloid leukemia.* Cancer Cell 2:117-125.
25. Azam M, Latek RR & Daley GO (2003). *Mechanism of autoinhibition and STI-571/imatinib resistance revealed by mutagenesis of BCR-ABL.* Cell 112:831-843.
26. Branford S, et al (2002). *High frequency of point mutations clustered within the adenosine triphosphate-binding region of BCR/ABL in patients with chronic myeloid leukemia or Ph-positive acute lymphoblastic leukemia who develop imatinib (STI571) resistance.* Blood 99:3472-3475.
27. Baccarani M, et al (2006). *Evolving concepts in the management of chronic myeloid leukemia. Recommendations from an expert panel on behalf of the European Leukemia Net.* Blood 108; 1809-1820.
28. Manley PW, Cowan-Jacob SW, & Mestan J (2005). *Advances in the structural biology, design and clinical development of Bcr-Abl kinase inhibitor for the treatment of chronic myeloid leukemia.* Biochim. Biophys. Acta 1754:3-13.
29. Verstovek S, et al (2006). *Effects of AMN 107, a novel aminopyrimidine tyrosine kinase inhibitor, on human mast cells bearing wild-type or mutated codon 816 c-kit.* Leukemia Res 30:1365-1370.
30. Weisberg E, et al (2005). *Characterization of AMN 107, a selective inhibitor of native and mutant BCR-ABL.* Cancer Cell 7:129-141.
31. O'Hare T, et al (2005). *In vitro activity of BCR-ABL inhibitors AMN 107 and BMS-354825 against clinically relevant imatinib-resistant ABL kinase domain mutants.* Cancer Res 65:4500-4505.
32. Kantarjian H, et al (2006). *Nilotinib in imatinib-resistant CML and Philadelphia chromosome-positive ALL.* N Engl J Med 354:2542-2551.
33. Kantarjian HM, et al (2007). *Nilotinib (formerly AMN 107), a highly selective BCR-ABL tyrosine kinase inhibitor, is effective in patients with Philadelphia chromosome-positive chronic myelogenous leukemia in chronic phase following imatinib resistance and intolerance.* Blood 110:3540-3546.

34. Das J, et al (2006). *2-aminothiazole as a novel kinase inhibitor template. Structure-activity relationship studies towards the discovery of N-(2-chloro-6-methylphenyl)-2[[6-[4-[2-hydroxyethyl)-1-piperazinyl)]-2-methyl-4-pyrimidinyl]amino)]-1,3-thiazole-5-carbixamide(dasatinib; BMS-354825) as a potent pan-src knase inhibitor.* J. Med. Chem. 49:6819-6832.

35. Tokarski, J, et al (2006). *The structure of dasatinib (BMS-354825) bound to activated ABL kinase domain elucidates its inhibitory activity against imatinib-resistant ABL mutants.* Cancer Res 66:5790-5797.

36. Shah NP, et al (2004). *Overriding imatinib resistance with a novel ABL kinase inhibitor.* Science 305:399-401.

37. Talpaz M, et al (2006). *Dasatinib in imatinib-resistant Philadelphia chromosome-positive leukemias.* N Engl J Med 354:2531-2541.

38. Hochhaus A, et al (2007). *Dasatinib induces notable hematologic and cytogenetic responses in chronic-phase chronic myeloid leukemia after failure of imatinib therapy.* Blood 109:2303-2309.

39. Hochhaus, A. et al (2006). *Dasatinib (Sprycel) 50 mg or 70 mg BID versus 100 mg or 140 mg QD in patients with chronic myeloid leukemia in chronic phase (CML-CP) resistant or intolerant to imatinib: results of the CA-180-034 Study.* Blood 108:166.

40. Puttini M, et al (2006). *In vitro and in vivo activity of SKI-606, a novel Src-Abl+ neoplastic cells.* Cancer Res 66;11314-11322.

41. Cortes J, et al (2006). *A phase 1/2 study of SKI-606, a dual inhibitor of Src and Abl kinases in adult patients with Philadelphia chromosome positive (Ph+) chronic myelogenous leukemia (CML) or acute lymphocytic (ALL) relapsed, refractory or intolerant of imatinib.* Blood 108:168a.

42. Kimura, S et al (2005). *NS-187, a potent and selective dual BCR-ABL/LYN tyrosine kinase inhibitor, is a novel agent for imatinib-resistant leukemia.* Blood 106:3948-3954.

43. Adrian, F.J., et al (2006). *Allosteric inhibitors of BCR-ABL-dependent cell proliferation.* Nature Chem. Biol. 2:95-102.

44. Harringtone, E.A. et al (2004). *VX-680, a potent and selective small-molecule inhibitor of the Aurora kinases suppresses tumor growth in vivo.* Nature Med 10:262-267.

45. Giles, F. et al (2007). *MK-0457, a novel kinase inhibitor, is active in patients with chronic myeloid leukemia or acute lymphocytic leukemia with T315I mutation.* Blood 109:500-502.

46. Michor F, et al (2005). *Dynamics of chronic myeloid leukemia.* Nature 435:1267-1270.

CHAPTER

6

Mechanism of Resistance to Imatinib Mesylate in Chronic Myeloid Leukemia (CML)

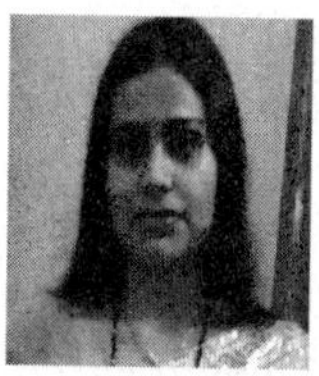

Pratibha Sharma, Lalit Kumar*, Sujata Mohanty and V. Kochupillai

Department of Medical Oncology, Institute Rotary Cancer Hospital, All India Institute of Medical Sciences, New Delhi 110029

ABSTRACT

Chronic myeloid leukemia(CML) is first human malignancy where molecular targeted therapy with imatinib mesylate has been successful. Imatinib mesylate is a tyrosine kinase inhibitor which specifically recognizes and binds to the ATP binding site of BCR-ABL fusion protein, a hallmark of CML. Therapy with this drug results in complete hematological (CHR,95-98%) and cytogenetic responses (CGR, 50-80%) in newly diagnosed chronic phase (CP) CML patients, however, response rates are low in Late CP or advanced phase of CML; CHR and CGR being 60-80% and 20%, respectively. Presence of primary resistance in advanced disease and development of secondary resistance to imatinib are major problems. Mechanisms for Imatinib resistance are multifactorial. Mutations in the BCR-ABL kinase domain or in Imatinib binding site or p loop mutations or amplification and overexpression of BCR-ABL protein are main BCR-ABL dependent mechanisms. In few cases, BCR-ABL independent mechanisms may also be responsible for resistance to imatinib. Early identification of such patients (with resistance to imatinib) can help to select appropriate therapy. Recently, two drugs Dasatinib and nilotinib have shown promising results. It appears that a combination of imatinib and second generation kinase inhibitors e.g. dasatinib, nilotinib may be more appropriate therapy atleast in some patients with multifactorial mechanism of resistance.

*email: lalitaiims@yahoo.com

INTRODUCTION

Chronic myeloid leukemia is a clonal myeloproliferative disorder of pluripotent hematopoietic stem cells and accounts for approximately 40% of all leukemia cases among adults in north India (1). The clinical course of CML typically progresses over time from an early chronic phase (CP) to blast crisis with an intermediate accelerated phase (AP). CML is characterized by the presence of Philadelphia chromosome which arises from the reciprocal translocation between chromosome 9 and 22. The resulting chimeric gene codes for BCR-ABL fusion protein, P210 with constitutively active tyrosine kinase activity which results in excessive proliferation , prevent apoptosis and decreased cellular adhesion . It has been shown that the enhanced tyrosine kinase activity of BCR-ABL is essential for CML pathogenesis and is likely to represent the initiating event (2,3). Thus, BCR-ABL fusion protein is an ideal target for molecular targeted therapy.

Though CML was described 100 years ago, Fowler solution (arsenic trioxide in potassium bicarbonate) and splenic radiations were the only treatment options available till the 1950s. Busulphan an alkylating agent was introduced in 1954 and was effective in controlling leucocytosis (4, 5). Hydroxyurea was introduced in the late 1960s, has a favourable toxicity profile and is effective in controlling the white cell count. Recombinant interferon –á became available in the early 1990s and was superior to hydroxyurea or busulfan in attaining higher complete hematological remission (CHR) , complete Cytogenetic responses (CGR) and prolonging survival (6). Experience with Allogeneic hematopoietic Stem Cell Transplant from an HLA-matched sibling or an unrelated donor suggests that it is the only potentially curative treatment for CML. Its limitations include - the availability of a matched sibling donor in less than one third of patients and the potential morbidity and mortality of the procedure (6).

Molecular Targeted Therapy: Imatinib Mesylate (STI-571, Gleevec)

Imatinib is a 2-phenylaminopyrimidine derivative and was approved for use in May 2001 for patients with CML. This drug specifically recognizes and binds to BCR-ABL ATP-binding site and stabilizes the inactive form of BCR-ABL, thereby preventing phosphorylation of substrate molecules. This ultimately results in switching off of the downstream signaling pathways that promote leukemogenesis.(7,8)

Hematological and Cytogenetic Responses to Imatinib

The initial landmark studies by Druker et al showed high response rates to Imatinib mesylate in patients with advanced CML and those pretreated with IFN-α.. Results of an International multicentric randomized trial (IRIS Group) showed that after follow up of 18 months the estimated major cytogenetic response (CGR) rate with imatinib was 87% compared with 34.7% in the IFN-á group. The estimated complete CGR was 76% as compare to 14.5 % in the IFN-á group (7,9) . This study confirmed that in terms of complete hematological response (CHR), major CGR and complete CGR and the likelihood of progression to AP/BC, Imatinib was superior to IFN-á and low dose Ara-C as first line therapy in newly diagnosed CP-CML patients. In addition, patients on Imatinib had a better quality of life. An update on the IRIS study has been published recently; at a median follow up of 42 months 98% patients were in CHR, 89% were in major CGR, 82% had complete CGR; 75% of the patients were still on Imatinib, 9% had progressed to AP/BC (10,11). Although response to Imatinib in CP-CML patients is significantly high yet responses in later stages of the disease are low. Among late CP patients who were intolerant or resistant to IFN- á or to other conventional chemotherapy complete CGR rates of 41% to 64% have been reported. For AP/BC patients CHR rates of 40 - 60% and major CGR rates of 20-30% have been reported (12-16).

Imatinib was introduced in India in 2001 through GIPAP (Gleevec International Patient Assistance Programme) where free drugs were provided to the patients. We have initial experience of this drug published from two major centers (AIIMS, Delhi and TMH, Mumbai) of India . Comparison of our response rates with two other major center of the world suggests that CHR rates are similar but complete CGR rates in our studies are relatively lower compared to IRIS trial. (17, 18). The possible reasons for the low CGR rates in the studies from India could be inclusion of a large number of patients in late CP and with advanced disease and of those pre-treated with IFN-α. (Table 6.1). Now more than 3000 patients are receiving Imatinib all over the country and about 500 patients at our center are on Imatinib therapy.

Table 6.1 Comparison of Responses of Imatinib mesylate in CML Patients

	Present study (2003-2006) (unpublished data)	**AIIMS Study(17)**	**TMH, Mumbai(18)**	**German study(16)**	**IRIS Trial (10)**
Total No of pts	**100**	**110**	**174**	**300**	**553**
Median Age (range) in years	CP=37.2 (11-60) AP + BC= 34.6(15-62)	CP=38(11-65) AP+BC=36 (13-60)	38(4-79)	CP= 56 (18.5-77)	50(18-70)
Sex M:F	68:32	84:34	122:52	78:61	341:212
Median interval from diagnosis to starting imatinib (months)	24 (6-96)	CP=25 (2-204) AP+BC=37 (6.5-120	36	31(2-312)	2.1
Disease status: CP/ AP/BC	88/10/2	79/23/16	97/47/30	139/80/81	All CP
Complete Hemato-logical Response (%)	CP=97.7 AP+BC=75	CP=95.8A P+BC=35	Early CP=100% Late CP=89% AP=55.5% BC=36.7%	CP=97% AP=61% BC=18%	95.3
Complete/major Cytogenetic response (%)	CP=40/7 AP+BC= 8.3/8.3	CP=24.5/30% AP+BC=6.7/13.4	Early CP=41.7/20.8% Late CP=27/19% AP=6.4/15% BC=13/10%	CP=49/61% AP=26/31% BC=8/12%	73.8/85.2

Resistance to Imatinib

Despite high rates of hematological and Cytogenetic responses to therapy, the emergence of resistance to Imatinib has been recognized as a major problem in the treatment of patients with CML. In the IRIS trial an estimated 5% of patients with newly diagnosed chronic phase failed to achieve CHR at 3 months 16 % failed to achieve a major CGR at 12 months and 24% failed to achieve complete CGR at 18 months and relapse rates was 17 % and another 7 % patients developed disease progression (10,19). Incidence of resistance - relapse is higher in later stages of the disease. In blast crisis almost all patients relapse after an initial response and 40-50% of patients with accelerated phase CML develop resistance after 2 years of treatment with an increase to 75% after 4 years of treatment (20).

Imatinib Resistance in Indian Patients

At our center about 500 patients have been enrolled on Imatinib therapy and we have observed development of resistance to Imatinib either in the beginning or during the course of the disease in a subset of patients. This prompted us to look into the mechanism of resistance responsible for resistance and eventually to apply strategies to overcome resistance.

100 CML patients on imatinib therapy coming to out patient department (OPD) at our institute were included in the study. 87 of 100 patients were in chronic phase and 13 were in accelerated / blast phase of the disease. Mean age of the patients was 34.42 years (range, 11 to 62 years) with male to female ratio being 2: 1. 30 CP patients were treated with imatinib as upfront therapy and 70 patients (57: CP;13 :AP/BC) were pretreated with IFN- α and/or Hydrea for mean time period of 28 months (Range 9-96 months) and patients who showed IFN intolerance and/or failure were treated with Imatinib mesylate (Dosage : 400mg/day for chronic phase patients and 600mg/day for accelerated/blast phase patients). Patients were monitored for hematological and cytogenetic responses on imatinib therapy and categorized as resistant or responders as per standard criteria (table-6.2 & 6.3).

Frequency of Resistance

23 of 58 (40%) previously treated CP patient and 90 % (11/12) (AP/BC) patients had evidence of primary hematological or cytogenetic resistance to Imatinib. 20% (6/30) newly diagnosed CP patients had cytogenetic resistance to Imatinib. We observed that resistance to Imatinib is higher in patients who were previously treated with IFN-α and/or hydroxyurea (40%) and those who had advanced phase of CML (90%) compared to patients treated with imatinib as up front therapy (20%). Duration of IFN-α and/or hydroxyurea pre-treatment was also found to be associated with development of resistance to Imatinib mesylate ($p=0.003$) where duration of pre-treatment was longer in resistant patients compared to responders.

Mechanism of Resistance

Mechanisms for Imatinib resistance are multifactorial but can be categorized as two broad groups BCR-ABL dependent and BCR-ABL independent.

Table 6.2 Criteria for Response to Imatinib mesylate (adapted from ref 21)

Response	Definition
Complete Hematological Response(CHR)	• TLC<10000/cmm, platelets counts <450000/cmm. • Differential count without immature granulocytes and < 5% basophils • No palpable spleen
Partial Hematological Response (PHR)	• More than 50% decrease in TLC from pretreatment levels to 20,000/cmm· Persistence of immature forms on differential counts • Persistent splenomegaly.
Cytogenetic response (CGR)	Category : Ph +ve metaphases No CGR : >95% Minimal CGR : 66%-95% Minor CGR : 36%-65% Partial CGR : 1%-35% Complete CGR : 0%
Molecular Response	Major : ≤0.10(BCR-ABL to control gene ratio according to international scale) Complete : BCR-ABL transcript nonquantifiable and nondetectable

Table 6.3 Criteria for Resistance to Imatinib mesylate (adapted from ref 21)

Resistance	Definition
Primary resistance	• No complete hematological response after 3 months • No cytogenetic response after 6 months. • No Major Cytogenetic response after 12 months.
Secondary resistance	• Loss of complete hematological response • Loss of Major cytogenetic response. • Progression to accelerated/ Blast phase of the disease.

1. BCR-ABL –dependent: It has been demonstrated BCR-ABL kinase activity inhibited at response but is reactivated in resistant patients.

Mutations of the BCR-ABL kinase domain: Initial study by Gorre et al revealed that point mutations in BCR-ABL fusion gene interfere with the binding of drug with BCR-ABL protein (22). We studied point mutations in the kinase domain in 40 resistant patients by direct sequencing of entire kinase domain after semi-nested RT-PCR. 12 different point mutations were detected in 18 (45%) patients (unpublished data). None of the mutation was detected in baseline samples (before Imatinib initiation). So far approximately 90 mutation at 57 residues have been reported at a frequency ranging from 40% to 90% (23-26). The regions of the kinase domain where mutations are detected fall into following four groups (27).

Mutations in Imatinib binding site (IB-site): Mutations at IB site interact directly with Imatinib and presumably impair drug binding without significantly affecting the binding of ATP. In our study 3 mutations (F317V, F317L, T315I) were detected in this region in 5 patients. T315I mutation within this region, detected in only one patient is completely resistant to Imatinib as amino acid 315 is critical for drug binding (unpublished data). Detection of this mutations influences therapeutic decisions as this mutation is also highly resistant to other new generation BCR-ABL kinase inhibitors such as nilotinib and Dasatinib (26).

P-loop mutations: The second group includes mutations in the ATP- binding loop (P-loop). Of all the mutations detected to date the most frequently occurring are those of P-loop which have been demonstrated to confer high levels of resistance. We found 6 mutations (Y253F,G250E, L248V,Q252H,M244V,Y253H) within this region in one patient each (unpublished data) In kinase assays p-loop mutants were found to be 70 to 100 fold less sensitive to Imatinib versus native BCR-ABL (26). Two separate studies evaluating the frequency and prognostic significance of BCR-ABL mutations in Imatinib resistant patients showed that patients harbouring P-loop mutations had particularly poor outcomes.(28, 29,30). However more recent reports showed contrasting results (28). In our study, we did not find any significant difference (p=0.274) in progression -free survival of resistant patients with p-loop mutations and those with mutation outside the p-loop (unpublished data).

Mutations in other regions: Other Imatinib resistant mutations are those with in the A*ctivation loop* .Closed conformation of activation loop is required for stabilizing the Imatinib binding. L387M mutation in this region was detected in 3 resistant patients. Another cluster of mutations located in the *Catalytic domain* of the kinase region provides a platform for the base of the activation loop. We detected 2 mutation (F359V,L364I) with in this region in 4 resistant patients(unpublished data) . Mutations in these regions confer low level of resistance and are therefore considered to be of lesser clinical importance .Studies have shown that some BCR-ABL mutations confer only intermediate resistance to Imatinib and therefore may respond to increased doses of Imatinib (26,31).

Amplification and overexpression of BCR-ABL: Mechanism of Imatinib resistance other than point mutations include increased production of BCR-ABL either at genomic level (amplification of gene) or transcript/ protein level (over expression).We detected amplification of BCR-ABL fusion gene in 4 of 40 (10%) resistant patients. Overexpression of BCR-ABL transcript was also detected at RNA level in majority of Imatinib resistant patients Mean BCR-ABL/ABL % values of resistant patients was significantly higher than responders (p=0.001) . High phosphorylation activity of BCR-ABL fusion protein was also detected in Imatinib resistant patients (unpublished data) .

2. BCR-ABL Independent: Although it has been shown that resistance to Imatinib can occur through restoration of BCR-ABL activity it had also been documented that Imatinib resistance can also occur through BCR-ABL independent mechanism. Phosphorylation activity of BCR-ABL kinase enzyme activates various multiple downstream substrates. Therefore constitutive activation of one of these downstream signaling molecules could result in activation of pathways regardless of BCR-ABL inhibition resulting in imatinib resistance. The SRC family kinases (SFKs) may be one such example of substrates which are essential mediators of BCR-ABL signaling that regulate cell proliferation and survival and have been implicated in the development of imatinib resistance. In vitro studies showed that CML cell lines overexpress LYN and HCK and dual inhibition of these

SFKs and BCR-ABL results in enhanced apoptotic response (34). Other BCR-ABL independent mechanism involves mechanism that decreases the intracellular concentrations of Imatinib. The plasma protein α-1 acid glycoprotein (AGP) is found to bind Imatinib in vitro blocking inhibition of the ABL kinase in a dose dependent manner but the causative role of AGP in human Imatinib resistance is yet to be described (35). *In vitro* studies have also showed that over expression of multidrug resistance P-glycoprotein (Pgp) may contribute to imatinib resistance. Imatinib is a substrate for Pgp and expression of this protein has been shown to mediate resistance (36).

Strategies to Overcome Resistance

It is now well established that patients with resistance to Imatinib or those who relapse after initial response have a poor prognosis, several new approaches are being attempted to overcome resistance.

(i) **High -dose Imatinib:** Imatinib in higher dosage from 400mg to 600 or 800mg daily have been shown to induce cytogenetic responses; 35-40% resistant patients have achieved major CGR but the durability of such response in generally limited . Higher doses of imatinib are also associated with increased toxicity (26).

(ii) **Alternative ABL inhibitors in clinical development:** Various new agents are now in early stages of development but following represent important advances in CML therapy.

Dasatinib(BMS-354825) is an orally available ABL kinase inhibitor that differs from Imatinib in that it can bind both to the active and in active conformations of the ABL kinase domain and also inhibits Src family kinases including Src and Lyn (37). This is structurally unrelated and about 300 times more active than Imatinib and *in vitro* active against most of the Imatinib resistant mutations with an exception of T315I and probably also to F317L mutant clone. Its use in CML was approved in 2006 in US and Europe (37, 38). In phase 2 clinical studies CHR rates were seen in 90% and major CGR in 52% of imatinib resistant patients. Responses were maintained in 95% of responding patients (33). With recent results of studies on Dasatinib it can be speculated that early and continuous use of Dasatinib in CP-CML patients may result in improved patient outcome.

Nilotinib(AMN107): Nilotinib is an orally active aminopyrimidine derivative which resembles imatinib but is modified and has increased affinity (20-30 times) to ATP binding site of BCR-ABL oncoprotein (37). It can bind only to the inactive conformation of BCR-ABL but does not inhibit Src family kinases .It is active against all imatinib resistant cell lines with ABL kinase mutations with the exception of T315I. The Y253H mutant clone may also be relatively resistant to this drug (33, 39). In recently reported phase-II trials in CML-CP patients, major CGR were observed in 56% patients of which 40 % were in complete CGR. However the durability of responses remains to be proven. The overall survival was approximately 95% at 12 months. (40)

Thus, both *Dasatinib* and *nilotinib* seems to be equally active in patients deemed to have failed imatinib but none of them is recommended for patients with T315I mutation. And the long term durability of responses with these agents remains undefined. *Bosutinib(SKI-606)* :_Bosutinib is a 4-anilino-3-quinolinecarbonitrile SRC/ABL kinase inhibitor that has undergone relatively limited phase 1/2 clinical testing to date. It is very much more active than Imatinib against CML cell lines. The experience of 76 patients with chronic-phase CML with resistance or intolerance to imatinib was recently presented. With a median follow-up of less than 3 months, fewer than half of the patients have been evaluated for a cytogenetic response. Of 31 evaluable patients, 32% have achieved a complete cytogenetic remission. Longer follow-up is necessary to obtain a more accurate assessment of this agent's toxicity and efficacy profiles (33, 41).

Conclusion and Future Directions

The introduction of imatinib has revolutionized the management of CML with higher hematological and cytogenetic response rates. A substantial number of patients are either initially resistant or acquire resistance after achieving initial response. To study the mechanism responsible for resistance is important as it may provide insight into appropriate therapeutic intervention .With new treatment options coming up, early identification of resistance becomes increasingly important in order to select the most appropriate therapy for our patients. Since mechanism of resistance may be multifactorial in many patients, it would be more appropriate to use a combination of BCR-ABL inhibitors. Treatment with combination between Dasatinib, nilotinib and imatinib may have better therapeutic efficacy than either agent alone. Combining second generation kinase inhibitors with agents that are active against the T315I mutant i.e. MK-0457 is also an attractive approach that may improve treatment outcomes in future.

REFERENCES

1. Bhutani M, Kumar L, Kochupillai V. Lympho-hemopoietic malignancies in India. Med Oncology 2002;19:141-150
2. Sawyers CL. Chronic myeloid leukemia. New Eng J Med 1999;340:1330-40.
3. Deininger MW, Goldman JM, Melo JV. The molecular biology of chronic myeloid leukemia. Blood. 2000;96: 3343-3356.
4. Medical Research Council's working party for therapeutic trials in Leukemia. Chronic granulocytic leukemia : Comparision of radiotherapy and busulphan therapy. Br Med J 1968;1:201-208.
5. Socie G, Clift RA, Blaise D, et al. Busulfan plus cyclophosphamide compared with total-body irradiation plus cyclophosphamide before marrow transplantation for myeloid leukemia: long-term follow-up of 4 randomized studies. Blood. 2001 ;98(13):3569-74.
6. Kumar L. Chronic myelogenous leukemia(CML): An update. Nat Med J India.2006;19(5):255-263.
7. Druker BJ, Talpaz M, Resta DJ, et al. Efficacy and safety of a specific inhibitor of the BCR-ABL tyrosine kinase in chronic myeloid leukemia. New Eng J Med 2001;344:1031-7.
8. Savage DG and Antman KH. Drug therapy : Imatinib mesylate – A new oral targeted therapy . New Eng J Med 2002;346:683-693.
9. Drucker BJ, Sawyers CL, Kantarjian H, et al. Activity of a specific inhibitor of BCR-ABL tyrosine kinase in the blast crisis of chronic myelogenous leukemia and acute lymphoblastic leukemia with the Philadelphia chromosome. New Eng J Med 2001;344:1038-1042.
10. O'Brien SG, Guilhot F, Larson RA, et al. Imatinib compared with interferon and low-dose cytarabine for newly diagnosed chronic-phase chronic myeloid leukemia. N Engl J Med. 2003;348: 994-1004
11. Deininger MW, O'Brien SG, Ford JM, Druker BJ J Practical management of patients with chronic myeloid leukemia receiving imatinib Clin Oncol. 2003 15;21(8):1637-47

12. Kantarjian H, Sawyers S, Hochhaus A, et al. Hematologic and cytogenetic responses to Imatinib Mesylate in chronic phase myelogenous leukemia. New Eng J Med 2002;346; 645-52.
13. Kantarjian HM, O'Brien S, Cortes J, et al. Imatinib mesylate therapy improves survival in patients with newly diagnosed Philadelphia chromosome-positive chronic myelogenous leukemia in the chronic phase: comparison with historic data. Cancer. 2003;98: 2636-2642.
14. Kantarjian H, Talpaz M, O'Brien S, Giles F, Faderl S, Verstovsek S,et al. Survival benefit with imatinib mesylate therapy in patients with accelerated-phase chronic myelogenous leukemia—comparison with historic experience. Cancer 2005;103(10):2099-108.
15. Rosti G.Martinelli G,Bassi S,etal. Molecular response to imatinib in late chronic phase chronic myeloid leukemia.Blood.2004;103;2284-2290.
16. Lahaye T, Riehm B, Berger U, et al. response and resistance in 300 patients with BCR-ABL positive leukemias treated with imatinib in a single center.: a 4.5 years follow up. Cancer 2005;103:1659-69.
17. Arora B, Kumar L, Kumaru M, Sharma A, Wadhwa J & Kochupillai V. Therapy with imatinib mesylate for chronic myeloid leukemia. Ind J Med & Paed Oncology 2005;26:5-18.
18. Deshmukh C, Saikia T, Bakshi A, Kadam PA, Baisane C and Parikh P. Imatinib mesylate in chronic myeloid leukemia: A prospective , single arm, non-randomized study. J Assoc Phys India 2005;53:290-295.
19. Druker BJ,Guilhot F,O'Brien SG,Gathmann I,Kantarjian H,Gattermann N et al. Five year follow-up of patients receiving imatinib for chronic myeloid leukemia.N Engl J Med 2006:355:2408-2417.
20. Silver RT,Talpaz M,Sawyers CL,et al. Four years follow –up of 1027 patients with late chronic phase(L-CP),accelerated phase (AP),or blast crisis (BC) chronic myeloid leukemia(CML) treated with imatinib in three large phase II trials. Blood 2004;104;abstract 23
21. Baccarni M,Sagio G,Goldman J,Hochhaus A,Simonsson B,Appelbaum F, et al.Evolving concepts in teh management of chronic myeloid leukemia: recommendations from an expert panel on behalf of the European leukemia Net. Blood 2006:108:1809-1820.
22. Gorre ME, Mohammed M, Ellwood K,et al. Clinical resistance to STI571cancer therapy caused by BCR-ABL gene mutation or amplification. Science.2001; 293:876- 880.
23. Branford S, Rudzki Z , Walsh S, et al. High frequency of point mutation clustered within adenosine triphosphate binding region of BCR/ABL in patients with chronic myeloid leukemia or Ph - positive acute lymphoblastic leukemia who develop imatinib (STI571) Resistance. Blood. 2002; 99: 3472-3475.
24. Hofmann WK , Jones LC, Lemp NA, etal. Ph(+)acute lymphoblastic leukemia resistant to the tyrosine kinase inhibitor STI571 has a unique BCR-ABL gene mutation. Blood.2002; 99: 1860-1862.
25. Von Bubnoff N, Schneller F, Peschel C,et al .BCR-ABL gene mutation in relation to clinical resistance of Philadelphia- chromosome positive leukemia to STI571:a prospective study. Lancet.2002; 359:487-491.
26. Kujawski L,Talpaz M. Strategies for overcoming imatinib resistance in chronic myeloid leukemia.Leukemia&Lymphoma 2007;48(12)2310-2322.
27. Branford S. Chronic myeloid leukemia: Molecular monitoring in clinical practiceHematology; 2007American Society of Hematology
28. Jabbour E, Kantarjian H, Jones D,Talpaz M,Bekele N,O'Brien S et al.Frequency and clinical significance of BCR-ABL mutations in patients with chronic myeloid leukemia treated with imatinib mesylate.Leukemia2006;20:1767-1773.

29. Branford S, Rudzki Z, walsh s, etal. Detection of BCR-ABL mutations in patients with CML treated with imatinib is virtually always accompanied by clinical resistance and mutations in ATP phosphate –binding loop(p-loop) are associated with a poor prognosis. Blood.2003;102;276-283.

30. Soverini s ,Martinelli G,rosti G, Bassi S, Amabile M,Poerio A, et al.ABL mutations in late chronic phase chronic myeloid leukemia with up front cytogenetic resistance to imatinib are associated with a greater likelihood of progression to blast crisis and shorter survival :a study by GIMEMA Working Party on Chronic Myeloid Leukemia.J Clin Oncol 2005;23:4100-4109.

31. Shah NP, Nicoll JM, Nagar B, Goree ME Paquette RL Kuriyan J, Sawyers CL. Multiple BCR-ABL kinase domain mutations confer polyclonal resistance to the tyrosine kinase inhibitor imatinib(STI571) in chronic phase and blast crisis chronic myeloid leukemia.2002 Cancer Cell; 2:117-125.

32. Hochhaus A, Kreil S, Corbin AS, La RP, Muller MC, Lahaye T, et al .Molecular and chromosomal mechanisms of resistance to imatinib (STI571) therapy.

33. Goldman JM. How I treat CML chronic myeloid leukemia in the imatinib era 2007. Blood.

34. Roginskaya V,Zuo S,Caudell E,Nambudiri G,Kraker AJ,Corey SJ. Therapeutic targeting of Src-kinase Lyn I myeloid leukemic cell growth.Leukemia 1999; 13:855-861.

35. Larghero J, Leguay T, Mourah S, Madelaine-Chambrin I, taksin AL,Raffoux E, et al .Relationship between elevated levels of the a-1 acid glycoprotein in chronic myelogenous leukemia in blast crisis and pharmacological resistnace to imatinib (Gleevec) in vitro and in vivo .Biochem Phamacol. 2003;66:1907-1913.

36. Illmer T,Schaich M, Platzbecker U et al .P-glycoprotein –mediated drug efflux is a resistance mechanism of chronic myelogenous leukemia cells to treatment with imatinib mesylate.2004;18:401-408.

37. O'hare T,Walters DK, Stoffregen EP,Jia T, Manley PW, Mestan J, et al . In vitro activity of BCR-ABL inhibitors AMN107 and BMS-354825 against clinically relevant imatinib –resistant Abl kinase domain mutants. Cancer Res.2005; 65:4500-4505.

38. Shah NP, Tran C, Lee FY, Chen P, Norris D, Sawyers CL. Overriding imatinib resistance with a novel ABL kinase inhibitor.Science 2004; 305:399-401.

39. Weisberg E Manley PW, Breitenstein W, Bruggen J, Cowan-Jacob SW, Ray A, et al. Charaterization of AMN107 a selective inhibitor of native and mutant Bcr-Abl. Cancer Cell.2005: 7: 129-141.

40. Rosti G, le Coutre P, Bhalla K, et al. A phase II study of nilotinib administered to imatinib resistant and intolerant patients with chronic myelogenous leukemia (CML) in chronic phase (CP) [abstract]. ASCO Meeting Abstracts. 2007; 25: abstract no. 7007.

41. Gambacorti-Passerini C, Brummerndorf T, Kantarjian H, et al. Bosutinib (SKI-606) exhibits clinical activity in patients with Philadelphia chromosome positive CML or ALL who failed imatinib [abstract]. ASCO Meeting Abstracts. 2007; 25: abstract no. 7006.

CHAPTER 7

Mechanisms of Multiple Forms of Tumorigenesis in LH/hCG Overexpressing Transgenic Mice

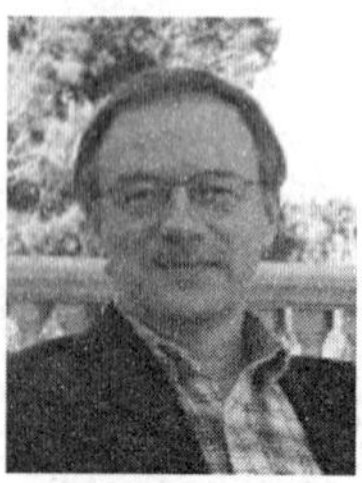

Susana B. Rulli[1], Petteri Ahtiainen[2], Matti Poutanen[2] and Ilpo T. Huhtaniemi[2,3]*

[1]Institute of Biology and Experimental Medicine-CONICET, Vuelta de Obligado 2490, Buenos Aires 1428, Argentina;
[2]Department of Physiology, University of Turku, Kiinamyllynkatu 10, FIN-20520 Turku, Finland; and
[3]Department of Reproductive Biology, Imperial College London, Hammersmith Campus, Du Cane Road, London W12 0NN, UK

INTRODUCTION

The two gonadotrophins, luteinizing hormone (LH) and follicle-stimulating hormone (FSH) are produced by the pituitary gland as heterodimers composed of a common α-subunit and the hormone- specific α-subunit. They have a key role in ovarian and testicular functions by acting through binding to their specific seven-transmembrane domain G-protein coupled receptors (Burger et al., 2004). In the gonads, LH receptors are located in testicular Leydig cells and in ovarian theca, granulosa and luteal cells (Ascoli et al., 2002). FSH receptors are expressed in testicular Sertoli cells and in granulosa cells of the ovary (Simoni et al., 1997). Although primarily expressed in gonads, LH receptors are also found in numerous extragonadal tissues (Rao, 2001; Filicori et al., 2005). However, their physiological significance is still unclear (Pakarainen et al., 2007). The placental analogue of LH, human chorionic gonadotrophin (hCG) interacts with the same LH/hCG receptor as LH, and functions as an LH agonist with a longer half-life and higher biopotency than its pituitary counterpart (Jameson and Hollenberg, 1993).

*email: ilpo.huhtaniemi@imperial.ac.uk

The physiological actions of LH and FSH are well characterised and are essential for folliculogenesis, ovulation and steroidogenesis in females, and for testicular growth, spermatogenesis and steroidogenesis in males. The existence of human diseases and mutant mouse models with deficient gonadotrophin secretion/action provides strong evidences that normal functions of gonadotrophins are needed for maintaning sex hormone production and fertility (Themmen and Huhtaniemi, 2000; Huhtaniemi and Themmen, 2005). On the other hand, there also exist physiological and pathophysiological conditions where gonadotrophin secretion and/or action are elevated. For instance, human pregnancy is characterized by a transient production of very high levels of hCG by the placenta during the first trimester, which is essential for the maintenance of progesterone production of the corpus luteum gravidarum, and to prepare the uterus for implantation and placental development (Jameson and Hollenberg, 1993). hCG is also needed to stimulate fetal testicular testosterone production for masculinization of the male fetus (Huhtaniemi, 1994). Postmenopause is a physiological situation where women are exposed to chronically elevated levels of gonadotrophins for decades, and this exposure is proposed to be a risk factor for developing ovarian tumours (Risch, 1998; Riman et al., 2004; Konishi, 2006). On the other hand, prolonged exposure to female sex hormones throughout the reproductive years has been associated with breast cancer (Russo and Russo, 1998; 2006). Finally, pathological conditions with high gonadotrophin secretion/action include pituitary tumours, activating gonadotrophin receptor mutations, polycystic ovarian syndrome, trophoblastic diseases and testicular germ cell tumors.

Studies on transgenic (TG) mouse models provide new insights into the pathophysiological role of LH/hCG in gonadal and extra-gonadal tumorigenesis. For instance, TG mice expressing the bovine bLHβ/hCGb-C-terminal peptide (CTP) fusion protein in the pituitary gland develop tumours of the granulosa cell lineage in certain genetic backgrounds (Risma et al., 1995; Keri et al., 2000). In TG mice expressing the Simian virus 40 T-antigen under the murine inhibin α-subunit promoter, elevated LH levels act as a tumour promoter, stimulating gonadal and adrenal tumorigenesis (Kananen et al. 1995; Mikola et al., 2003). In addition, mice deficient in the inhibin α-subunit gene develop mixed granulosa/Sertoli cell tumors in the presence of high LH and FSH levels (Kumar et al., 1996).

We have recently developed two TG mouse models overexpressing the α and/or β subunit of hCG that produce chronically elevated levels of bioactive LH/hCG (Rulli et al., 2002; 2003). Multiple gonadal and extragonadal tumours and altered endocrine functions were observed in these mice (Rulli et al., 2002; 2003; Ahtiainen et al., 2005; 2006; Huhtaniemi et al., 2005; 2006). The observations on these mice support the hypothesis that elevated LH/hCG exposure may have tumorigenic effects. We will smmarise below the main findings on these two TG mouse models.

GENERATION AND PHENOTYPIC CHARACTERISATION OF TRANSGENIC MICE PRODUCING HIGH LEVELS OF LH/HCG

We produced a TG mouse model harbouring the hCGβ subunit coding sequence under the human ubiquitin C promoter (hCGβ+ mice). The promoter used directs ubiquitous low level expression of the transgene in most tissues, both in fetal life and in adulthood (Schorpp et al., 1996). The TG hCGb associates with the endogenously expressed glycoprotein hormone common α-subunit (Cα) in the pituitary gland, and produces moderate levels of bioactive Cα/hCGβ dimers, mainly due to the limited availability of Cα for the dimerisation process. Circulating LH/hCG bioactivity was increased about 30-fold in females (Fig. 1A) (Rulli et al., 2002), but only a 3-4-fold in males (Rulli et al., 2003). The female hCGβ+ mice showed precocious puberty and infertility due to ovarian and uterine defects (Rulli et al., 2002). The hormone profile was severely affected, with high levels of sex steroids and prolactin (PRL). The hCGβ+ males were fertile and showed only a mild phenotype, in agreement with the moderately increased levels of hCG (Rulli et al., 2003).

We also developed a mouse model that produces pharmacological levels of hCG (hCGαβ+ mice; Fig 1, A) (Rulli et al., 2003). These mice were achieved by intercrossing the hCGβ+ mice with another TG mouse line overexpressing the Cα-subunit under the same ubiquitin promoter (hCGα+ mice). The double TG mice are able to co-express both subunits in various tissues, and in these mice the concentration of bioactive LH/hCG is 1000-fold in both sexes in comparison to wild-type (WT) animals (Fig. 7.1A) (Rulli et al., 2003; SB Rulli, P Ahtiainen, M Poutanen & I Huhtaniemi, unpublished observations). With this model, we observed that excessive levels of hCG lead to novel phenotypes in both males and females that were not revealed in conditions with only moderately elevated hormone production of the hCGβ+ mice.

The hCGα+ mice showed normal appearance and were fertile, confirming the absence of biological effects of the free gonadotrophin subunits. As will be described in the following paragraphs, the hCGαβ+ females presented with precoucious puberty and infertility, and their gonads and some extragonadal tissues were profoundly affected. In contrast to the single hCGβ+ model, the double hCGaβ+ males were infertile and their reproductive organs were severely affected (Rulli et al., 2003).

The Female Phenotype

Ovarian luteinisation

The ovaries of the hCGβ+ mice presented with active steroid biosynthesis as a consequence of direct hCG hyperstimulation. Accordingly, transiently high levels of oestradiol at peri-puberty, and persistently elevated levels of testosterone and progesterone in adulthood were found in the mice. The dominant steroidogenic pathway of the hCGβ+ ovaries was consequently altered, progesterone being the primary steroid hormone produced (Rulli et al., 2002). The ovaries presented with occasional haemorrhagic cysts and looked massively luteinised, resembling luteomas (Fig.7.1C). In addition, luteinised unruptured follicles are a frequent histological finding on th hCGβ + ovaries (Fig. 7.1 D).

The hCGαβ+ females also had enhanced steroidogenesis accompanied by elevated levels of oestradiol, testosterone and progesterone at early age, but the main difference with the hCGβ+ model was that they developed ovarian tumors resembling human teratomas at 6-8 weeks of age (SB Rulli, P Ahtiainen, M Poutanen & I Huhtaniemi, unpublished observations). Such tumors derive from the parthenogenetically activated oocytes within the ovaries, and consist of a variety of differentiated tissue types including digestive and respiratory epithelium, hair follicles, sebaceous glands, skin, cartilage and neural tissue (Mutter, 1997; Ulbright, 2004). They represent around 20% of all ovarian neoplasms in humans. They are benign tumors, however a malignant transformation occurs at an incidence of approximately 1.4-2% (Comerci et al., 1994). Since the molecular pathogenesis in humans has not been fully clarified, this model represents a good tool to unravel the mechanisms involved in tumor development. The mechanism that triggers the initial steps of teratogenesis in our model is unknown and is currently under investigation.

Another TG model for hCG has been reported, where either one or both subunits of hCG were overexpressed using the mouse metallothionein promoter (Matzuk et al., 2003). In this model, the double TG females were infertile and developed cystic ovaries, with hyperplastic theca cells.

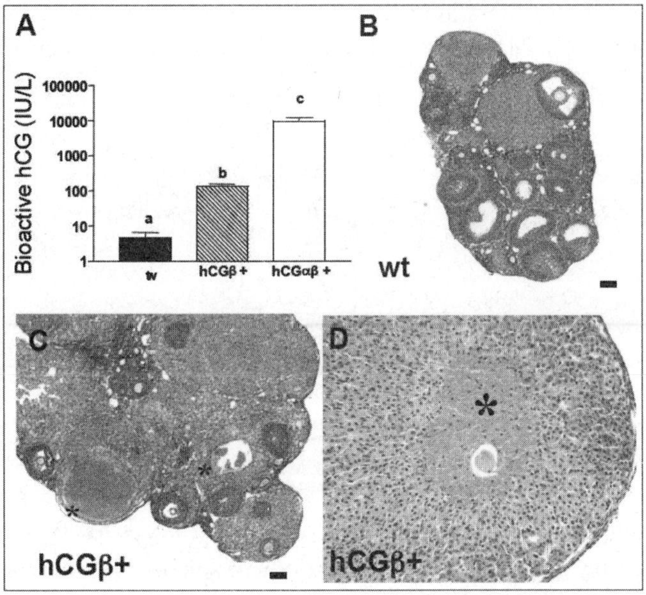

Fig. 7.1 Circulating bioactive LH/hCG and ovarian phenotype on wind-type (wt), hCGβ+, and hCGαβ+ mice. (A) Serum levels of bioactive LH/hCG in adult wt, hCGβ+, and hCGαβ+ female mice (n= 5-10). Different letters denote statistically significant differences, $p < 0.05$; (B) Histology of adult wt ovary; (C) The ovary of a hCGβ+ mouse showing massive luteinisation and hemorrhagic cysts (asterisks); (D) The ovary of a hCGβ+ mouse showing an oocyte entrapped within luteinised tissue (asterisk). Hematoxylin and eosin staining; scale bar = 50 mm.

Pituitary tumorigenesis

The hCGβ+ female mice presented with hyperplasia of pituitary lactotroph cells. The hyperplasia was obvious from the age of 2 months onwards, and progressed gradually into pituitary adenomas (Fig 7.2). By the age of 12 months, macroscopic prolactinomas with suprasellar expansion, distorted architecture and dilated blood-filled spaces were observed with 100% penetrance (Rulli et al., 2002). The neoplastic foci showed breakdown of the reticulin fiber network as a diagnostic sign of adenomas. Specific immunostaining for PRL in the tumorous areas, in association with severe hyperprolactinaemia, confirmed the lactotroph origin for the adenomas.

Ovariectomy, despite persistently high levels of hCG, prevented the development of the prolactinomas, indicating that ovarian factors are responsible for this pathological response. The LHβCTP transgenic mice (see Introduction) were reported to develop ovary-dependent functional adenomas restricted to cells of the Pit-1 lineage (Mohammad et al., 2003). Oestrogens are known to promote lactotroph hyperplasia (Freeman et al., 2000) and PRL producing pituitary tumours in certain inbred strain of rats sensitive to oestrogen (Heaney et al., 1999). In our model there was only a peripubertal rise of oestradiol with normal levels thereafter, suggesting that ovarian factors other than oestradiol are needed for the pituitary tumorigenesis. Interestingly, the high levels of progesterone coincide with the development of prolactinomas and could, therefore, contribute to the pathogenesis. In fact we have recently obtained convincing evidence that oestrogen and progesterone synergize in stimulating the proliferation of lactoroph cells in the female hCGβ+ mice (P Ahtiainen, SB Rulli, A Rivero-Müller, V Mamaeva, M Röyttä & I Huhtaniemi, submitted for publication).

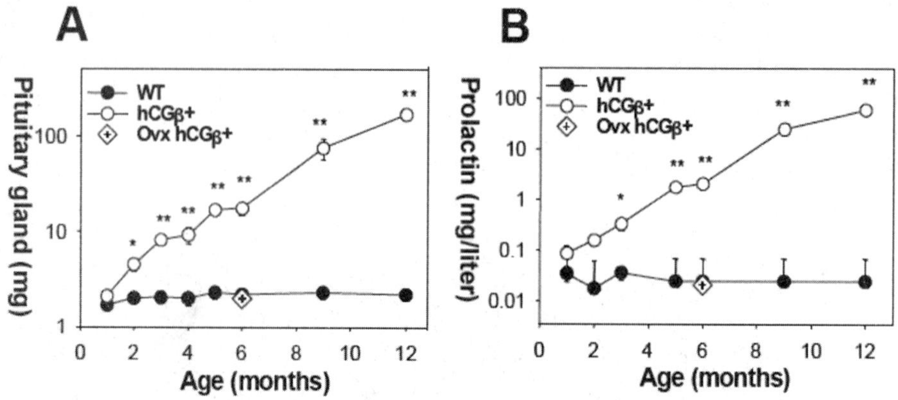

Fig. 7.2 Pituitary phenotype of the hCGβ+ transgenic mice. (A) Age-related changes in weights of the pituitary glands; B) Concentrations of serum PRL in wild-type (WT) (*filled circles*) and hCGβ+ females (*open circles*). The effects of ovariectomy (Ovx) on hCGβ+ females are indicated by a diamond-shaped symbol at 6 months of age (n = 6). *: $p < 0.05$; **: $p < 0.01$ *vs*. wt. (modified from Rulli et al., 2002).

Adrenal phenotype

We have demonstrated that chronically elevated LH in female bLHβCTP mice causes adrenal hyperplasia, and induces LH receptor expression in the adrenal gland, in association with high corticosterone production (Kero et al. 2000). Thus, these mice have a phenotype reminiscent of Cushing's syndrome, and they may provide a useful model to study human adrenal diseases. Furthermore, the effect of LH/hCG appears to be dependent on ovarian hyperfunction since gonadectomy abolishes the adrenal disturbances.

We have also observed that that the elevated post-gonadectomy levels of LH induce in the adrenal gland LH receptor expression and LH-dependent tumorigenesis in TG mice with the inhibin-α promoter driven SV40 T-antigen (Kananen et al. 1996; Mikola et al. 2003). A similar induction of LH receptor expression with subsequent adrenocortical hyperplasia occurs in certain inbred strains of WT mice. This response was revealed genetically to represent a complex trait driven by multiple epistatic loci (Bernichtein et al. 2008).

Mammary gland tumorigenesis

In addition to prolactinomas, the hCGβ+ female mice present with lobuloalveolar growth of the mammary gland, resembling the prelactating state. This is followed by the appearance of mammary gland adenocarcinomas at the age of 9 months (Fig. 7.3), with 90% penetrance at the age of 12 months (Rulli et al., 2002). The tumours also send aggressively metastases to several organs. The mammary tumours have similar histopathology as those observed in TG mice with activation of the wnt/β-catenin signalling pathway, showing accumulation of β-catenin accompanied by abnormal expression of the *Wnt* genes (Kuorelahti et al., 2007).

The role of PRL in mammary gland development and tumorigenesis in mice has been well established (Clevenger et al., 2003). Furthermore, increased sex steroid action has been associated with increased breast cancer risk, with numerous reports suggesting a proliferating role for oestradiol (Russo and Russo, 1998; 2006), and progesterone as a priming factor for the action of growth factors on breast cancer cells (Lange, 2004). In this respect, the high hCG production by the transgene, along with increased oestrogen, progesterone and PRL levels may be responsible for mammary gland proliferation and differentiation of the hCGβ+ mice. Ovariectomy abolishes the mammary gland phenotype, indicating the dependence of tumorigenesis on ovarian endocrine activity.

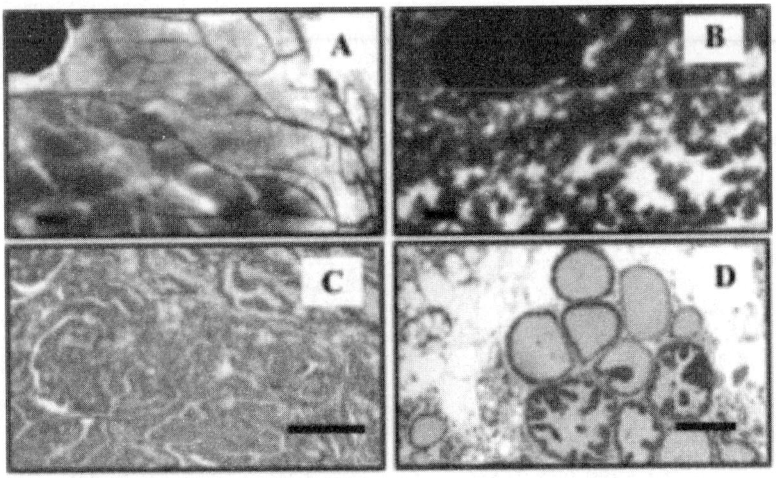

Fig. 7.3 Lobuloalveolar development and tumorigenesis in the hCGβ+ female mice. (A) whole-mount mammary gland from a WT mouse; (B) whole-mount mammary gland from a hCGβ+mouse at the age of 6 months; C and D) histology of adenocarcinoma in aged hCGβ+ females. Scale bars = 100 mm. (modified from Rulli et al., 2002).

The Male Phenotype

Accessory sex organs

Whereas the hCGβ+ males are fertile and present only with mild phenotypic responses, the hCGαβ+ males showed multiple reproductive defects, including infertility, increased testicular testosterone and progesterone production, reduced testis size and enlarged seminal vesicles and ventral prostates (Rulli et al., 2003). Abnormal function of the accessory sex organs and lower urinary tract was evident in these males, with functional obstruction of vasa deferentia, dilated urinary bladder and signs of hydronephrosis. The prostate and seminal vesicles were enlarged mainly due to distension of the glandular lumina, indicating either enhanced production of secretory fluids or impaired emptying of the glands. The epididymides were histologically normal in young adults, but sperm granulomas and abnormal sperm morphology were detected from the age of 8 months onwards. Most of the changes are likely to be caused by the high testosterone concentration in the mice. Since the males are infertile already in young adulthood, before any epididymal changes or ejaculatory duct obstruction, it is possible that their infertility is due to their abnormal aggressiveness and sex behaviour.

Testicular tumorigenesis

The adult hCGαβ+ males showed focal Leydig cell hyperplasia/hypertrophy, but no testicular tumours were observed. This is in agreement with previous studies with long-term LH/hCG treatments *in vivo* (Risbridger et al., 1982). Interestingly, we found in the hCGαβ+ males Leydig cell adenomas in postnatal age. The adenomas reached their maximum size at 10 days of age, followed by a regression and disappearance towards adulthood (Figure 7.4) (Ahtiainen et al., 2005). The expression pattern of fetal and adult Leydig cell markers suggested that the adenomas originated from the fetal Leydig cell population, indicating that the adult Leydig cells are resistant to development of gonadotrophin-induced adenomas.

The phenotypes observed in the prepubetal hCGαβ+ males are in agreement with the presence of Leydig cell adenomas in men with a specific somatic activating mutation of the *LH receptor* ($Asp^{578}His$) (Liu et al., 1999). Whether the activation of alternative intracellular signalling pathways of the LH receptor explains the early Leydig cell tumorigenesis in hCGαβ+ males remains to be elucidated.

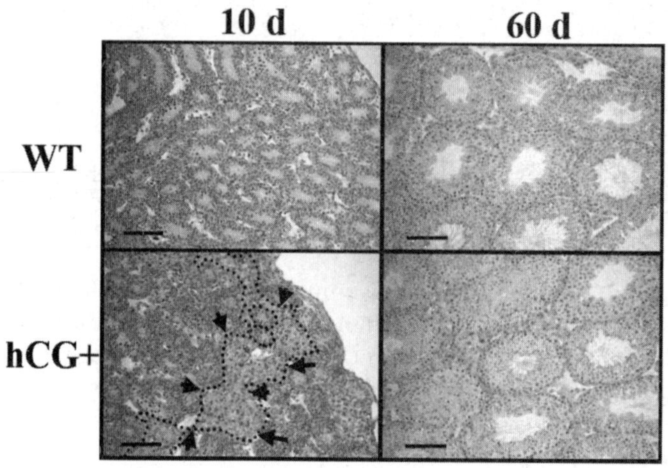

Fig. 7.4 Testicular histology of 10- (d) and 60 day-old wild-type (WT) and hCG+ transgenic mice.
Note the large Leydig cell adenomatous area (arrows and dotted lines) in the young transgenic mouse testis, and the absence of such areas in the adult testis. Scale bars = 100 mm.

CONCLUSIONS

Our findings on the LH/hCG overexpressing TG mice show clearly that chronically elevated levels of this hormone bring about in mice a multitude of endocrine anomalies that are accompanied with benign or malignant tumours in the gonads and in several extragonadal tissues. The ovaries show profound luteinisation of the somatic cell compartment, as the consequence of strong LH/hCG stimulation. Young female mice show precocious puberty and peripubertal elevation of oestrongen production, but later on their oestrogen levels return to the control range. This is apparently due to the strong ovarian luteinisation and highly elevated progesterone production. Extragonadal tumorigenic responses are observed in the mice in the pituitary, adrenal and mammary glands, and the ovarian endocrine activity is needed for these responses, because no extragonadal phenotypes are observed in gonadectomised mice, despite their persistently elevated levels of hCG. The pituitary tumours are lactotroph adenomas, and the highly elevated progesterone production synergises with normal oestrogen levels in the induction of these neoplasms. The adrenal response is cortical hyperplasia with elevated corticosterone production and obesity, and it occurs apparently due to direct stimulation of the adrenal tissue by LH/hCG. The mammary gland tumours are of the papillary adenocarcinoma type with frequent metastasis to other organs.

The only clear tumorigenic response observed in TG male mice were the neonatal Leydig cell adenomas originating from the fetal growth phase of these cells. Conspicuously, the adult males were remarkably resistant to the elevated LH/hCG stimulation in spite of the concomitant strong stimulation of testicular testosterone production.

The relevance of the findings to tumorigenesis in humans remains to be studied in conditions with elevated gonadotrophic stimulation, such as pregnancy, the postmenopausal state, polycystic ovary syndrome, gonadotrophin treatments of infertility and hypergonadotrophic hypogonadism. Although the mouse data are in favour of the ovarian hyperstimulation being the indirect cause of the extragonadal tumours, the possibility of direct extragonadal actions of LH/hCG should also be considered.

REFERENCES

1. Ahtiainen P, Rulli S, Pakarainen T, Zhang FP, Poutanen M, Huhtaniemi I (2006) *Phenotypic characterisation of mice with exaggerated and missing LH/hCG action.* Mol Cell Endocrinol **260-262**: 255-263.
2. Ahtiainen P, Rulli S, Pelliniemi LJ, Toppari J, Poutanen M, Huhtaniemi I (2005) *Fetal but not adult Leydig cells are susceptible to adenoma formation in response to persistently high hCG level; a study on hCG overexpressing transgenic mice.* Oncogene **24**: 7301-7309.
3. Ascoli M, Fanelli F, Segaloff DL (2002) *The lutropin/choriogonadotropin receptor, a 2002 perspective.* Endocr Rev **23**: 141-174.
4. Bernichtein S, Petretto E, Jamieson S, Goel A, Aitman T, Mangion JM, Huhtaniemi IT (2008) *Adrenal tumorigenesis after gonadectomy in mice is a complex genetic trait driven by epistatic loci.* Endocrinology: in press.
5. Burger LL, Haisenleder DJ, Dalkin AC, Marshall JC (2004) *Regulation of gonadotropin subunit gene transcription.* J Mol Endocrinol. **33**: 559-584.
6. Clevenger CV, Furth PA, Hankinson SE, Schuler LA (2003) *The role of prolactin in mammary carcinoma.* Endocr Rev **24**: 1-27.
7. Comerci JT Jr, Licciardi F, Bergh PA, Gregori C, Breen JL (1994) *Mature cystic teratoma: a clinicopathologic evaluation of 5'7 cases and review of the literature.* Obstet Gynecol. **84**: 22-28.
8. Filicori M, Fazleabas AT, Huhtaniemi I, Licht P, Rao ChV, Tesarik J, Zygmunt M.(2005) *Novel concepts of human chorionic gonadotropin: reproductive system interactions and potential in the management of infertility.* Fertil Steril **84**:275-284.
9. Freeman ME, Kanyicska B, Lerant A, Nagy G (2000) *Prolactin: structure, function, and regulation of secretion. Physiol Rev* **80:** 1523–1631.

10. Heaney AP, Horwitz GA, Wang Z, Singson R, Melmed S (1999) *Early involvement of estrogen-induced pituitary tumor transforming gene and fibroblast growth factor expression in prolactinoma pathogenesis.* Nat Med **5**: 1317-1321.
11. Huhtaniemi I (1994) *Fetal testis—a very special endocrine organ.* Eur J Endocrinol **130**:25-31.
12. Huhtaniemi I, Ahtiainen P, Pakarainen T, Rulli SB, Zhang FP, Poutanen M (2006) *Genetically modified mouse models in studies of luteinising hormone action.* Mol Cell Endocrinol. **252**: 126-135.
13. Huhtaniemi I, Rulli S, Ahtiainen P, Poutanen M 2005 *Multiple sites of tumorigenesis in transgenic mice overproducing hCG.* Mol Cell Endocrinol. **234**: 117-126.
14. Huhtaniemi IT, Themmen AP (2005) *Mutations in human gonadotropin and gonadotropin-receptor genes.* Endocrine **26**: 207-217.
15. Jameson JL, Hollenberg AN (1993) *Regulation of chorionic gonadotropin gene expression.* Endocr Rev **14**: 203-221.
16. Kananen K, Markkula M, Mikola M, Rainio E-M, McNeilly A, Huhtaniemi I (1996) *Gonadectomy permits adrenocortical tumorigenesis in mice transgenic for the mouse inhibin a-subunit promoter/ simian virus 40 T-antigen fusion gene: evidence for negative autoregulation of the inhibin a-subunit gene.* Mol Endocrinol **10**:1667-1677.
17. Kananen K, Markkula M, Rainio E, Su J-G, Hsueh AJW, Huhtaniemi IT (1995) *Gonadal tumorigenesis in transgenic mice bearing the mouse inhibin a-subunit promoter/Simian Virus T-antigen fusion gene: characterization of ovarian tumors and establishment of gonadotropin-responsive granulosa cell lines.* Mol Endocrinol **9**: 616-627.
18. Keri RA, Lozada KL, Abdul-Karim FW, Nadeau JN, Nilson JH (2000) *Luteinizing hormone induction of ovarian tumors: oligogenic differences between mouse strains dictates tumor disposition.* Proc Natl Acad Sci USA **97**: 383–387.
19. Kero J, Poutanen M, Zhang FP, Rahman N, McNicol AM, Nilson JH, Keri RA, Huhtaniemi IT (2000) *Elevated luteinizing hormone induces expression of its receptor and promotes steroidogenesis in the adrenal cortex.* J Clin Invest **105:** 633–641.
20. Konishi I (2006) *Gonadotropins and ovarian carcinogenesis: a new era of basic research and its clinical implications.* Int J Gynecol Cancer **16**: 16-22.
21. Kumar TR, Wang Y, Matzuk MM (1996) *Gonadotropins are essential modifier factors for gonadal tumor development in inhibin-deficient mice.* Endocrinology **137**: 4210-4216.
22. Kuorelahti A, Rulli S, Huhtaniemi I, Poutanen M (2007). *hCG upregulates wnt5b and wnt7b in the mammary gland and hCG{beta} transgenic female mice present with mammary gland tumors exhibiting characteristics of the Wnt/{beta}-catenin pathway activation.* Endocrinology **148**: 3694-3703.
23. Lange CA (2004) *Making sense of cross-talk between steroid hormone receptors and intracellular signaling pathways: who will have the last word?* Mol Endocrinol **18**: 269-278.
24. Liu G, Duranteau L, Carel JC, Monroe J, Doyle DA, Shenker A (1999) *Leydig-cell tumors caused by an activating mutation of the gene encoding the luteinizing hormone receptor.* N Engl J Med **341**: 1721-1736.
25. Matzuk MM, DeMayo FJ, Hadsell LA, Kumar TR (2003) *Overexpression of human chorionic gonadotropin causes multiple reproductive defects in transgenic mice.* Biol. Reprod **69:** 338–346.
26. Mikola M, Kero J, Nilson JH, Keri RA, Poutanen M, Huhtaniemi I (2003) *High levels of luteinizing hormone analog stimulate gonadal and adrenal tumorigenesis in mice transgenic for the mouse inhibin-alpha-subunit promoter/Simian virus 40 T-antigen fusion gene.* Oncogene **22**: 3269-3278.

27. Mohammad HP, Abbud RA, Parlow AF, Lewin JS, Nilson JH. (2003) *Targeted overexpression of luteinizing hormone causes ovary-dependent functional adenomas restricted to cells of the Pit-1 lineage.* Endocrinology **144**: 4626-4636.

28. Mutter GL (1997) *Role of imprinting in abnormal human development.* Mutat Res. **396**: 141-147.

29. Pakarainen T, Ahtiainen P, Zhang F-P, Rulli S, Poutanen M, Huhtaniemi I (2007) *Extragonadal LH/hCG action – not yet time to rewrite textbooks.* Mol Cell Endocrinol 2**269**: 9-16.

30. Rao CV (2001) *An overview of the past, present, and future of nongonadal LH/hCG actions in reproductive biology and medicine.*Semin Reprod Med **19**: 7-17.

31. Riman T, Nilsson S, Persson IR (2004) *Review of epidemiological evidence for reproductive and hormonal factors in relation to the risk of epithelial ovarian malignancies.* Acta Obstet Gynecol Scand **83:** 783-795.

32. Risbridger GP, Robertson DM, de Kretser DM (1982) *The effects of chronic human chorionic gonadotropin treatment on Leydig cell function.* Endocrinology **110**: 138-145.

33. Risch HA (1998) *Hormonal etiology of epithelial ovarian cancer, with a hypothesis concerning the role of androgens and progesterone.* J Natl Cancer Inst. **90**: 1774-1786.

34. Risma KA, Clay CM, Nett TM, Wagner T, Yun J, Nilson JH (1995) *Targeted overexpression of luteinizing hormone in transgenic mice leads to infertility, polycystic ovaries, and ovarian tumors.* Proc Natl Acad Sci USA **92**: 1322–1326.

35. Rulli SB, Ahtiainen P, Makela S, Toppari J, Poutanen M, Huhtaniemi I (2003) *Elevated steroidogenesis, defective reproductive organs, and infertility in transgenic male mice overexpressing human chorionic gonadotropin.* Endocrinology **144:** 4980–4990.

36. Rulli SB, Kuorelahti AI, Karaer O, Pelliniemi L, Poutanen M, Huhtaniemi IT (2002) *Reproductive disturbances, pituitary lactotrope adenomas, and mammary gland tumors in transgenic female mice producing high levels of human chorionic gonadotropin.* Endocrinology **143:** 4084–4095.

37. Russo IH, Russo J (1998) *Role of hormones in mammary cancer initiation and progression.* J Mammary Gland Biol Neoplasia **3**:49-61.

38. Russo J, Russo IH (2006) *The role of estrogen in the initiation of breast cancer.* J Steroid Biochem Mol Biol **102**: 89-96.

39. Schorpp M, Jager R, Schellander K, Schenkel J, Wagner EF, Weiher H, Angel P (1996) *The human ubiquitin C promoter directs high ubiquitous expression of transgenes in mice.* Nucleic Acids Res **24**: 1787-1788.

40. Simoni M, Gromoll J, Nieschlag E (1997). *The follicle-stimulating hormone receptor: biochemistry, molecular biology, physiology, and pathophysiology.* Endocr Rev **18**: 739-773.

41. Themmen APN, Huhtaniemi IT (2000) *Mutations of gonadotropins and gonadotropin receptors: elucidating the physiology and pathophysiology of pituitary-gonadal function.* Endocr Rev **21**: 551–583.

42. Ulbright TM (2004) *Gonadal teratomas: a review and speculation.* Adv Anat Pathol. **11**:10-23.

8

CHAPTER

Targeted Therapy of β-hCG Expressing Cancers

G. P. Talwar[1], Hemant Kumar Vyas[1], Rafi Shiraz Kabeer[1], Rita Singh[2], Rahul Pal[3], Ram A. Vishwakarma[3], Shilpi Purswani[1], Pooja Arora[3], Prem Chopra[4], Lalit Kumar[5] and Ritu Gupta[5]

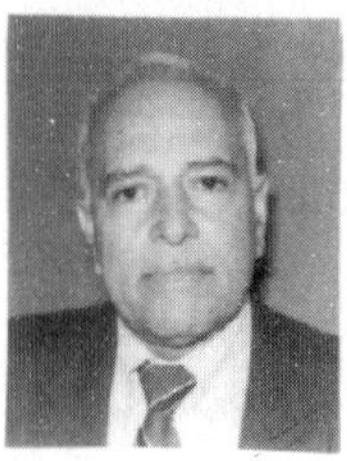

[1] Talwar Reasearch Foundation, E-8, Neb Valley, Neb Sarai, New Delhi 110 068
[2] Department of Zoology, University of Delhi, New Delhi 110007
[3] National Institute of Immunology, New Delhi 110067
[4] Department of Histopathology and Cytology, Sir Gangaram Hospital, New Delhi 110060
[5] B.R.Ambedkar Intitute and Rotary Cancer Research Hospital, All India Insitute of Mdical Sciencs, New Delhi 1100 29

ECTOPIC EXPRESSION OF β-hCG IN CANCERS

Human chorionic gonadotropin (hCG) is serving universally as a reliable and early index of pregnancy. Employing sensitive methods it is titerable in blood and in urine of women around or before the expected day of menstruation. Non-pregnant females and normal males do not secrete hCG in blood or urine in measurable amounts.

As hCG is made by trophoblasts during pregnancy, it is expected that trophoblastic cancers i.e. choriocarcinomas make and secrete hCG in amounts proportional to their mass. Since the past two decades however, reports have appeared on ectopic expression of hCG or its subunits by a variety of non-trophoblastic cancers: lung cancer [1], bladder carcinoma [2,3], colon adenocarcinoma [4], gastric carcinoma [5,6], pancreatic carcinoma [7,8], breast cancer [9], cervical carcinoma [10,11], oral cancers [12,13], head and neck cancers [14], vulva/vaginal cancers [15,16], prostate cancer [17] and renal carcinoma [18,19]. Moreover it is observed that the prognosis and the survival of the patients carrying a given cancer expressing β–hCG is poorer than the patients carrying the same cancer not expressing β–ηCG [2,4,10,19]. It can be postulated that at advanced stage, the dediffer-

email: gptalwar@gmail.com

entiation of cancer cells proceeds to an extent that they assume embryonic character and they start making embryonic proteins such as hCG.

Kabeer carried out immunohistological studies on 61 advanced stage tumors of various types in collaboration with Dr. Prem Chopra at Sir Ganga Ram Hospital. They found that 45 out of 61 such tumors belonging to intestine, breast, gall bladder, stomach, oesophagus, kidney, cervix, urinary bladder, parotid gland, testis and ovarian cancers were positive for immuno-reactivity with the highly specific antibody cPiPP. It was further observed that while *β*-hCG was expressed in 50% of the early stage tumors, 79% of advanced stage tumors were *β*-hCG positive.

BINDING OF CHIMERIC RECOMBINANT ANTIBODY WITH CELL LINES FROM RELAPSE CASES

We extended these studies on two cell lines obtained from ATCC. These were MOLT-4 T-lymphoblastic leukemia and U937 histiocytic lymphoma, both developed from relapse cases. Both MOLT-4 and U937 cells demonstrated binding with cPiPP, a chimeric antibody engineered from a *β*-specific monoclonal. The live tumor cells bound the antibody on the membrane (Figure 8.1). Permeablized cells showed internal presence of *β*–hCG binding with this antibody, implying thereby that the cells synthesize hCG and its subunits, and these are then displayed on their membranes [20]. It was also observed that the peripheral blood mononuclear cells from healthy donors did not bind cPiPP (Figure 8.2).

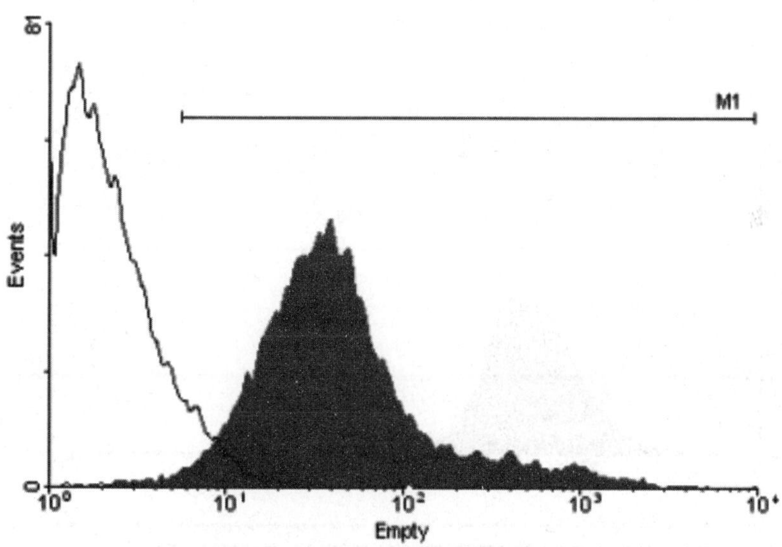

System: Log Parameter Means: Geometric

Param	M	Low,High	Events	%Total	%Gated	GMean	CV
FL1	0	0,1023	10000	100.00	100.00	45.42	31.14
	1	193,1023	9824	98.24	98.24	47.64	29.56

Fig. 8.1 Surface binding of anti-*β*-hCG (cPiPP) antibody to MOLT-4 cells. 98% of the cells show binding with the antibody

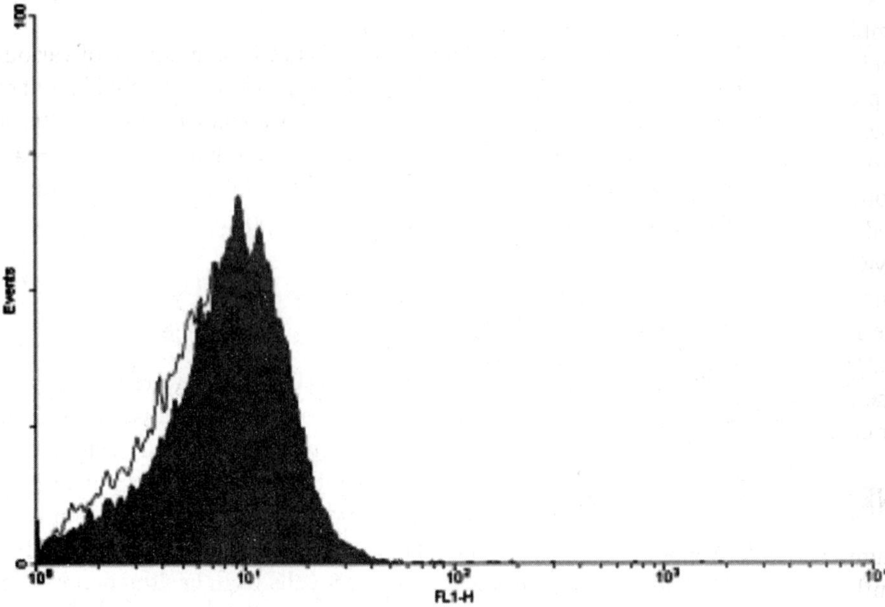

Fig. 8.2 Lack of binding of cPiPP with Peripheral Blood Mononuclear Cells (PBMC) isolated from healthy donor. [From Kabeer et al., 2005]

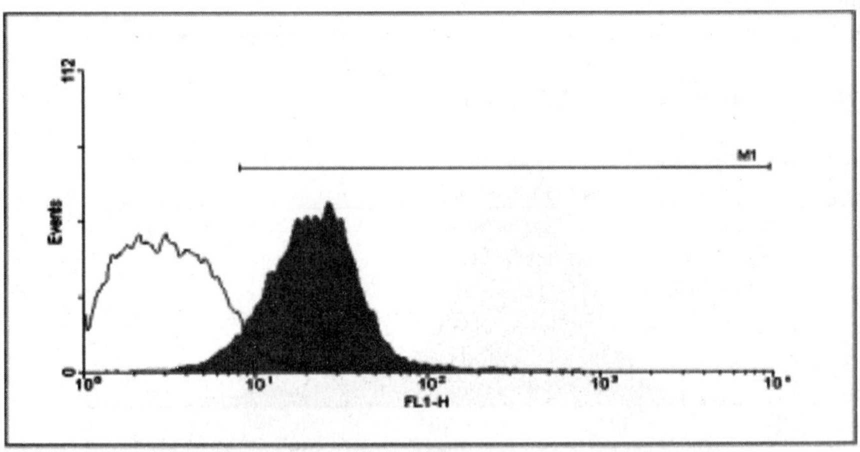

System: Log Parameter Means: Geometric

Param	M	Low,High	Events	%Total	%Gated	GMean	CV
FL1-	0	0,1023	10000	100.00	100.00	22.46	24.17
	1	234,1023	9359	93.59	93.59	24.75	20.80

Fig. 8.3 Surface binding of anti-β-hCG (cPiPP) antibody to U 937 cells. 93 % of the cells show binding with the antibody.

With these observations, the next obvious question was, whether the antibody binding to these cells exercised any cytotoxic action on tumor cells. Antibodies are toxic to cells either in presence of complement which kills the cells by complement mediated cytolysis or kill by antibody-dependent-cell-cytotoxicity (ADCC). No significant lysis of these cells was observed in presence of complement, presumably due to the decay accelerating factor CD55, which is believed to inhibit the complement action. The ADCC requires an *in vivo* system for evaluation and the current investigations are *in vitro*. We explored also the possibility that hCG or its subunits may have an autocrine growth promoting role as was the case for Chago lung cell carcinoma which secreted a-hCG and anti-α-antibodies prevented the proliferation of these cells *in vitro* and *in vivo* [21]. This was not the case with MOLT-4 cells as the cells did not increase nor was there any inhibition of cell multiplication in presence of anti-hCG antibody.

The fact that the antibody bound with more than 90% of MOLT-4 and U937 cells (Figure 8.1 and 8.3) as determined by Flow cytometery and had no binding with PBMC (Figure 8.2) suggested that the antibody can be used as a selective vehicle for delivery of anti-cancerous compounds to the tumor cells.

LINKAGE OF CURCUMIN TO cPiPP

Curcumin (diferuloyl methane) the active principle of curcuma longa has been reported to have anti-inflammatory [22] and anti-cancerous properties [23]. Curcumin is highly safe and intake upto 8g orally per day in a Phase I clinical trial was well tolerated and showed no side-effects in humans [24]. We therefore chose curcumin for linkage to our recombinant chimeric antibody. This was achieved by creating an amino linker on terminal hydroxyl group of curcumin which was condensed with carboxylic acid of acidic amino acids of the antibody. We were able to obtain a conjugate of the curcumin with the antibody which did not compromise to any significant extent the antigen binding capacity of the antibody.

EFFECT OF cPiPP-CURCUMIN ON MOLT-4 AND U-937 CELLS IN VITRO

The tumor cells were seeded in cell culture microtitre plates. Fresh medium with cPiPP-curcumin conjugate at different concentrations i.e. 10 μg, 50 μg and 100 μg was added to these cultures and the cells incubated for 48 hrs at 37^0 C. Parallel controls without the immuno-conjugate were taken. Cytotoxicity on tumor cells was assessed by 4 methods i.e. 3-(4,5-dimethylthiazol-2-yl)-2,5-diphenyl tetrazolium bromide (MTT) assay, Propidium iodide (PI) staining Fluorescent assisted cell sorting, Trypan Blue exclusion and microscopy.

The results were coincident by all methods. Nearly 100% of both types of tumor cells were killed in culture at and above 50mg of cPiPP-curcumin. The cPiPP-curcumin had no deleterious effect on PBMCs of healthy donors.

EXTENSION OF STUDIES TO LEUKEMIA PATIENTS

We examined peripheral blood cells of 22 patients, 14 of them were diagnosed as Acute Myeloid Leukemia (AML) patients. Out of these, peripheral blood lymphocytes of 7 patients showed binding with cPiPP as observed by flow cytometery. The percentage of cells expressing β-hCG in bleeds of patients expressing β-hCG varied from 20-64.8 %. Reactivity with antibodies against tumor markers CD-33 and CD-13 were also determined with cells of a few β-hCG positive patients. In some patients the percentage of cells expressing β-hCG were of the same order as those carrying CD-33 marker. In others there was discrepancy. Reactivity with a panel of tumor marker antibodies would have to be investigated, to draw firm conclusions as to whether the cells expressing β-hCG are tumor cells belonging to one or the other sub-population.

In the Acute Lymphoblastic Leukemia category three out of four patients were positive for β-hCG. The percentage of cells expressing β-hCG ranged from 27 to 80%.

The study is continuing and we trust that with bleeds of more patients, a clear idea will be available on the presence of β-hCG expressing tumor cells in various types of leukemias.

ACKNOLEDGEMENTS

This work is supported by a research grant given by Department of Biotechnology, Govt. of India. HKV acknowledges senior research fellowship from CSIR, Govt. of India.

REFRENCES

1. Yokotani T, Koizumi T, Taniguchi R, et al. Expression of alpha and beta genes of human chorionic gonadotropin in lung cancer. Int J Cancer 1997; 71: 539-44.
2. Iles RK, Persad R, Trivedi M, et al. Urinary concentration of human chorionic gonadotrophin and its fragments as a prognostic marker in bladder cancer. Br J Urol 1996; 77: 61-9.
3. Nishimura R, Koizumi T, Norisue k, et al. Expression and secretion of the beta subunit of human chorionic gonadotropin by bladder carcinoma in vivo and in vitro. Cancer Res 1995; 55: 1479-4.
4. Lundin M, Nordling S, Carpelan-Holmstrom M, et al. A comparison of serum and tissue hCG beta as prognostic markers in colorectal cancer. Anticancer Res 2000; 20: 4949-51.
5. Rau B, Below C, Liebrich W, von Schilling C and Schlag PM. Significance of serum b-hCG as a tumor marker for stomach carcinoma. Langenbecks Arch Chir 1995; 380: 359-64.
6. Louhimo J, Nordling S, Alfthan H, von Boguslawski K, Stenman UH and Haglund C. Specific staining of human chorionic gonadotropin beta in benign and malignant gastrointestinal tissues with monoclonal antibodies. Histopathology 2001; 38: 418-4.
7. Syrigos KN, Fyssas I, Konstandoulakis MM, et al. Beta human chorionic gonadotropin concentrations in serum of patients with pancreatic adenocarcinoma. Gut 1998; 42: 88-1.
8. Alfthan H, Haglund C, Roberts P and Stenman UH. Elevation of free beta subunit of human chorionic gonadotropin and core beta fragment of human chorionic gonadotropin in the serum and urine of patients with malignant pancreatic and biliary diseases. Cancer res 1992; 52: 4628-3.
9. Bièche I, Lazar V, Noguès C, et al. Prognostic value of chorionic gonadotropin beta gene transcripts in human breast carcinoma. Clin Cancer Res 1998; 4: 671-6.
10. Crawford RA, Iles RK, Carter PG, Caldwell CJ, Shepherd JH and Chard T. The prognostic significance of beta human chorionic gonadotrophin and its metabolites in women with cervical carcinoma. J Clin Pathol 1998; 51: 685-8.
11. Grossmann M, Hoermann R, Gocze PM, Ott M, Berger P and Mann K. Measurement of human chorionic gonadotropin-related immunoreactivity in serum, ascites and tumour cysts of patients with gynaecologic malignancies. Eur J Clin Invest 1995; 25: 867-3.

12. Hedström J, Grenman R, Ramsay H, et al. Concentration of free hCGbeta subunit in serum as a prognostic marker for squamous-cell carcinoma of the oral cavity and oropharynx. Int J Cancer 1999; 84: 525-8.

13. Bhalang K, Kafrawy AH and Miles DA. Immunohistochemical study of the expression of human chorionic gonadotropin-beta in oral squamous cell carcinoma. Cancer 1999; 85: 757-62.

14. Scholl, PD, Jurco S and Austin JR. Ectopic production of beta-HCG by a maxillary squamous cell carcinoma. Head Neck 1997; 19:701-5.

15. de Bruijn HW, ten Hoor KA, Krans M and van der Zee AG. Rising serum values of beta-subunit human chorionic gonadotrophin (hCG) in patients with progressive vulvar carcinomas. Br J Cancer 1997; 75: 1217-8.

16. Carter PG. Iles RK, Neven P, Ind TE, Shepherd JH and Chard T. Measurement of urinary beta core fragment of human chorionic gonadotrophin in women with vulvovaginal malignancy and its prognostic significance. Br J Cancer 1995; 71: 350-3.

17. Sheaff MT, Martin JE, Badenoch, DF and Baithun SI. Beta hCG as a prognostic marker in adenocarcinoma of the prostate. J Clin Pathol 1996; 49: 693-4.

18. Jiang Y, Zeng F, Xiao C and Liu J. Expression of beta-human chorionic gonadotropin genes in renal cell cancer and benign renal disease tissues. J Huazhong Univ Sci Technolog Med Sci 2003; 23: 291-3.

19. Hotakainen K, Ljungberg B, Paju A, Rasmuson T, Alfthan H and Stenman U H. The free beta-subunit of human chorionic gonadotropin as a prognostic factor in renal cell carcinoma. Br J Cancer 2002; 86:185-9.

20. Kabeer RS, Pal R, and Talwar GP. Human acute lymphoblastic leukemia cells make human pregnancy hormone hCG and expose it on the membrane: A case for using recombinant antibody against hCG for selective delivery of drugs and/or radiations Curr Sci 2005; 89: 1571-6.

21. Kumar S, Talwar GP, Biswas DK. Necrosis and inhibition of growth of human lung tumor by anti α-human chorionic gonadotropin antibody. J Natl Cancer Inst. 1992; 84; 42-7.

22. Abe Y, Hashimoto S, Horie T. Curcumin inhibition of inflammatory Cytokine production by human peripheral blood monocytes and alveolar macrophages. Pharmacol Res 1999; 39: 41-7.

23. Mukhopadhyay A, Bueso-Ramos C, Chatterjee D, Pantazis P and Aggarwal BB. Curcumin down regulates cell survival mechanisms in human prostate cancer lines. Oncogene 2001; 20: 7597-09.

24. Cheng AL, Hsu CH, Lin JK, et al. Phase I clinical trial of curcumin, a chemopreventive agent, in patients with high-risk or pre-malignant lesions. Anticancer Res 2001; 21: 2895-900.

9

CHAPTER

The Next Generation of Recombinant Immunotoxins: Targeting CD30 Receptor

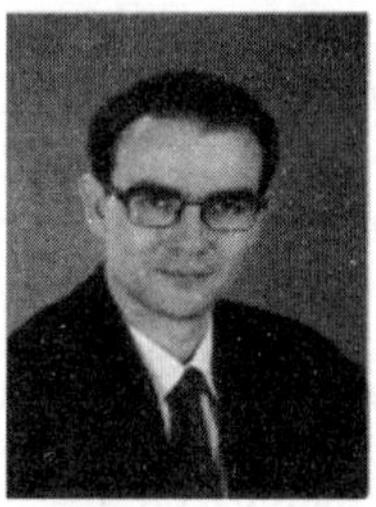

Theo Thepen[2], Michael Huhn[3] and Stefan Barth[1]

[1]Helmholtz-Institute for Applied Medical Engineering, Department of Experimental Medicine and Immunotherapy, University Hospital RWTH Aachen, Pauwelsstr. 20, 52074 Aachen, Germany

[2]Fraunhofer IME, Department of Pharmaceutical Product Development, Forckenbeckstr. 6, 52074 Aachen, Germany

[3]Institute for Molecular Biotechnology, RWTH Aachen University, Worringer Weg 1, 52074 Aachen, Germany

In the fight against cancer the major aim is to kill off the malignant cells. To this several avenues have been explored, in principle all based on a higher sensitivity of the malignant cells for the treatment as opposed to other cells of the body. The balance between wanted and unwanted effects has been the major problem medical science has faced regarding cancer treatment. In addition, although the body has been ineffective in preventing and fighting the cancer itself, it is still able to potentially mount a response against the therapy. In therapeutic development it is therefore essential to increase efficacy and specificity of the therapeutics, while remaining obscured for e.g. the immune system.

Chemotherapy and radiation rely on the high sensitivity of the cancer cells, but have no intrinsic targeting properties. The development of antibody techniques has been one of the major advantages allowing for specific, targeted therapy. Therefore, if an antibody, used as targeting moiety, is combined with a toxin, a so-called immunotoxin is created. The very first generation immunotoxins were composed of a complete, often mouse, antibody and a chemically-linked plant or bacterial toxin. These were not very successful, mainly due to their non-specific toxicity, which was already observed in animal models. Several improvements, like exclusively using the toxic domain of the toxin, antibody fragments like Fab, and humanization of the antibodies, diminished many side effects and resulted in the first clinical trials albeit with limited success. A major advancement was the application of DNA techniques and genetic engineering. Firstly, his made it possible to very specifically remove all redundant parts of the molecule reducing it to its bare essentials for a fully functional immunotoxin, thereby further reducing the size and side effects. Secondly, this opened new channels for optimizing immunotoxins to specific requirements by addition of supplementary sequences to the molecule. Thirdly, these recombinant proteins can be produced in a number of expression systems, ranging from small scale in culture flasks, to large scale in bacteria, yeast, mammalian cells, and even in plants allowing for cheap, very large scale production, reducing costs. Finally, to allow repeated administration, new immunotoxins with greatly reduced immunogenicity need to be developed. This will also be realized by a series of novel constructs encoding different human enzymes to induce targeted apoptosis. Thus, an overall future objective will be the development of tailor-made immunotoxins, not only in terms of the targeting component, but also carrying appropriate cytotoxic agents to specifically destroy tumor cells.

Development of The First Pseudomonas Exotoxin A-based Recombinant Anti-CD30 Immunotoxin

Although patients with Hodgkin lymphoma or anaplastic large-cell lymphoma can be cured by polychemotherapy and extended field radiotherapy, less than 30% of those whose lymphoma relapses remain disease-free after second-line treatment. The major reason for this poor outcome is the persistence of residual tumor cells surviving standard therapy.1-3 Thus, the selective elimination of minimal residual disease using monoclonal antibody-based immunoconjugates after standard treatment might improve the outcome in malignant lymphoma.

One of the most promising target antigens for immunotherapy of malignant lymphoma is the CD30 receptor. This antigen was originally discovered on cultured Hodgkin/Reed–Sternberg (H-RS) cells using the monoclonal antibody (mAb) Ki-1 (Engert et al., 1997). The gene encoding for the CD30 receptor molecule (Schnell et al 2000) is located on chromosome 1p36. The naturally occurring CD30 ligand also has been identified and cloned (Pasqualucci et al., 1995). The CD30/CD30 ligand system triggers cytolytic cell death in malignant lymphoma cell lines and induces proliferation and cytokine production in T cells or neutrophils (Klimka et al., 2000). The CD30 antigen is overexpressed on hematologic malignancies such as Hodgkin lymphoma, anaplastic large-cell lymphoma, peripheral T-cell lymphoma (Stein et al. 1985), virally transformed cell lines (Stein et al., 1985, Froese et al., 1987), and latently HIV-infected CD4 T cells (McDonald et al.,1995). The CD30 Receptor is a member of the TNF receptor family and activates nuclear factor kB(NFkB) via TNF receptor-associated factors (TRAF) 2 and 5, leading to pleitropic effects *in vitro* ranging from cell proliferation to cell death. It is also expressed on lymphocytes infected with HIV, HTLV-1 or EBV, and crosslinking of HIV-infected T cells is involved in the activation of HIV production. Its selective expression in lymphomas gave rise to hopes of repeating the success of antibody therapy seen with B-cell non-Hodgkin's lymphomas (Dübel, 2007).

In the late 90s, a number of chemically linked immunotoxins was evaluated for clinical application (Schnell et al., 2000; Engert et al., 1997). One of the constructs, Ki-4.dgA (Schnell et al., 1995) was based on the anti-CD30 mAb Ki-4, which has been demonstrated to inhibit the shedding of the extracellular part of the CD30 molecule (Horn-Lohrens et al., 1995). Our group subsequently used phage display technology to isolate a specific, high affinity Ki-4 scFv from its corresponding hybridoma (Klimka et al., 1999). For the construction of the first recombinant anti-CD30 immunotoxin, this scFv was genetically fused to a modified *Pseudomonas aeruginosa* exotoxin A gene (ETA') (Matthey et al., 1999). Recombinant immunotoxins expressed so far under standard conditions remained primarily associated with inclusion bodies (FitzGerald et al., 1998) and were purified after careful denaturation and renaturation procedures (Buchner et al., 1992). Under optimized conditions, only 5% to 10% of the input protein was properly folded and active. Thus, we developed a new protocol for the periplasmic expression of recombinant proteins under osmotic stress conditions in the presence of compatible solutes resulting in more than 95% functional activity in terms of specific *in vitro* binding and cytotoxic activity (Barth et al., 2000a). This method was successfully applied to different immunotoxins with an average yield of approximately 1 mg protein/4 g cell paste from bacterial shaking cultures (Barth et al., 2000b). This expression system has been further standardized, delivering functional protein within 3 weeks from cloning to expression. Using the periplasmic expression strategy followed by a 2-step purification of Ki-4(scFv)–ETA', we can now easily produce significant amounts of functional rIT in a short time. In accordance with published data for other rITs (Engert et al., 1997; Bera et al., 1998; Reiter et al., 1994), purified Ki-4(scFv)–ETA' demonstrated to be stable in terms of binding and cytotoxic activity in mouse serum at 37°C for at least 24 hours. Recombinant immunotoxins have a much shorter half-life in mouse serum compared to IgG-based chemical conjugates. (Bera et al., 1998) Blood distribution times range from 20 to 30 minutes after challenge with 10 ìg rIT or more (Wels et al., 1992; Reiter et al., 1994; Kreitman et al., 1999). The calculated distribution time t1D 2a of 19 minutes determined for Ki-4(scFv)–ETA' matches these results. The stability in mouse serum indicates functional activity of the protein during serum elimination time t1D 2b of 193 minutes resulting in excellent antitumor activity against disseminated growing human tumors in SCID mice. The effects of Ki-4(scFv)–ETA' against disseminated growing L540 lymphomas was evaluated by gross macroscopy, immunohistopathology, and measurement of soluble CD30 receptor in serum. A high degree of correlation in detecting L540 tumors was documented by these methods. Tumors identified by gross macroscopy were confirmed by immunohistology of tumor sections stained for human CD30. In addition, soluble CD30 directly correlated with tumor burden. These results compared favorably with those obtained using chemically linked immunotoxins.

After the initial report by our group (Barth et al., 2000b), CD30 has attracted increasing attention for immunotherapy. This is at least in part attributable to the fact that CD30 is an attractive tumor-associated antigen expressed in high copy number on malignant cells compared to its low expression on normal immune cells (Kasamon et al., 2007).

Besides being a excellent tumor-associated antigen for targeted therapy, CD30 is also shedded from its surface and is representing a perfect marker directly correlating to severity of disease (Zanotti et al., 2002). Having had access to a set of different antibodies targeting the extracellular part of CD30, we chose Ki-3 as an antibody which enhances the constitutive cleavage of CD30 leading to a downregulation of CD30 and increase of soluble CD30 in the cellular environment. By the use of a specific metalloproteinase inhibitor (BB-3644), shedding of CD30 was not only blocked but also significantly increased the cytotoxic activity of recombinant Ki-3(scFv)-ETA' by a factor of 2.75 (Hansen et al., 2002). The application of Ki-3(scFv)-ETA' alone in the same disseminated L540 tumor model as described above showed no tumor-free survival in any of the treated animals. Nevertheless, additional application of BB-3644 increased the mean survival time from 35 days

(Ki-3(scFv)-ETA' alone) to 93 days (p = 0.0017) (Matthey et al., 2004). These results clearly demonstrate that besides having identified a good tumor-associated antigen, successful therapy is clearly dependent from the molecular behavior of the target receptor in response to the antibody chosen for therapy. Additionally, concomitant application of metalloproteinase inhibitors might become clinically relevant in antibody-based therapeutic approaches targeting these kind of receptors.

Development of The First Recombinant Human Anti-CD30 Immunotoxin

These encouraging data with the recombinant antibody fragment-based ETA' construct spurred us to design a novel genetically engineered construct this time not using a murine antibody fragment. For development of this new immunotoxin we used the extracellular part of the natural human CD30 ligand in combination with ETA'. Again, the recombinant fusion protein showed CD30-specific binding and toxicity (Barth et al., 1999).

Having shown all the adaptations from a crude, complete antibody based immunotoxin towards a new CD30-specific immunotoxin, the next logical step was to exchange the bacterial toxin for a new, preferably human enzyme with cytotoxic activity upon internalization into diseased target cells. One such candidate family are the human RNases which include e.g. angiogenin (hANG). This small protein, with a molecular weight of 14.1 kDa, belongs to the pancreatic ribonuclease A (RNase A) superfamily that normally induces neovascularization (Fett et al., 1985). There is a 33% sequence identity with bovine pancreatic RNase. The essential sequences for the enzymatic activity, including the catalytic site residues, are also conserved in hANG (Strydom et al., 1985; Kurachi et al., 1985; Acharya et al., 1994). Functionally important regions of the protein include the catalytic residues, a nuclear localization sequence, a putative receptor-binding region and a region important for immunomodulation (Shapiro et al., 1989b; Moroianu et al., 1994a; Moroianu et al., 1994b; Hu et al., 1997; Tschesche et al., 1994; Matousek et al., 1995). ANG orthologues exhibit a high degree of conservation at the amino acid level (Adams et al., 1999; Subramanian et al., 2008) and in the case of hANG and mouse ANGs, the very weak ribonucleolytic activity (Shapiro et al., 1986) was found to be necessary for their angiogenic function (Shapiro et al., 1989; Crabtree et al., 2007). hANG was originally isolated from HT29 conditioned medium (Fett et al., 1985) indicating that it is secreted by this tumor derived cell line. It is believed that tumor cells secrete hANG which then stimulates endothelial cells leading to neovascularization. hANG promotes the organization of endothelial cells in culture into tube-like structures, induces secondary messengers and supports endothelial cell migration during neovascularization (Bicknell et al., 1989; Hu et al., 1994; Jimi et al., 1995; Subramanian et al., 2008).

We constructed a completely human fusion gene, which was subsequently inserted into a pET-based expression plasmid (Huhn et al., 2001). Transformed *Escherichia coli* BL21(DE3) were grown under osmotic stress conditions in the presence of compatible solutes. After isopropyl ß-D-thiogalactoside induction, the 37 kDa His10-tagged Ang-CD30L was directed into the periplasmic space and functionally purified by a combination of metal ion affinity followed by enterokinase cleavage of the His10-Tag and molecular size chromatography. The characteristics of the recombinant protein were assessed by ELISA, flow cytometry, and toxicity assays showing specific activity against CD30-positive Hodgkin-derived cells. CD30 receptor-specific binding of Ang-CD30L was verified by competition with anti-CD30 monoclonal antibody Ki-4 and commercially available CD30L-CD8 chimeric protein. Ang-CD30L showed RNase activity *in vitro*. The completely human recombinant immunotoxin showed significant toxicity toward several CD30-positive cell lines (HDLM-2, L1236, KM-H2, and L540) and exhibited highest cytotoxicity against L540 cells (IC_{50} = 8 ng/ml) as determined by cell proliferation assays. CD30-specificity was again confirmed by competitive toxicity assays.

The Next Generation of Recombinant Immunotoxins

The set of experiments described in this overview, demonstrate that there is a gradual, yet steady development in the development of immunotoxins. The early immunotoxins, at that time sometimes coined as the 'magic bullets' turned out to have many drawbacks like non-specific toxicity and poor tolerability due to the induction of defense mechanisms like immune responses against these proteins. Step by step these problems have been addressed, reaching the present stage at which we can produce genetically engineered constructs that are relatively easy to modify and produce in large amounts at low cost. The next developments will most likely focus on the discovery of suitable targets, their corresponding ligands, as well as human enzymes to be used for the next generation of recombinant immunotoxins (Barth, 2007).

REFERENCES

1. Acharya., K.R., Shapiro, R., Allen, S.C., Riordan, J.F., and Vallee, B.L. - Crystal structure of human angiogenin reveals the structural basis for its functional divergence from ribonuclease. Proc. Natl. Acad. Sci. USA, 91, 2915–2919. (1994).
2. Adams, S.A., and Subramanian, V. - The angiogenins: an emerging family of ribonuclease related proteins with diverse cellular functions. Angiogenesis, 3, 189–199. (1999).
3. Barth S. – The next generation of recombinant immunotoxins. Pharma Focus Asia 5: 29-31 (2007).
4. Barth S., Huhn M., Matthey B., Klimka A., Galinski E.A., Engert A. - Compatible solute-supported periplasmic expression of functional recombinant proteins under stress conditions. Appl. Environm. Microbiol. 66(4): 1572-1579 (2000a).
5. Barth S., Huhn M., Matthey B., Tawadros S., Schnell R., Diehl V., Engert A. - Ki-4(scFv)-ETA', a new recombinant anti-CD30 immunotoxin with highly specific cytotoxic activity against disseminated Hodgkin tumors in SCID mice. Blood 95 (12): 3909-3914 (2000b).
6. Barth S., Huhn M., Matthey B., Schnell R., Tawadros S., Schinköthe T., Lorenzen J., Diehl V., Engert A. - Recombinant anti-CD25 immunotoxin RFT5(scFv)-ETA' demonstrates successful elimination of disseminated human Hodgkin´s lymphoma in SCID mice. Int. J. Cancer 86: 718-724 (2000c).
7. Barth S., Matthey B., Huhn M., Diehl V., Engert A. - CD30L-ETA': A new recombinant immunotoxin based on the CD30 ligand for possible use against human lymphoma. Cytok. Cell. Molec. Ther. 5: 69-78 (1999).
8. Barth S., Schnell R., Diehl V., Engert A. - Development of immunotoxins for potential clinical use in Hodgkin's disease. Ann Oncol.;7(suppl 4): 135. (1996).
9. Bicknell, R., and Vallee, B.L. - Angiogenin activates endothelial cell phospholipase C. Proc. Natl. Acad. Sci. USA, 85, 5961–5965. (1988).
10. Bera T.K., Pastan I. - Comparison of recombinant immunotoxins against LeY antigen expressing tumor cells: influence of affinity, size, and stability.Bioconjug Chem.;9:736. (1998).

11. Bicknell, R., and Vallee, B.L. - Angiogenin stimulates endothelial cell prostacyclin secretion by activation of phospholipase A2. Proc. Natl. Acad. Sci. USA, 86, 1573–1577. (1989).
12. Bruell D., Bruns C.J., Yezhelyev M., Huhn M., Müller J., Ischenko I., von der Decken V., Fischer R., Finnern R., Jauch K.W., Barth S. – Recombinant anti-EGFR immunotoxin 425(scFv)-ETA' demonstrates strong anti-tumor effect against disseminated human pancreatic cancer in nude mice. Int. J. Molec. Med. 15(2): 305-313 (2005).
13. Buchner J., Pastan I., Brinkmann U. A method for increasing the yield of properly folded recombinant fusion proteins: single-chain immunotoxins from renaturation of bacterial inclusion bodies. Anal Biochem.;205:263. (1992).
14. Crabtree, B., Holloway, D.E., Baker, M.D., Acharya, K.R., and Subramanian, V. - Biological and structural features of mouse angiogenin-4, an angiogenic protein. Biochemistry, 46, 2431–2443. (2007).
15. Dübel S. - In therapeutic proteins; Antibodies in Phase I/II/III: Cancer Therapie 593-672 Thieme (2007).
16. Engert A., Diehl V., Schnell R., Radzuhn A., Hatwig M.T., Drillich S., Schön G., Bohlen H., Tesch H., Hansmann M.L., Barth S., Schindler J., Ghetie V., Uhr J., Vitetta E.S. - A phase-I study of an anti-CD25 ricin A chain immunotoxin (RFT5-SMPT-dgA) in patients with refractory Hodgkin´s lymphoma. Blood 89: 403-410 (1997).
17. Falini B., Bolognesi A., Flenghi L., Tazzari P.L., Broe M.K., Stein H., et al.. - Response of refractory Hodgkin's disease to monoclonal anti-CD30 immunotoxin. Lancet;339:1195–6. (1992).
18. Fett, J.W., Strydom, D.J., Lobb, R.R., Alderman, E.M., Bethune, J.L., Riordan, J.F. Vallee, B.L. - Isolation and characterization of angiogenin, an angiogenic protein from human carcinoma cells. Biochemistry, 24, 5480–5486. (1985).
19. FitzGerald D., Pastan I., Robertus J. - Clinical applications of immunotoxins. Intro Curr Top Microbiol Immunol.;234:1. (1998).
20. Froese P., Lemke H., Gerdes J., Havsteen B., Schwarting R., Hansen H., Stein H. - Biochemical characterization and biosynthesis of the Ki-1 antigen in Hodgkin-derived and virus-transformed human B and T lymphoid cell lines. J Immunol.; 139:2081.(1987).
21. Hansen H.P., Matthey B., Barth S., Kisseleva T., Mokros T., Davies S.J., Beckett R.P., Foelster-Holst R., Lange H.H., Engert A., Lemke H. - Inhibition of metalloproteinases enhances the internalization of anti-CD30 antibody Ki-3 and the cytotoxic activity of Ki-3 immunotoxin. Int. J. Cancer 98(2): 210-215 (2002).
22. Horn-Lohrens O, Tiemann M, Lange H, Kobarg J, Hafner M, Hansen H, Sterry W. - Shedding of the soluble form of CD30 from the Hodgkin-analogous cell line L540 is strongly inhibited by a new CD30-specific antibody (Ki-4). . J Cancer. Feb 8;60(4):539-44. (1995).
23. Huhn M., Sasse S., Tur M.K., Matthey B., Schinköthe T., Rybak S., Barth S., Engert A. - Human angiogenin fused to human CD30 ligand (Ang-CD30L) exhibits specific cytotoxicity against CD30-positive lymphoma. Cancer Res. 61(24): 8737-8742 (2001).
24. Parwaresch R.M., Lemke H. - Shedding of the soluble form of CD30 from the Hodgkin-analogous cell line L540 is strongly inhibited by a new CD30-specific antibody (Ki-4). Int J Cancer. 1995;60:539. (1995).
25. Hu, G., Riordan, J.F., and Vallee, B.L. - Angiogenin promotes invasiveness of cultured endothelial cells by stimulation of cell-associated proteolytic activities. Proc. Natl. Acad. Sci. USA, 91, 12096–12100. (1994).

26. Hu, G.F., Riordan, J.F., and Vallee, B.L. - A putative angiogenin receptor in angiogenin-responsive human endothelial cells. Proc. Natl. Acad. Sci. USA, 94, 2204–2209. (1997).

27. Jimi, S., Ito, K., Kohno, K., Kuwano, M., Itagaki, Y. Ishikawa, H. - Modulation by bovine angiogenin of tubular morphogenesis and expression of plasminogen activator in bovine endothelial cells. Biochem. Biophys. Res. Commun., 211, 476–483. (1995).

28. Kasamon Y.L., Ambinder RF - Immunotherapies for Hodgkin's lymphoma. Crit Rev Oncol Hematol. 2007.

29. Klimka A., Barth S., Matthey B., Roovers R.C., Lemke H., Hansen H., Arends J.W., Diehl V., Hoogenboom H.R., Engert A. - An anti-CD30 single-chain Fv selected by phage display and fused to Pseudomonas exotoxin A (Ki-4(scFv)-ETA') is a potent immunotoxin against a Hodgkin-derived cell line. Brit. J. Cancer 80(8): 1214-1222 (1999).

30. Klimka A., Matthey B., Roovers R., Barth S., Bot F., Arends J.W., Engert A., Hoogenboom H.R. - Human anti-CD30 recombinant antibodies by guided phage antibody selection using cell panning. Brit. J. Cancer 83: 252-260 (2000).

31. Kreitman R., Wang Q., FitzGerald D., Pastan I. - Complete regression of human B-cell lymphoma xenografts in mice treated with recombinant anti- CD22 immunotoxin RFB4(dsFv)-PE38 at doses tolerated by cynomolgus monkeys. Int J Cancer.;81:148 (1999).

32. Kurachi, K., Davie, E.W., Strydom, D.J. and Vallee, B.L. - Sequence of the cDNA and gene for Angiogenin, a human angiogenesis factor. Biochemistry, 24, 5494–5499. (1985).

33. Matousek J., Soucek J., Ríha J., Zankel T.R., Benner S.A. - Immunosuppresive activity of angiogenin in comparison with bovine seminal ribonuclease and pancreatic ribonuclease. Comp. Biochem. Physiol. B Biochem. Mol. Biol., 112, 235–241. (1995).

34. Matthey B., Borchmann P., Schnell R., Tawadros S., Lange H., Huhn M., Klimka A., Tur M.K., Barth S., Engert A., Hansen H.P. – Metalloproteinase inhibition augments anti-tumor efficacy of the anti-CD30 immunotoxin Ki-3(scFv)-ETA' against human lymphomas in vivo. Int. J. Cancer 111(4): 568-574 (2004).

35. Matthey B., Klimka A., Diehl V., Engert A., Barth S. - A new series of pET-derived vectors for high efficiency expression of Pseudomonas exotoxin-based fusion proteins. Gene 229: 145-153 (1999).

36. McDonald P.P., Cassatella M.A., Bald A., Maggi E., Romagnani S., Gruss H.J., Pizzolo G. - Activation of HIV expression by CD30 triggering in CD41 T cells from HIV-infected individuals. Immunity. ;3:251; (1995).

37. Moroianu, J., and Riordan, J.F. - Nuclear translocation of angiogenin in proliferating endothelial cells is essential to its angiogenic activity. Proc. Natl. Acad. Sci. USA, 91, 1677–1681. (1994a).

38. Moroianu, J., and Riordan, J.F. - Identification of the nucleolar targeting signal of human angiogenin. Biochem. Biophys. Res. Commun., 203, 1765–1772. (1994b).

39. Falini B., Kadin M.E. - Antitumor activity of anti-CD30 immunotoxin (Ber-H2/ saporin) in vitro and in severe combined immunodeficiency disease mice xenografted with human CD301 anaplastic large-cell lymphoma. Blood. 85::2139. (1995).

40. Reiter Y., Pai L., Brinkmann U., Wang Q., Pastan I. - Antitumor activity and pharmacokinetics in mice of a recombinant immunotoxin containing a disulfide- stabilized Fv fragment. Cancer Res.; 54:2714. (1994).

41. Schnell R., Vitetta E., Schindler J., Borchmann P., Barth S., Ghetie V., Hell K., Drillich S., Diehl V., Engert A. - Treatment of refractory Hodgkin's lymphoma patients with an anti-CD25 ricin A-chain immunotoxin. Leukemia. 14(1):129-35.(2000).

42. Schnell R, Linnartz C, Katouzi AA, Schön G, Bohlen H, Horn-Lohrens O, Parwaresch RM, Lange H, Diehl V, Lemke H, et al.– Development of new ricin A-chain immunotoxins with potent anti-tumor effects against human Hodgkin cells in vitro and disseminated Hodgkin tumors in SCID mice using high-affinity monoclonal antibodiesdirected against the CD30 antigen. Int J Cancer. 1995;63:238.

43. Shapiro, R., Riordan, J.F., and Vallee, B.L. - Characteristic ribonucleolytic activity of human angiogenin. Biochemistry, 25, 3527–3532. (1986).

44. Shapiro, R., and Vallee, B.L. - Site-directed mutagenesis of histidine-13 and histidine-114 of human angiogenin. Alanine derivatives inhibit angiogenin-induced angiogenesis. Biochemistry, 28, 7401–7408. (1989).

45. Shapiro, R., Fox, E.A., and Riordan, J.F. - Role of lysines in human angiogenin: chemical modification and site-directed mutagenesis. Biochemistry, 28, 1726–1732. (1989).

46. Shapiro, R., Weremowicz, S., Riordan, J.F. and Vallee, B.L - Ribonucleolytic activity of angiogenin: essential histidine, lysine, and arginine residues. Proc. Natl. Acad. Sci. USA, 84, 8783–8787. (1987).

47. Soncin, F. - Angiogenin supports endothelial and fibroblast cell adhesion. Proc. Natl. Acad. Sci. USA, 89, 2232–2236. (1992).

48. Stein H, Mason DY, Gerdes J, O'Connor N, Wainscoat J, Pallesen G, Gatter K, Falini B, Delsol G, Lemke H, et al. - The expression of the Hodgkin's disease associated antigen Ki-1 in reactive and neoplastic lymphoid tissue: evidence that Reed–Sternberg cells and histiocytic malignancies are derived from activated lymphoid cells. Blood.;66:848. (1985).

49. Stöcker M., Tur M.K., Sasse S., Krüßmann A., Barth S., Engert A. – Secretion of functional anti-CD30 angiogenin immunotoxins into the supernatant of transfected 293T cells. Prot. Expr. Purif 28 (2): 211-219 (2003).

50. Strydom, D.J., Fett, J.W., Lobb, R.R., Alderman, E.M., Bethune, J.L., Riordan, J.F. Vallee, B.L. - Amino acid sequence of human tumor derived angiogenin. Biochemistry, 24, 5486–5494. (1985).

51. Subramanian V., Crabtree B., Acharya K.R. - Human angiogenin is a neuroprotective factor and amyotrophic lateral sclerosis associated angiogenin variants affect neurite extension/pathfinding and survival of motor neurons. Hum Mol Genet.;17(1):130-49 (2008).

52. Tschesche, H., Kopp, C., Horl, W.H. Hempelmann, U. - Inhibition of degranulation of polymorphonuclear leukocytes by angiogenin and its tryptic fragment. J. Biol. Chem., 269, 30274–30280. (1994).

53. Tur M.K., Huhn M., Thepen T., Stöcker M., Krohn R., Vogel S., Jost E., Osieka R., van de Winkel J.G., Fischer R., Finnern R., Barth S. - Recombinant CD64-specific single chain Immunotoxin exhibits specific cytotoxicity against acute myeloid leukemia cells. Cancer Res. 63 (23): 8414-8419 (2003); 64: 3725 (2004).

54. Tur M.K., Sasse S., Stöcker M., Djabelkhir K., Huhn M., Matthey B., Gottstein C., Engert A., Barth S. – An anti-GD2 single chain Fv selected by phage display and fused to Pseudomonas exotoxin A develops specific cytotoxic activity against neuroblastoma derived cell lines. Int. J. Molec. Medicine 8(5): 579-584 (2001).

55. Wels W., Harwerth I., Mueller M., Groner B., Hynes N. - Selective inhibition of tumor cell growth by a recombinant single-chain antibody-toxin specific for the erbB-2 receptor. Cancer Res., 52: 6310 (1992).

56. Zanotti U., Trolese A., Ambrosetti A., Nadali G., Visco C., Ricetti M.M., Benedetti F., Pizzolo G. – Serum levels of soluble CD30 improve International Prognostic Score in predicting the outcome of advanced Hodgkin's lymphoma. Ann. Oncol. 13: 1908-1914 (2002).

10

CHAPTER

CD40 and Cancer Therapy

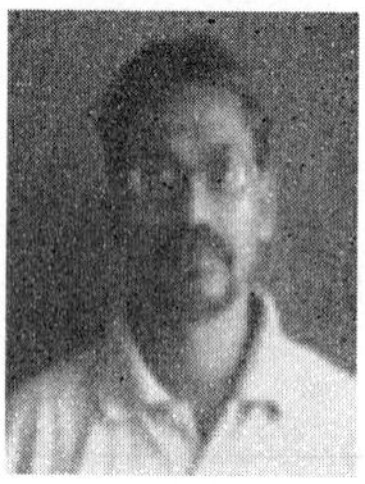

Bhaskar Saha

National Centre for Cell Science, Ganeshkhind, Pune 411007

ABSTRACT

A benign tumor results from the loss of contact inhibition whereas its transformation to a cancerous form results from the gain in metastatic potential whereby it disseminates to distant organs. Such a scenario implies a minimum of two key alterations in cellular physiology: first, the loss of contact inhibition implies alteration in cellular signaling originating from the molecules involved in intercellular adhesion that connects to cell cycle control; second, the loss in adhesion of the cells to the basement membrane and other supportive matrices so that they can acquire the metastatic potential. While the latter function may be viewed as an adaptation to the changing nutritional need of the growing tumor mass, this may also indicate to the immune cells a way to reach the altered self - that a cancer tissue is- and destroy it. It is intriguing to observe that CD40, originally known as a B cell survival molecule but later shown to be expressed on macrophages, dendritic cells and endothelial cells, performs paradoxical roles in cancer cell dissemination and cancer cell destruction by promoting angiogenesis and tumor-specific T cell functions, respectively. Knowing the finer regulation of these two processes will help formulate a better CD40-based anti-cancer immunotherapy.

CD40 - a Glycoprotein Receptor That Plays a Dual Role in Angiogenesis and Immune Response

CD40 was originally found to be expressed on B cells. It was observed that the B cells, which would otherwise undergo apoptosis following Ig cross-linking by anti-Ig antibodies, survived by the CD40-

email: sahab@nccs.res.in

induced costimulation. Later on, CD40 was reported to play roles in germinal centre formation, antibody class switching and affinity maturation. At the same time, it was also observed that the activated T cell membrane could essentially provide the same help to the B cells as delivered by an agonistic anti-CD40 antibody suggesting that the ligand for CD40 might be present on T cells. Later studies characterized the molecule as CD40-ligand (CD40-L) and designated it as CD154. CD40-L is expressed not only on T cells but also on platelets. While platelets outnumber T cells in circulation, T cells outnumber platelets in lymphoid tissues. Therefore, it is possible that platelet expressed CD40-L serves as a major ligand for endothelial cell-expressed CD40 whereas T cell expressed CD40-L interacts primarily with CD40 expressed on antigen-presenting cells. However, there is no indication how such a restriction can be enforced in practice.

In macrophages, dendritic cells and endothelial cells, CD40 signaling leads to production of both pro-inflammatory and anti-inflammatory mediators. Some of these mediators, such as vascular endothelial growth factor (VEGF) help in angiogenesis, the process of forming new capillaries. Although these capillaries can function as conduits for tumor-cell metastasis, these same vessels can also be a gateway for entry of activated tumor-specific effector cells that eliminate tumors. How such countercurrent processes can be turned in favor of anti-tumor immunity is discussed below.

Antigen-presenting Cell-expressed CD40 Plays a Dual Role in Anti-tumor Immunity

Anti-tumor immunity is crucially dependent on CD40–CD40-ligand interactions (1). CD40, a trans-membrane glycoprotein on endothelial cells (ECs) and antigen-presenting cells (APCs) such as B cells, macrophages and dendritic cells (DCs) (2, 3), binds to CD40-ligand (CD40-L), expressed primarily on T cells and platelets (4). The APC-T cell interactions via CD40–CD40-L results in IL-12-dependent tumor-specific cytotoxic T cells (CTLs) and T helper 1 (Th1) cells that mediate tumor regression (5-7). On the other hand, CD40–CD40-L interactions also result in angiogenesis (8, 9), the process of generating new blood vessels from pre-existing ones, and thereby promote tumor growth. Angiogenesis is mediated primarily by VEGF and transforming growth factor-b (TGF-b), which can all be induced by CD40 ligation. The intra-tumoral neovascularization presents a functional paradox, as these vessels facilitate both tumor cells metastasis and infiltration of tumor-eliminating immunocompetent cells, such as DCs, macrophages, natural killer (NK) cells and T cells. Thus, as a principle of anti-tumor therapy, CD40-CD40-L interactions need to be tipped toward inducing anti-tumor immunity, while minimizing tumor metastasis.

CD40-L expressed on T cells binds to APC-expressed CD40 and triggers CD40 signals in macrophages and DCs, inducing cytokines that have crucial roles in T-cell activation and differentiation to functional subsets, which can modulate anti-tumor immune responses counteractively. For example, CD40 signaling through p38 mitogen-activated protein (MAP) kinase induces expression of IL-12 (10), which promotes CTL responses and differentiation of Th1 cells (5-7, 11). Immature and mature DCs also respond to IL-12 by up-regulation of MHC class I and II and costimulatory molecules (12). IL-12 reverses immune suppression by inducing apoptosis of regulatory T cells (Treg cells) and aids the infiltration of $CD8^+$ effector T cells (13). IL-12-induced apoptosis of Treg cells is crucially important, as they interfere with the boosting of tumor-primed $CD4^+$T cells with IFN-g-dependent anti-angiogenic activity and peptide-elicited long-lasting tumor immunity (14).

Paradoxically, CD40 can also promote tumor growth. For example, CD40 signals through extracellular signal regulated kinase (ERK-1/2), inducing expression of IL-10 in macrophages and

DCs (10). IL-10 exerts its autocrine or paracrine suppressive effects on the DC during differentiation from its progenitors, maturation and subsequent function (15) and affects the cells involved in both the innate and adaptive arms of anti-tumor immunity. We demonstrated that in mice expressing less CD40-L, vaccination with tumor antigens induced an IL-10-dominated pro-tumor T-cell response, whereas in higher CD40-L-producing mice, the antigen priming resulted in anti-tumor effector T cells (16). Similarly, vaccination with prostrate tumor antigen-pulsed DC expressing higher levels of CD40 resulted in efficient anti-tumor immune responses, whereas the lower CD40-expressing DCs resulted in an IL-10-dominated pro-tumor immune response (17). The tumor-derived IL-10 also down-regulates CD40 expression and CD40-triggered DC functions (18). The pro-tumor effect of IL-10 is mediated by inhibition of CD40 signaling (10) through p38 MAP kinase, which might otherwise lead to the production of inflammatory mediators, inhibition of Th1 cells (19), IFN-γ receptor signaling (20) and reduced IL-12 receptor β2 subunit production (21). However, direct effects of IL-10 on tumor growth or even elimination cannot be ruled out. Indeed, an IL-10 promoter polymorphism study associated high IL-10 production with an anti-tumor effect, whereas low IL-10 production with increased risk of tumor growth (22). These observations indicate that CD40 signaling in macrophages and DCs triggers counter-regulatory effects on tumor-specific immune responses. Thus, the combination of CD40-triggered events in APCs results in either anti-tumor immunity or suppressive pro-tumor effector functions. Because CD40 is also expressed on ECs, we have assessed how CD40 differentially regulates their functions in tumorigenesis and tumor regression.

Endothelial Cell-expressed CD40 Contributes to Angiogenesis and Tumor Metastasis

As the tumor cells proliferate and grow to a solid mass of tissue, the cells in the core of the tissue develop a spatial restriction for diffusion of nutrients from the peripheral vasculature. Therefore, the physiological adaptation requires vascular growth into the tumor mass. Indeed, it is shown that CD40 induces signaling through phosphatidylinositol-3 kinase (PI-3K) and Akt in ECs, resulting in less apoptosis and increased proliferation (23), eventuating in vitro the formation of vessel-like tubular structures. Besides its direct effects on the proliferation of ECs, CD40 also induces VEGF, which binds to VEGF receptors to induce EC proliferation and angiogenesis (24-27). VEGF neutralization by an anti-VEGF antibody reduces neovascularization and prevents tumor metastasis (28), indicating that the capillaries formed under the influence of VEGF are conduits for tumor-cell metastasis. Thus, although VEGF-mediated angiogenesis is a crucial physiological process, as VEGF-deficiency is embryonically lethal, the same process contributes to the patho-physiology of tumor growth and metastasis.

The pro-tumor functions of CD40 by way of promoting angiogenesis and metastasis are executed by induction of interstitial collagenase (MMP-1), gelatinase A (MMP-2), stromylase (MMP-3), and gelatinase B (matrix metalloprotease, MMP-9) that help ECs penetrate the extracellular matrix (29). In addition, CD40 signaling upregulates expressions of various integrins in ECs (30). Just as natural Treg cells express a specific class of integrin and chemokine receptor, such as CD103 and CCR7, tumor cells also express a group of integrin ligands and chemokines. These factors, alone or in combination, might target these regulatory cells to the tumor where they can mitigate anti-tumor immunity. By contrast, because the tumor tissues have infiltrates of immune cells that include T cells, NK cells, monocytes, macrophages and DCs (among others) (31), these same vessels can be the gateway for immune cells to access the core of tumor tissues. Thus, CD40 signaling in EC can direct the extent and cellular composition of the leukocyte infiltrate in the tumor and influence angiogenesis resulting in an altered microenvironment and modified tumor-specific immune responses (32–38).

CD40 Plays a Paradoxical Role By Antagonizing Angiogenesis

CD40 induces its anti-angiogenic effects by at least two different mechanisms. Firstly, it induces reactive oxygen species in ECs resulting in inhibition of angiogenesis (39). Secondly, CD40 induces IL-10 and IL-12 and in various experimental settings, both the cytokines are shown to inhibit angiogenesis, tumor growth and dissemination (40- 43). The anti-angiogenic activity of IL-10 could be due to downregulation of VEGF, tumour necrosis factor-alpha (TNF-α) and IL-6 (42) and the inhibition of tumor stroma whereas the anti-angiogenic activity of IL-12 could be due to EC apoptosis. However, as IL-12 induces overproduction of IFN-γ, which has toxic side effects (44), the therapeutic use of the cytokine is restricted.

Because CD40 exerts both anti-tumor and pro-tumor effects, it is postulated that such functions may depend on the stage of tumor growth. For example, in transgenic model of breast cancer, deficiency of CD40 before tumor development inhibited tumor growth, whereas deficiency of CD40 at later stages increased the tumorigenicity, demonstrating that the differential outcome of CD40 on tumor growth depends on the stage of tumor development (45). Mechanistically, as the type and quantity of chemokines released at the site of the tumor may vary at different stages of tumor growth, the functional phenotypes of the tumor-infiltrating cells can also be counteractive. One of these functional phenotypes can be the differential levels of CD40 expression on ECs (46) and DCs (17). Because the effector functions of these cells are dependent on intracellular signaling, it is possible that CD40 expression levels regulate downstream signaling pathways to modulate CD40-induced angiogenesis and other effector functions. Although supporting evidence does not exist at present, it is possible that the pro-tumor or anti-tumor outcome is a combination of all these CD40-induced regulators operating in tandem.

Angiopoietins and TGF-β are Dual Regulators Induced by CD40 in EC

Secreted by the EC, angiopoietins bind to the endothelium-specific tyrosine-kinase receptor (Tie-2) inducing phosphorylation and dimerization of the known domains (47) and as a consequence, regulate angiogenesis by both an autocrine and a paracrine manner. Of the four angiopoietins described till date, angiopoietin-1 and angiopoietin-2 are the best characterized. Although angiopoietin-1 stabilizes the existing blood vessels, angiopoietin-2 (expressed at the site of vascular remodeling) is thought to counteract the actions of angiopoietin-1. With VEGF, angiopoietin-2 promotes angiogenesis, whereas in the absence of VEGF, angiopoietin-2 leads to vessel regression (48). However, the relationship between CD40-induced regulation of angiopoietins and VEGF remains unclear (49, 50).

The CD40–VEGF/Angiopoietin loop that modulates angiogenesis includes another angiogenic factor, TGF-β. CD40-induced and cancer cell-secreted TGF-β also induces VEGF (51-53) and thereby, promotes VEGF-mediated angiogenesis. TGF-β increases the receptivity of ECs to VEGF by enhanced expression of VEGF receptor (54). In addition to its role in VEGF induction, TGF-β also supports the proliferation of stromal cells, including fibroblasts (55), which might help develop and stabilize the vascular tube. By contrast, TGF-β reduces the malignant behavior by activation of the phosphatase PP-2A, which results in increased mobility of ECs.

An Integrated View of the Duality of CD40 in Angiogenesis and Anti-tumor Immunity

Current literature indicates that CD40 has dual roles in immune responses against tumors. This could result from various combinations of the functional properties of the patho-physiological adjustments of the growing tumor and the altered stress on the immune system. On one hand, as tumor cells grow into a solid mass and devoid of oxygen at the core, the local hypoxic stress induces VEGF that initiates angiogenesis. The neovascularization draws in the CD40-L expressing platelets and T cells that interact with EC expressed CD40, promoting further angiogenesis. The intratumoral angiogenesis provides not only the nutrition for tumor growth and the escape route for the tumor cells, but also the channel through which the immune cells can attack the relatively inaccessible tumor cells at the core of the solid tumor mass, constituting a local effect. On the other hand, the cancer antigens are now released into circulation and trapped in different lymphoid organs for presentation to T cells by CD40 expressing APCs, constituting the central effect by tumoral stress on the immune system. Such a distinction between the local and central effects of CD40 during tumor growth implies that reinforcing CD40 activation centrally and neutralizing VEGF locally in the tumor may lead to a combined immunotherapeutic regimen. For example, VEGF and IL-10 inhibition might prevent tumor metastasis and immunosuppression, and therapeutic vaccination with high levels of CD40 expressing DC might help tumor regression more efficiently than that observed earlier.

REFERENCES

1. Toes, R.E. et al. (1998) CD40-CD40Ligand interactions and their role in cytotoxic T lymphocyte priming and anti-tumor immunity. Semin. Immunol. 10, 443–448.
2. Hollenbaugh, D. et al. (1994) The role of CD40 and its ligand in the regulation of the immune response. Immunol. Rev. 138, 23–37.
3. Quezada, S.A. et al. (2004) CD40/CD154 interactions at the interface of tolerance and immunity. Annu. Rev. Immunol. 22, 307–328.
4. Schonbeck, U. and Libby, P. (2001) The CD40/CD154 receptor/ligand dyad. Cell. Mol. Life Sci. 58, 4–43.
5. Alexandroff, A.B. et al. (2000) Role for CD40-CD40 ligand interactions in the immune response to solid tumors. Mol. Immunol. 37, 515–526.
6. Colombo, M.P. and Trinchieri, G. (2002) Interleukin-12 in anti-tumor immunity and immunotherapy. Cytokine Growth Factor Rev. 13, 155-168.
7. Mackey, M.F. et al. (1998) The role of CD40/CD154 interactions in the priming, differentiation, and effector function of helper and cytotoxic T cells. J. Leukoc. Biol. 63, 418–428.
8. Reinders, M.E. et al. (2003) Proangiogenic function of CD40 ligand-CD40 interactions. J. Immunol. 171, 1534–1541.

9. Bergmann, S. and Pandolfi, P.P. (2006) Giving blood: a new role for CD40 in tumorigenesis. J. Exp. Med. 203, 2409–2412.
10. Mathur, R.K. et al. (2004) Reciprocal CD40 signals through p38MAPK and ERK-1/2 induce counteracting immune responses. Nat. Med. 10, 540–544.
11. Knutson, K.L. and Disis, M.L. (2005) Tumor antigen-specific T helper cells in cancer immunity and immunotherapy. Cancer Immunol. Immunother. 54, 721–728.
12. Belardelli, F. and Ferrantini, M. (2002) Cytokines as a link between innate and adaptive antitumor immunity. Trends Immunol. 23, 201–208.
13. Kilinc, M.O. et al. (2006) Reversing tumor immune suppression with intra-tumoral IL-12: activation of tumor-associated T effector/memory cells, induction of T suppressor apoptosis, and infiltration of CD8+ T effectors. J. Immunol. 177, 6962–6973.
14. Casares, N. et al. (2003) CD4+/CD25+ regulatory cells inhibit activation of tumor-primed CD4+ T cells with IFN-gamma-dependent anti-angiogenic activity, as well as long-lasting tumor immunity elicited by peptide vaccination. J. Immunol. 171, 5931–5939.
15. Murugaiyan, G. et al. (2006) Reversal of tumor induced dendritic cell paralysis: a treatment regimen against cancer. Curr. Immunol. Rev. 2, 261–272.
16. Murugaiyan, G. et al. (2007) Differential CD40/CD40L expression results in counteracting antitumor immune responses. J. Immunol. 178, 2047–2055.
17. Murugaiyan, G. et al. (2007) Levels of CD40 expression on the immunizing DC dictate tumor growth or regression. Clin. Exp. Immunol. 149, 194–202.
18. Shurin, M.R. et al. (2002) Inhibition of CD40 expression and CD40-mediated dendritic cell function by tumor-derived IL-10. Int. J. Cancer 101, 61–68.
19. Bashyam, H. (2007) Th1/Th2 cross-regulation and the discovery of IL-10. J. Exp. Med. 204, 237.
20. Ding, Y. et al. (2003) Suppressor of cytokine signaling 1 inhibits IL-10-mediated immune responses. J. Immunol. 170, 1383–1391.
21. Romano, C.C. et al. (2005) The role of interleukin-10 in the differential expression of interleukin-12p70 and its beta2 receptor on patients with active or treated paracoccidioidomycosis and healthy infected subjects. Clin. Immunol. 114, 86–94.
22. Howell, W.M. et al. (2001) IL-10 promoter polymorphisms influence tumour development in cutaneous malignant melanoma. Genes Immun. 2, 25–31.
23. Deregibus, M.C. et al. (2003) CD40-dependent activation of phosphatidylinositol 3-kinase/Akt pathway mediates endothelial cell survival and in vitro angiogenesis. J. Biol. Chem. 278, 18008–18014.
24. Flaxenburg, J.A. et al. (2004) The CD40-induced signaling pathway in endothelial cells resulting in the overexpression of vascular endothelial growth factor involves Ras and PI3-kinase. J. Immunol. 172, 7503– 7509.
25. Melter, M. et al. (2000) Ligation of CD40 induces the expression of vascular endothelial growth factor by endothelial cells and monocytes and promotes angiogenesis in vivo. Blood 96, 3801–3808.
26. Byrne, A.M. et al. (2005) Angiogenic and cell survival functions of vascular endothelial growth factor (VEGF). J. Cell. Mol. Med. 9, 777–794.
27. Shibuya, M. and Claesson-Welsh, L. (2006) Signal transduction by VEGF receptors in regulation of angiogenesis and lymphangiogenesis. Exp. Cell Res. 312, 549–560.
28. Zhang, W. et al. (2002) A monoclonal antibody that blocks VEGF binding to VEGFR2 (KDR/Flk-1) inhibits vascular expression of Flk-1 and tumor growth in an orthotopic human breast cancer model. Angiogenesis 5, 35–44.

29. Ottaiano, A. et al. (2002) CD40 activation as potential tool in malignant neoplasms. Tumori 88, 361–366.
30. Kotowicz, K. et al. (2000) Biological function of CD40 on human endothelial cells: costimulation with CD40 ligand and interleukin-4 selectively induces expression of vascular cell adhesion molecule-1 and P-selectin resulting in preferential adhesion of lymphocytes. Immunology 100, 441–448.
31. Bronte, V. et al. (2006) Leukocyte infiltration in cancer creates an unfavorable environment for antitumor immune responses: a novel target for therapeutic intervention. Immunol. Invest. 35, 327–357.
32. Opdenakker, G. and van Damme, J. (2004) The countercurrent principle in invasion and metastasis of cancer cells. Recent insights on the role of chemokines. Int. J. Dev. Biol. 48, 519–527.
33. Burger, J.A. and Kipps, T.J. (2006) CXCR4: a key receptor in the crosstalk between tumor cells and their microenvironment. Blood 107, 1761–1767.
34. Vicari, A.P. et al. (2004) In vivo manipulation of dendritic cell migration and activation to elicit anti-tumor immunity. Novartis Found. Symp. 256, 241–254.
35. Ishida, T. and Ueda, R. (2006) CCR4 as a novel molecular target for immunotherapy in cancer. Cancer Sci. 97, 1139–1146.
36. Roodman, G.D. et al. (2004) MIP-1 alpha and myeloma bone disease. Cancer Treat. Res. 118, 83–100.
37. Girouard, J. et al. (2005) Requirement of the extracellular cysteine at position six for CD40/CD40 dimer formation and CD40-induced IL-8 expression. Mol. Immunol. 42, 773–780.
38. Altenburg, A. et al. (1999) CD40 Ligand-CD40 interaction induces chemokines in cervical carcinoma cells in synergism with IFNgamma. J. Immunol. 162, 4140–4147.
39. Urbich, C. et al. (2002) CD40-ligand inhibits endothelial cell migration by increasing production of endothelial reactive oxygen species. Circulation 106, 981–986.
40. Kohno, T. et al. (2003) Interleukin-10-mediated inhibition of angiogenesis and tumor growth in mice bearing VEGF-producing ovarian cancer. Cancer Res. 63, 5091–5094.
41. Kundu, N. and Fulton, A.M. (1997) Interleukin-10 inhibits tumor metastasis, down-regulates MHC class I, and enhances NK lysis. Cell. Immunol. 180, 55–61
42. Moore, K.W. et al. (2001) Interleukin-10 and the interleukin-10 receptor. Annu. Rev. Immunol. 19, 683–765.
43. Coughlin, C.M. et al. (1998) Interleukin-12 and interleukin-18 synergistically induce murine tumor regression which involves inhibition of angiogenesis. J. Clin. Invest. 101, 1441–1452.
44. Rakhit, A. et al. (1999) Down-regulation of the pharmacokinetic–pharmacodynamic response to interleukin-12 during long-term administration to patients with renal cell carcinoma and evaluation of the mechanism of this adaptive response in mice. Clin. Pharmacol.Ther. 65, 615–629.
45. Chiodoni, C. et al. (2006) Triggering CD40 on endothelial cells contributes to tumor growth. J. Exp. Med. 203, 2441–2450.
46. Vowinkel, T. et al. (2006) Differential expression and regulation of murine CD40 in regional vascular beds. Am. J. Physiol. Heart Circ. Physiol. 290, H631–H639.
47. Maisonpierre, P.C. et al. (1997) Angiopoietin-2, a natural antagonist for Tie2 that disrupts in vivo angiogenesis. Science 277, 55–60.
48. Peters, K.G. (1998) Vascular endothelial growth factor and the angiopoietins: working together to build a better blood vessel. Circ. Res. 83, 342–343.

49. Zhang, L. et al. (2003) Tumor-derived vascular endothelial growth factor up-regulates angiopoietin-2 in host endothelium and destabilizes host vasculature, supporting angiogenesis in ovarian cancer. Cancer Res. 63, 3403–3412.
50. Tai, Y-T. et al. (2002) CD40 activation induces p53-dependent vascular endothelial growth factor secretion in human multiple myeloma cells. Blood 99, 1419–1427.
51. Wikstrom, P. et al. (2001) Role of transforming growth factor-beta 1 in prostate cancer. Microsc. Res. Tech. 52, 411–419.
52. Breier, G. et al. (2002) Transforming growth factor-beta and Ras regulate the VEGF/VEGF-receptor system during tumor angiogenesis. Int. J. Cancer 97, 142–148.
53. Wang, L. et al. (2004) Transforming growth factor-1 stimulates vascular endothelial growth factor-1 via mitogen-activated protein kinase kinase-3, and p38 mitogen-activated protein kinase-dependent pathway in murine mesangial cells. J. Biol. Chem. 279, 33213–33219.
54. Shih, S-C. et al. (2003) Transforming growth factor b induction of vascular endothelial growth factor receptor 1: Mechanism of pericyte-induced vascular survival in vivo. Proc. Natl. Acad. Sci. U. S. A. 100, 15859–15864.
55. Huang, X. and Lee, C. (2003) Regulation of stromal proliferation, growth arrest, differentiation and apoptosis in benign prostatic hyperplasia by TGF-beta. Front. Biosci. 8, s740–s749.

11

CHAPTER

Optimization of Antigens for use in Anti-Cancer Vaccines

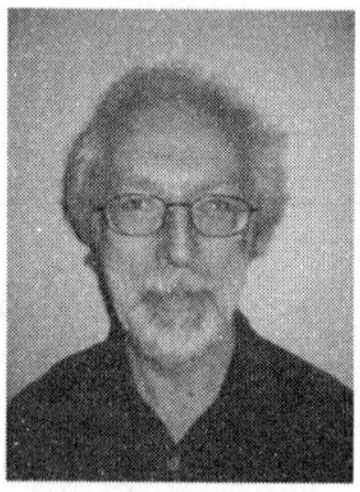

Peter J. Delves

Division of Infection and Immunity, University College London, UK.

INTRODUCTION

Vaccination against infectious agents is a very successful preventative measure aimed at combating human disease. A number of human cancers are now known to be linked to infection, including cervical carcinoma (human papilloma viruses 16 and 18), gastric cancer (*Helicobacter pylori*), liver cancer (hepatitis B and C viruses) and nasophayngeal cancer (Epstein-Barr virus). In these cases, potentially preventative vaccines are either currently available or under development. However, the majority of human cancers do not have a defined infectious agent known to be associated with them, and many are likely to have a non-infectious trigger. For these cancers the development of prophylactic vaccines may be limited by the fact that the vaccine target would likely be an autoantigen. Unless a unique variant of the autoantigen is specifically associated with the cancer, then prophylactic vaccination would stand a substantial risk of provoking autoimmune disease in the vaccinated individual. Whilst in an extreme life-threatening situation some measure of mild autoimmune disease may be deemed an acceptable 'trade-off' for eradicating a malignant tumor, this would certainly not be acceptable in a preventative vaccine program. The infrequency of tumor-specific, as opposed to tumor-associated, antigens implies that anti-cancer vaccines would often need to be designed for therapeutic rather than prophylactic use.

So far, vaccination against tumors has had limited success (Rosenberg *et al.*, 2004). In general, vaccines have traditionally been much better at provoking antibody responses than cytotoxic T lymphocyte (CTL) activity. Thus, extracellular bacteria or their products have been relatively easy to combat with vaccines. Viruses can be neutralised before they enter cells, but antibodies are of considerably less use once the virus hides inside the cell. In animal studies, DNA vaccines have often proved to be potent inducers of CTL responses, but the pre-clinical success of this approach to vaccination has yet to be broadly translated to human disease (Lowe *et al.*, 2007). Anti-cancer vaccines would often be optimal if they are capable of activating both arms of the adaptive immune response.

Desirable Anti-tumor Responses

Tumor-associated antigens may be soluble and present in the extracellular environment, present in a native form on the tumor cell surface, present as processed antigen together with antigen-presenting molecules (for example, peptides with MHC or glycolipids with CD1) on the tumor cell surface, or restricted to the intracellular milieu of the cell. The form, location, and biological function of the antigen will dictate the type of therapeutic immune response that needs to be stimulated. Thus, glycolipids presented by CD1 may require a T-cell with cytotoxic capability bearing a specific gamma-delta TCR, whereas intracellular protein antigens may only reveal themselves as peptides in complex with MHC class I on the cell surface and be recognised by a CTL bearing an alpha-beta TCR.

As in the case of an immune response to infection, the production of specific effector and memory cells to a tumor-associated antigen has multiple requirements. The absolute minimum goal of the vaccine will be to contain a tumour-associated antigen in a form that has the ability to enter the antigen-processing pathway of dendritic cells, to activate the dendritic cell to express sufficient levels of costimulatory molecules such as CD80/CD86 and necessary cytokines such as (for example) IL-12, the ability of the antigen to be processed in a way that generates peptide(s) capable of binding the host MHC class II molecules with an adequate affinity, and the ability of the peptide-MHC complex to be transported to the cell surface and then be capable of being recognised by a $CD4^+$ helper T-cell with a cognate TCR. Such a T-cell, if of the Th1 phenotype, could secrete interferon-gamma with subsequent activation of tumoricidal macrophages. However, in most cases additional arms of the immune response are likely to be essential to control the tumor – namely cytotoxic T-cells, and/or B-cells that can give rise to antibody-secreting plasma cells.

Taking the above as a starting point, an anti-cancer vaccine will therefore need to comprise:

1. A tumor-associated antigen which contains components which can be recognised by protective host B-cells and/or (after processing) host CTL.
2. A protein (part of, or additional to, the antigen) capable of being processed into peptides that can bind host MHC class II molecules to form a complex capable of being recognised by host helper T-cells of an appropriate phenotype (Th1, Th2 or Th17, etc).
3. Molecules capable of activating dendritic cells into modes which enable antigen processing, migration to germinal centers in secondary lymphoid tissues, upregulation of costimulatory molecules, and so forth.

In addition to these minimal requirements, ideally the vaccine should be able to:

4. Induce long-term, preferably life-long, immunological memory.
5. Generate memory cells with high affinity antigen-receptors.
6. Only stimulate a response to the tumor-associated antigen, with no cross-reaction with other antigens.
7. Mimic as closely as possible the native conformation and post-translational modifications of the tumor-associated antigen.
8. Stimulate a response against tumor-associated antigens whose expression is maintained on metastatic cells in the face of the immune response, e.g. do not become modulated off the surface of the tumor cells.

Other, generic, requirements of vaccines will also need to be met (safety, ability to manufacture sufficient amounts of the vaccine, stability, etc).

Some of the above concepts can be illustrated using the tumor-associated antigen human chorionic gonadotropin (hCG) as an example.

hCG

Human CG is required to maintain the corpus luteum, and thus the secretion of oestrogens and progesterone, during pregnancy. Indeed, the essentially requirement of hCG for a successful pregnancy has led to the development of family planning vaccines aimed at producing neutralising antibodies to this hormone (Talwar, 1999; Stevens, 1996). The hormone is a heterodimer, comprising an alpha chain that is also utilised by the other 3 members of the glycoprotein hormone family (follicle-stimulating hormone [FSH], luteinising hormone [LH] and thyroid-stimulating hormone [TSH]), and an hCG-unique beta chain. Both the alpha and beta chain bear two N-linked oligosaccharides, with the beta chain additionally possessing four O-linked carbohydrate structures. The hCG alpha chain is encoded by a single gene, whereas there are six genes with the potential to encode the hormone-unique beta chain. It has been known for a long time that the hormone is expressed by tumors of germ cell origin (Vaitukaitis, 1973). More recently it has become apparent that the aberrant expression of hCG, particularly of the beta-chain in the absence of the alpha chain, is associated with a number of non-germ cell cancers, including bladder cancer, colorectal cancer, ovarian cancer, lung cancer, pancreatic cancer, cervical cancer, prostate cancer and breast cancer (Stenman *et al.*, 2004). In non-germ cell cancers it is usually just a subset of patients that aberrantly express readily detectable amounts of hCG, and the hCGbeta 3/9, 5 and 8 genes are upregulated compared to the hCGbeta 6/7 genes (Hotakainen *et al.*, 2007).

Natural immune Responses to hCG

It is perhaps noteworthy that the paucity of reports of autoimmunity to hCG suggests that spontaneously occurring autoantibodies to this hormone are rather rare. Indeed, it has very recently been proposed that natural hCG is capable of inducing immunological tolerance in pregnancy by upregulating immunosuppressive indoleamine 2,3-dioxygenase in dendritic cells (Ueno *et al.*, 2007). Thus, a requirement of anti-hCG vaccines is that they are able to overcome immunological tolerance to the antigen.

Expression *in vivo*

During pregnancy, hCG is produced initially by the pre-implantation blastocyst and subsequently by the syncytiotrophoblast of the placenta. When aberrantly expressed in tumors it is generally assumed that the hormone is produced by the malignant cells themselves, although it remains a formal possibility that in some tumors expression may represent activation of some other, nontransformed, cell by products of the malignant cell. In such cases an anti-cancer vaccine based upon hCG would most likely be ineffective. However, there is strong evidence from several studies that the malignant cells themselves are often the source of the hCG beta chain (Iles, 2007).

Choice of *in vitro* Expression System for Production of Recombinant hCG beta Chain

The hCG beta chain has been expressed in a wide variety of cells types including *E.coli*, hamster ovary, monkey kidney fibroblasts and insect cells. The glycoforms borne by the protein will differ dependent upon the particular expression system chosen. Indeed, even changes in culture conditions of a particular cell type can lead to alterations in the carbohydrate structures, and such changes might cause protein to multimerise or might change protein folding. More prosaically, different expression systems vary greatly in the efficiency of protein production. All of these factors need to be taken into account when selecting the expression system. In our own studies, we explored several different cell types (*E.coli*, CHO, COS, sf9) and found the baculovirus expression system in sf9 cells to be relatively efficient, although the amount of protein produced varied between wild-type and mutated hCG-beta sequences, with mutated proteins sometimes produced at higher levels than the wild-type.

Purification

Efficient isolation of the vaccine antigen in a non-denatured state is required, and for recombinant proteins is often facilitated by the introduction of a tag, such as His_6 or c-myc, to the protein. Not only does the particular tag, if any, need to be chosen, but it is also necessary to decide where to place the tag. Although it is possible to place tags at any location within the sequence of the protein, the C-terminus or N-terminus is often selected in order to minimise structural alterations. Placing a His_6 tag at the C-terminus of wild-type and mutated hCG-beta proteins does not appear to affect their conformation (Chiesa *et al.*, 2001). The isolation conditions also need to be carefully selected to avoid aggregation of the protein. With respect to hCG-beta, large aggregates are virtually impossible to re-solubilise and therefore conditions must be chosen that avoid this.

T-cell Help

CTLs, B-cells and macrophages can all be activated by helper T-cells. Indeed, in the absence of T-cell help, most adaptive immune responses are unable to occur. Thus, given that most helper T-cells are $CD4^+$ and therefore MHC class II-restricted, vaccines need to include epitopes that can be presented to the TCR by this class of MHC. This requirement is essential in order to generate immunological memory, and is illustrated by the case of carbohydrate antigens of either infectious or tumor origin which are unable to induce immunological memory unless they are associated with a protein. Thus meningococcal group C and pneumococcal vaccines consist of specific carbohydrates conjugated to, for example, tetanus toxoid as an immunological carrier possessing helper T-cell epitopes (Finn, 2004). The polymorphism of the MHC also requires the epitopes to be promiscuous, i.e. capable of binding to a broad range of MHC haplotypes, as illustrated for hCG by Gupta and colleagues (2001). Unlike vaccines aimed at combating infectious disease or for use as family planning agents, anti-cancer vaccines can perhaps be less constrained by such considerations and to an extent 'tailored' to particular groups of patients. With respect to epitopes recognised by cytotoxic T-cells, the HLA-A2 molecule is relatively highly represented in some populations and vaccines have been developed specifically to target patients who are HLA-A2. Thus, a NY-ESO-1 testis antigen peptide vaccine has undergone a Phase I clinical trial in patients with a variety of cancers (Bender *et al.*, 2007).

It also needs to be borne in mind that regulatory T-cells have the potential to dampen down the response to anti-cancer vaccines (Zhou *et al.*, 2006), and therefore any epitopes preferentially triggering these types of cells should be eliminated. Indeed, it was reported some time ago that hCG can induce immunosuppressive T-cells (Fuchs *et al.*, 1982). A recent study by Nair and colleagues (2007) has provided evidence that it is possible to deplete regulatory T-cells by vaccinating against Foxp3, with the generation of CTL that kill Foxp3$^+$ regulatory T-cells.

Dendritic Cell Activation

Naive T-cells require particularly potent costimulation in order to ensure their activation. Interdigitating dendritic cells, when activated, express high levels of MHC class II to ensure efficient antigen-specific stimulation, but crucially also express high levels of costimulatory molecules including CD80 and CD86 (B7.1 and B7.2) which engage CD28 on the T-cell. Thus, this cell type needs to be activated by the vaccine in order to obtain the required adaptive response. This is also particularly important given the fact that non-activated dendritic cells can be tolerogenic (Morelli and Thomson, 2007), switching off the response rather than initiating it. During natural infections, microbial components such as lipopolysaccharides, peptidoglycans, nucleic acids, etc activate dendritic cells via Toll-like receptors and other types of pattern recognition receptors (Kabelitz and Medzhitov, 2007). Vaccines, including anti-cancer vaccines, need to mimic this effect by including either microbial or synthetic components capable of activating dendritic cells. One such potential component, mycobacterium tuberculosis hsp70, has proved to be effective as both a carrier which provides helper T-cell epitopes and as an adjuvant able to activate pro-inflammatory NFkB activity via TLR4 and TLR2 (Bulut *et al.*, 2005).

Cross-reaction

Any vaccine should ideally produce an immune response only against the desired target. Regarding the hCG beta chain, there is a high degree of sequence homology with the beta chain of luteinising hormone. This causes a cross-reaction between these two molecules, such that the antibody-response provoked by the native hCG beta chain recognises epitopes that are also present on LH. Although in practice this does not appear to lead to any undesirable side effects of hCG vaccines (Talwar *et al.*, 1994), it would be preferable to have a vaccine that only targets the tumor-associated hormone rather than additionally targeting other hormones. One way to address this is to use only the C-terminal amino acids 109-145 as this part of the molecule is unique to hCG (Stevens, 1996).

However, there are other hCG-specific amino acids which fold to provide hCG-unique discontinuous epitopes in the rest of thc molecule and which potentially provide important targets for the anti-tumor response. In order to address this issue, we used oligonucleotide-directed site-specific mutagenesis to make rational amino acid replacements in the hCG beta chain wild-type sequence. Using this approach we were able to remove cross-reactive epitopes whilst maintaining the folding of the molecule to retain the hormone-specific conformational-dependent B-cell epitopes (Jackson *et al.*, 1996; Delves *et al.*, 2007).

Route and form of Administration

Most vaccines are given by intradermal or intramuscular injection. Alternative, less invasive, routes have been explored more recently, including transdermal and intranasal. With our hCG vaccines we have found that intranasal administration together with *E.coli* heat-labile enterotoxin led to specific antibody production not only at remote mucosal sites but also systemically (Chiesa *et al.*, 2001). Particularly in cancer patients, who already are being subjected to many invasive procedures, a less invasive route of anti-cancer vaccine administration would be welcome.

Acknowledgments

Research in the author's laboratory has been supported in part by grants from The Wellcome Trust, Sir Jules Thorn Charitable Trust, and The Cleveland General and Immunological Trust.

REFERENCES

1. Bender A, Karbach J, Neumann A, Jäger D, Al-Batran SE, Atmaca A, Weidmann E, Biskamp M, Gnjatic S, Pan L, Hoffman E, Old LJ, Knuth A, Jäger E. (2007) *LUD 00-009: phase 1 study of intensive course immunization with NY-ESO-1 peptides in HLA-A2 positive patients with NY-ESO-1-expressing cancer.* Cancer Immun. **7**: 16.
2. Bulut Y, Michelsen KS, Hayrapetian L, Naiki Y, Spallek R, Singh M, Arditi M. (2005) *Mycobacterium tuberculosis heat shock proteins use diverse Toll-like receptor pathways to activate pro-inflammatory signals.* J Biol Chem. **280**: 20961-20967.
3. Chiesa MD, Martensen PM, Simmons C, Porakishvili N, Justesen J, Dougan G, Roitt IM, Delves PJ, Lund T. (2001) *Refocusing of B-cell responses following a single amino acid substitution in an antigen.* Immunology **103**: 172-178.
4. Delves PJ, Iles RK, Roitt IM, Lund T. (2007) *Designing a new generation of anti-hCG vaccines for cancer therapy.* Mol Cell Endocrinol. **260-262**: 276-281.
5. Gupta A, Pal R, Ahlawat S, Bhatia P, Singh O. (2001) *Enhanced immunogenicity of a contraceptive vaccine using diverse synthetic carriers with permissible adjuvant.* Vaccine **19**: 3384-3389.
6. Finn A. (2004) *Bacterial polysaccharide-protein conjugate vaccines.* Br Med Bull. **70**: 1-14.
7. Fuchs T, Hammarström L, Smith CI, Brundin J. (1982) *Sex-dependent induction of human suppressor T cells by chorionic gonadotropin.* J Reprod Immunol. **4**: 185-190.
8. Hotakainen K, Lintula S, Jarvinen R, Paju A, Stenman J, Rintala E, Stenman UH. (2007) *Overexpression of human chorionic gonadotropin beta genes 3, 5 and 8 in tumor tissue and urinary cells of bladder cancer patients.* Tumour Biol. **28**: 52-56.

9. Iles RK. (2007) *Ectopic hCGbeta expression by epithelial cancer: malignant behaviour, metastasis and inhibition of tumor cell apoptosis*. Mol Cell Endocrinol. **260-262**: 264-270.
10. Jackson AM, Klonisch T, Lapthorn AJ, Berger P, Isaacs NW, Delves PJ, Lund T, Roitt IM. (1996) *Identification and selective destruction of shared epitopes in human chorionic gonadotropin beta subunit.* J. Repro. Immunol. **31**: 21-26.
11. Kabelitz D, Medzhitov R. (2007) *Innate immunity—cross-talk with adaptive immunity through pattern recognition receptors and cytokines.* Curr Opin Immunol. **19**: 1-3.
12. Lowe DB, Shearer MH, Jumper CA, Kennedy RC. (2007) *Towards progress on DNA vaccines for cancer.* Cell Mol Life Sci. **64**: 2391-2403.
13. Morelli AE, Thomson AW. (2007) *Tolerogenic dendritic cells and the quest for transplant tolerance.* Nat Rev Immunol. **7**: 610-621.
14. Nair S, Boczkowski D, Fassnacht M, Pisetsky D, Gilboa E. (2007) *Vaccination against the forkhead family transcription factor Foxp3 enhances tumor immunity.* Cancer Res. **67**: 371-380.
15. Rosenberg SA, Yang JC, Restifo NP. (2004) *Cancer immunotherapy: moving beyond current vaccines.* Nat Med. **10**: 909-915.
16. Stenman UH, Alfthan H, Hotakainen K. (2004) *Human chorionic gonadotropin in cancer.* Clin Biochem. **37**: 549-561.
17. Stevens VC (1996) *Progress in the development of human chorionic gonadotropin antifertility vaccines.* Am. J. Reprod. Immunol. **35**: 148-155.
18. Talwar GP, Singh O, Pal, R, Chatterjee N, Sahai P, Dhall K, Kaur, J, Das SK, Suri S, Buckshee K, Saraya L, Saxena BN (1994) *A vaccine that prevents pregnancy in women.* Proc. Natl. Acad. Sci. USA **91**: 8532-8536.
19. Talwar GP (1999) *Vaccines and passive immunological approaches for the control of fertility and hormone-dependent cancers.* Immunol. Rev. **171**: 173-192.
20. Ueno A, Cho S, Cheng L, Wang J, Hou S, Nakano H, Santamaria P, Yang Y. (2007) *Transient upregulation of indoleamine 2,3-dioxygenase in dendritic cells by human chorionic gonadotropin downregulates autoimmune diabetes.* Diabetes **56**: 1686-1693.
21. Vaitukaitis JL (1973) *Immunologic and physical characterization of human chorionic gonadotropin (hCG) secreted by tumors.* J Clin Endocrinol Metab. **37**: 505-514.
22. Zhou G, Drake CG, Levitsky HI. (2006) *Amplification of tumor-specific regulatory T cells following therapeutic cancer vaccines.* Blood. **107**: 628-636.

12

CHAPTER

Immune Targeting of Oncogenic Proteins of High Risk Human Papilloma Virus Type 16 (HPV 16)

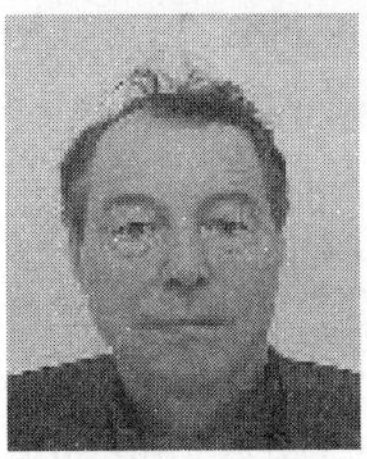

C.J.M. Melief [1], M.J.P. Welters[1], M.J.G. Löwik[2], A.P.G. Vloon[1], J.W. Drijfhout[1], A.R.P.M. Valentijn[3], A.R. Wafelman[3], G.J. Fleuren[4], R. Offringa[1], S.H. van der Burg[5] and G.G. Kenter[2]

Depts. of [1]Immunohematology and Blood Transfusion, [2]Gynaecology, [3]Pharmacy, [4]Pathology and [5]Clinical Oncology, Leiden University Medical Center, Leiden, the Netherlands.

ABSTRACT

Activation of Dendritic Cells (DC) that have processed tumor-associated antigens rescues therapeutic CD8 T-cell activity in vivo (1). A therapeutic vaccine was designed based on long overlapping peptides covering the complete amino acid sequence of the HPV16 E6 and E7 oncogenic proteins, thereby harboring all potential T helper and CTL epitopes. The peptides were between 27 and 35 amino acids in length and need to be processed in vivo by DC for presentation of T-cell epitopes by the available MHC class I and II molecules. Previously, we demonstrated that HPV16 specific T-cell immunity induced by this vaccine,delivered in Montanide ISA 51 adjuvant was able to terminate persistent infections and eradicate established HPV16+ tumors in mice and rabbits (2)(3). This principle was used to vaccinate patients with end-stage cervical cancer and with pre-malignant HPV 16-induced lesions, because we have found that such patients have impaired T helper 1 immunity against HPV 16 (4). In patients with end-stage cervical cancer the HPV 16 E6 and E7 synthetic long peptide vaccine is highly immunogenic in that it markedly increases the number and activity of HPV 16-specific T-cells. Injection of the E6 and E7 peptides at two different sites increases the E7 response but did not affect the magnitude of the E6-induced response (5). This vaccine moreover induced HPV 16-specific CD4+ and CD8+ T-cell responses to a broad array of T-cell epitopes in each patient. The expansion of both CD4- and CD8 T-cells indicates the immunotherapeutic potential of this vaccine (6)

Currently, 20 patients with histologically proven HPV16+ vulvar intraepithelial neoplasia (VIN) grade III were vaccinated 4 times with a 3-week interval by s.c. injection of the long peptides emulsified in Montanide ISA 51. Immunological monitoring was performed at the systemic level by the analysis of blood samples, drawn before each vaccination and after the last vaccination, and at the local level by the analysis of HPV16-specific T-cells in tissue biopsies of the VIN lesion (before and after vaccination) as well as a biopsy from the last vaccination site.

In all 20 patients, already after 2 vaccinations, strong and broad vaccine-induced systemic proliferative responses, accompanied with the production of IFNg and IL-5 were detected. This type of response is similar to the memory T-cell responses observed in healthy individuals with HPV16-specific immunity. Importantly, circulating HPV16 E6 and E7 specific T-cells produced IFNg upon stimulation with naturally processed and presented antigen. Notably, vaccination resulted in the induction of both CD4+ and CD8+ HPV16-specific T-cells. Multiple epitopes were recognized in each patient. Analysis of the local immune response demonstrated the presence of HPV16-specific Th1/Th2 cells infiltrating both the vaccination site and the VIN lesion after vaccination in 6 out of 9 patients analyzed. A complete clinical response was seen in 5 out of 20 patients, as determined by complete clearance of lesions by macroscopy and microscopy. In 4 of these patients HPV 16 was also cleared as determined by PCR. Many of the remaining 15 patients experienced a partial remission of lesions and substantial improvement of disease-associated complaints.

In conclusion, our peptide-based vaccine elicits a strong and broad HPV16-specific T-cell response that displays the capacity to migrate into the persistently HPV16-infected lesion of patients with high grade VIN and causes complete regressions in a substantial proportion of patients. The reason for the marked effectiveness of the synthetic long peptide HPV 16 vaccine is the capacity of such long peptides to deliver specific antigens to professional antigen-presenting cells (Dendritic Cells, DC) (7,8). Appropriate DC activation subsequently elicits the therapeutic CD4+ and CD8+ responses that cause regression of established pre-malignant VIN lesions induced by high risk HPV (7,8). In patients with end stage cervical cancer, those patients that received immunotherapy prior to standard chemotherapy appeared to respond better to the chemotherapy than patients that had not received immunotherapy (5). These results now need to be confirmed in randomized clinical trials.

REFERENCES

1. Antigen presentation by an immature myeloid dendritic cell line does not cause CTL deletion in vivo, but generates CD8+ central memory-like T cells that can be rescued for full effector function. Dumortier H., van Mierlo G.J., Egan D., van Ewijk W., Toes R.E., Offringa R., Melief C.J. J Immunol 175: 855-863, 2005.
2. Established human papillomavirus type 16-expressing tumors are effectively eradicated following vaccination with long peptides. Zwaveling S., Ferreira Mota S.C., Nouta J., Johnson M., Lipford G.B., Offringa R., van der Burg S.H., Melief C.J. J Immunol 169: 350-358, 2002.
3. Therapeutic vaccination with papillomavirus E6 and E7 long peptides results in the control of both established virus-induced lesions and latently infected sites in a pre-clinical cottontail rabbit

papillomavirus model. Vambutas A., DeVoti J., Nouri M., Drijfhout J.W., Lipford G.B., Bonagura V.R., van der Burg S.H., Melief C.J. Vaccine 23: 5271-5280, 2005.

4. Human papillomavirus type 16-positive cervical cancer is associated with impaired CD4+ T-cell immunity against early antigens E2 and E6. de Jong A., van Poelgeest M.I., van der Hulst J.M., Drijfhout J.W., Fleuren G.J., Melief C.J., Kenter G., Offringa R., van der Burg S.H. Cancer Res 64: 5449-5455, 2004.
5. Phase I Immunotherapeutic Trial with Long Peptides Spanning the E6 and E7 Sequences of High-Risk Human Papillomavirus 16 in End-Stage Cervical Cancer Patients Shows Low Toxicity and Robust Immunogenicity. Kenter G.G., Welters M.J.P., Valentijn A.R.P.M., Lowik M.J.G., Berends-van der Meer T.M.A., Vloon A.P.G., Drijfhout J.W., Wafelman A.R., Oostendorp J., Fleuren G.J., Offringa R., van der Burg S.H., Melief C.J.M. Clin Cancer Res 14(1):1-9, 2008.
6. Induction of tumor-specific CD4+ and CD8+ T-cell immunity in cervical cancer patients by an HPV16 E6 and E7 long-peptide vaccine. Welters M.J.P., Kenter G.G., Piersma S.J., Vloon A.P.G., Löwik M.J.G., Berends-van der Meer T.M.A., Drijfhout J.W., Valentijn A.R.P.M., Wafelman A.R., Oostendorp J., Fleuren G.J., Offringa R., Melief C.J.M., van der Burg S.H. Clin Cancer Res 14: 178-187, 2008.
7. Immune pact with the enemy. Melief C.J.M., Nature 450:803-804, 2007.
8. Immunotherapy of established (pre-)malignant disease by synthetic long peptide vaccines. Melief Cornelis J.M., Sjoerd H. van der Burg Nature Reviews Cancer 8: 531, 2008.

13

CHAPTER

Elimination of HPV and Control of Viral Oncogene Expression in Cervical Cancer Cells by Herbal Compounds

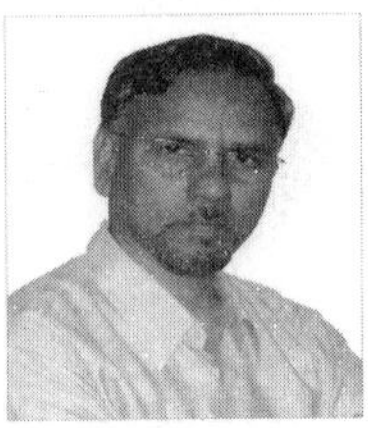

Sutapa Mahata, Shirish Shukla, Saurabh Maru, Suresh Hedau, Alok C. Bharti and Bhudev C. Das*

[1]Division of Molecular Oncology, Institute of Cytology and Preventive Oncology (ICMR), I-7, Sector-39, Noida

INTRODUCTION

Chronic inflammation and cancer are strongly linked. Although much research has been devoted to understanding cancer and its causes, the role of persistent infections leading to chronic inflammation and carcinogenesis is of major concern. According to WHO, up to 23% of malignancies in developing countries are caused by infectious agents whereas, in developed countries, it amounts to nearly 8% of all malignancies. Of variety of infectious agents, mainly viruses are among the few known causes of cancer that contribute to a variety of malignancies worldwide (**Table 13.1**) (Das *et al.* 2006).

Human Papillomaviruses (HPVs) is a large group of epitheliotropic viruses with more than 111 types, 30 of which effect the anogenital tract and other anatomic sites of the body. About 15 types are designated as defined highly oncogenic HPV types and are considered as the major etiological agents associated with the development of cervical cancer (Das *et al.* 2008). In addition, various

*email: bcdas48@hotmail.com

cofactors such as early marriage, high parity, promiscuity, smoking, and other reproductive tract infections may also modify the risk of developing cancer in women following infection with HPV(Das *et al.* 2000). Of all high risk HPV types, HPV16 & 18 collectively have been found to be associated with more than 70% cervical cancers globally and more than 80% cases in Indian scenario (Kailash *et al.* 2006, Parkin and Bray 2006).

Table 13.1 Biological agents that cause cancer

Virus/Bacteria	Type	Tumor/cancer
Retrovirus	HTLV-1	Adult T-cell Leukemia, Lymphoma
Hepatitis Virus	HBV, HCV	Liver Cancer
Herpes Virus	EBV HHB	Nasopharyngeal Carcinoma Lymphoma
Papillomavirus	HPV	Cervical Cancer, Oral Cancer
HIV	HIV-1/-2	Kaposi sarcoma
Helicobactor	*Helicobactor pylori*	Stomach Cancer

Infection and cancer often provides unique models of pathogenesis in relation to diagnosis, screening, therapy and prevention. Infection-associated cancer provides opportunity in cancer prevention and cure as the pathogen is known and can be treated. There are efforts for prophylactic therapy as well as other chemotherapeutics for the treatment of cancers. Vaccinations, a key to preventing some of these cancers that are associated with infection. HBV vaccination has already been shown to prevent liver cancer in high-incidence countries and it is likely that human papillomavirus (HPV) vaccination will become a reality in 3 to 5 years. However, at present there is no therapeutics for the treatment of HPV. The present article briefly describes HPV, transcriptional regulation of the viral oncogene expression and targeting the expression of these viral oncogenes using herbal derivatives with the main aim of discovering their therapeutic efficacy.

Cervical Cancer and Human Papillomaviruses

Cervical cancer is the most common women cancer in developing countries including India. The worldwide annual incidence rate of cervical cancer was estimated to be 493,000 and mortality of 274,000 per year. More than two thirds of these cases are from developing countries (Parkin *et al.* 2005). The areas of the highest incidence are sub-Saharan Africa, Latin America, the Caribbean, South Central Asia, and Southeast Asia. In India more than 130,000 cases, comprising one fourth of total world annual incidence, are diagnosed in India and about 74,000 deaths occur every year. It constitutes 24% of the total cancer incidence in Indian women.

The pathological effect of HPV is primarily confined to the epithelium and there exists a close association between viral replication and squamous epithelium differentiation. All HPVs infect keratinocytes in the basal layers of epidermis, but they replicate only in the differentiating epithelium and thus depend on the cellular DNA replication proteins thereof, the viral gene expression is also strongly regulated by the differentiation status of the infected keratinocytes. When the virus enters the basal stem cells of epithelium the viral early genes are amplified leading to the establishment of viral genome as a stable episome in the host cell nucleus. Expression of early genes also stimulates cell growth and differentiation in basal layer and later viral replication and late gene expression are activated in the upper layer of the fully differentiated epithelial cells leading to the production of infectious viral particles (Howley 1996). During chronic HR-HPV infection the HPV genomes which initially are in episomal form get integrated at multiple sites in the host genome through disruption of its E2 ORF sequence but sparing the E6 and E7 genes which remains transcriptionally active. This integration thus contributes to progression of the disease. Therefore, the expression of these genes in host cells becomes the primary target for any intervention strategies aimed towards development of anti-HPV therapeutics.

Genomic Organization of Human Papillomavirus

Papillomaviruses are small, double-stranded ~8kb DNA viruses enclosed in a protein capsid. The viral genome usually exists in an episomal (circular) configuration that can be divided into three regions: the upstream regulatory region (URR), the early region (E), and the late region (L) (**Figure 13.1**). The URR is responsible for regulation of viral replication and controls transcription of some sequences in the early region (E). The early region encodes predominantly for proteins that are important in viral replication, which occurs "early" in the viral life cycle. The late region encodes for viral structural proteins that are necessary for capsid production, which occurs "late" in

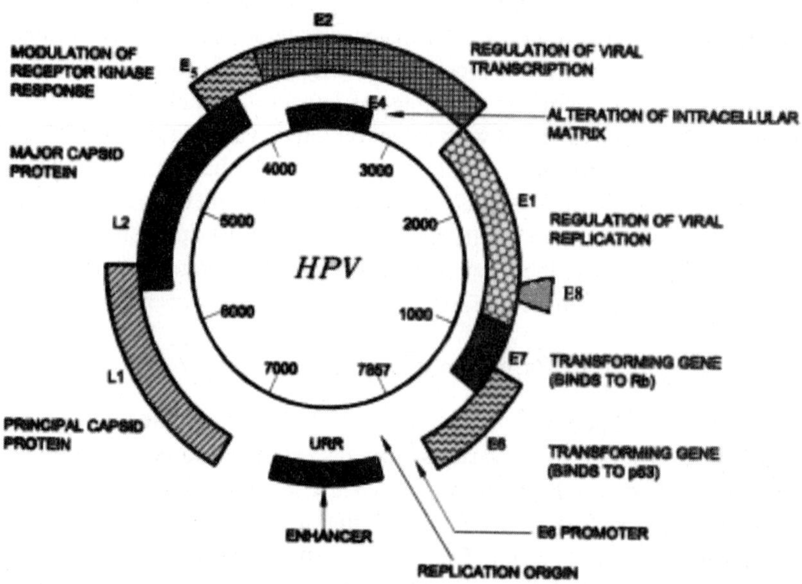

Fig. 13.1 Genomic organization of Human papillomavirus. All papilloma viruses have a similar genome organization with an 8Kb circular DNA genome and is divided into nine open reading frames.E6, E7, E8, E1, E2, E4, E5, L1 and L2- coding for 'early'(E) or 'Late'(L)genes.

the viral life cycle. These proteins, L1 & L2 are the most conserved regions and thus have been utilized for development of anti HPV vaccines. Seven different early regions that can encode for proteins have been identified and are designated E1, E2, E3, E4, E5, E6, and E7. Regions E2, E4, and E5 are involved in reproduction of the virus and its properties of infectivity. Whereas, regions

E6 and E7 are crucial in the process of oncogenesis as they produce the proteins that target the critical cell cycle proteins and hence are necessary for "transformation" of the cell. Low-risk HPVs have a much lower capacity to induce malignant transformation than do high-risk HPVs due to functional differences between their E6 and E7 proteins. The oncogenic potential of the virus can be attributed to the E6 and E7 open reading frames, whose gene products functionally interfere with the cell cycle control by interacting with tumor suppressor proteins such as p53 (Werness *et al.* 1990) and the retinoblastoma proteins (Rb) (Dyson *et al.* 1989) and interfere with the host cell cycle control, which leads to uncontrolled cell cycle proliferation and neoplastic growth.

HPV Infection and Transcription Factors

Similar to other virus HPV also does not have its own transcriptional machinery for which it is entirely dependent on the host transcription factors. Though E6 and E7 possess some intrinsic trans-activation capacity on their homologous promoters (Desaintes *et al.* 1992), their constitutive ex-pression is mainly dependent on the availability of a defined set of transcription factors of the infected host cell. A number of transcription factor binding sites have been identified in the URRs of the various papillomaviruses that have been studied. The transcription factors that bind to and activate the transcriptional enhancer elements includes AP-1(Offord and Beard 1990, Butz and Hoppe-Seyler 1993), NF-kB (Fontaine *et al.* 2000), NF-1 (Chong *et al.* 1991, Butz and Hoppe-Seyler 1993) SP-1, Oct-1, YY-1, TEF-1, TEF-2, STAT-3, KRF-1 (Mack and Laimins 1991) as well as glucocorticoid responsive elements etc. Most of these factors bind to the central region of the LCR, the *enhancer-region.* They regulate the transcription of the E6/E7 promoter located at the 3'-terminus of the LCR. Although many of these factors stimulate the promoter, some of them (specifi-cally YY-1) have a dual function and repress as well as stimulate the viral promoter (Bauknecht *et al.* 1992, Bauknecht *et al.* 1995). Besides the cellular regulation, intragenomic regulation of the E6/E7 gene activity by the viral E2 protein plays an important role in activating or suppressing these oncogenes. Some of the major transcription factors like AP-1 and NFkB which independently can promote carcinogenesis were found to be highly expressed in cervical cancer tissues (Prusty and Das 2005, Prusty *et al.* 2005). Since these transcription factors play a major role in the transcrip-tional regulation of almost all HPV ORF the host transcription factors also become primary targets for anti-HPV therapeutics strategies.

Targeting HPV and Its Oncogenes Expression Using Herbal Derivatives: Development Of Potential Anti-HPV therapeutics

Cervical cancer remains one of the greatest killers of women worldwide. It is difficult to foresee a dramatic increase in cure rate even with the most optimal combination of cytotoxic drugs, surgery, and radiation as well as development of prophylactic or therapeutic vaccine which will be highly type-specific. Therefore, testing of molecular-targeted therapies against HPV in general is highly desirable to prevent as well as treat HPV-associated malignancy. Considering low toxicities and their pharmacological safety, we looked for herbal derivatives with respect to two different thera-peutic aspects: (a) to target the expression of viral oncoproteins, E6 and E7, as their elimination may limit the propagation of established tumor cells and tumorigenic progression of lesion, and (2) to eliminate of HPV sequences from lesions at an early precancer stage where pathological changes in the cervical lesions are reversible and HPV DNA is in the episomal form. On these lines, our group has been actively working on various herbal entities, some of which showed remarkable anti-HPV properties and are under active investigation. Some of these leads are being described below.

(a) Targeting of HPV oncoproteins by curcumin

Curcumin, (1, 7-bis (4-hydroxy-3-methoxyphenyl)-1, 6-heptadiene- 3, 5-dione) the major yellow pigment of turmeric, is a commonly used spice derived from the rhizome of the plant *Curcuma longa* has been reported to have anti-inflammatory, antioxidant, and anti-proliferative properties(Aggarwal *et al.* 2003). Our investigation showed a transcriptional regulatory role of a curcumin in cervical cancer cells and demonstrates that curcumin is not only a potent inhibitor of AP-1, it selectively suppresses HPV transcription in cervical cancer cells (Prusty and Das 2005). Incubation of HeLa cells with curcumin showed a decline in HPV18-specific mRNA expression resulting in complete loss of HPV 18 E6 transcription by 4–5 hr (**Figure 13.2**). This abolition of HPV transcription was found to be selective and virus-specific and not the consequence of a general transcriptional blockage, since curcumin has no effect on the expression of the endogenous control

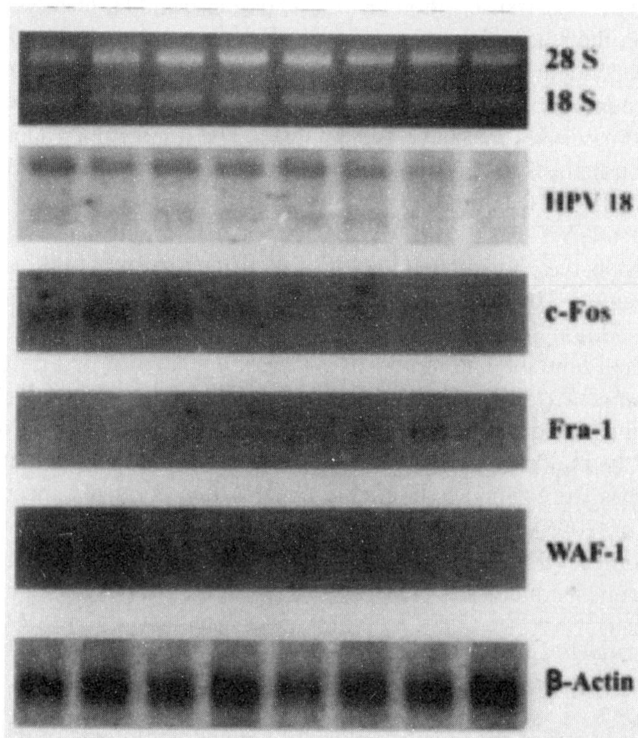

Fig. 13.2 Time-dependent downregulation of HPV 18 transcription in presence of curcumin. Northern blot analysis showing selective downregulation of HPV-18, c-fos and WAF-1 mRNA expression in HeLa cells and upregulation of Fra-1 mRNA expression after 100 M curcumin treatment at different time intervals. Lane a, untreated cells; Lanes b–h, 15 min, 30 min, 1 hr, 2 hr, 3 hr, 5 hr and 6 hr of incubation in the presence of 100 μM curcumin, respectively. To confirm equal RNA loading, the filters were reincubated with β-actin probes. The positions of the 28S and 18S rRNAs are indicated.

gene β-actin (**Figure 13.2**). To gain further insight into the effects of curcumin, we performed immunoblot analysis, which revealed a time-dependent downregulation of c-fos expression matching the downregulation of AP-1 activity; but most interestingly, curcumin upregulated fra-1 expression to a level generally observed in normal cervical cells (Figure 13.3). This antioxidant-induced abolition of HPV oncogene expression, coupled with the downregulation of AP-1 binding activity, represented a novel mechanism that can control pathogenic HPV expression during keratinocyte differentiation and progression of cervical cancer. This study revolutionized the field of anti-HPV research and was immediately picked for National Multicentric clinical trials by Department of Biotechnology, Government of India.

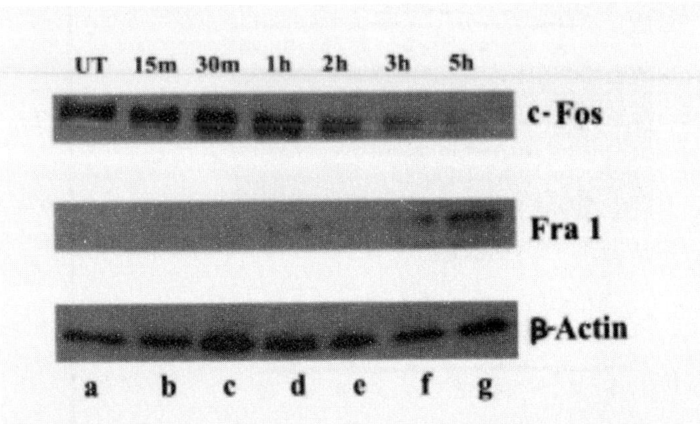

Fig. 13.3 Time-dependent downregulation of c-fos protein expression and upregulation of Fra-1 expression in presence of 100 μM curcumin. HPV-18 positive HeLa cells were treated with 100 μM curcumin for different periods and protein was extracted at each time-point. Separation of 30 μg protein was done in a 10% SDSPAGE gel. After electrotransfer, the filters were consecutively incubated with c-Fos and Fra-1 antibodies. Lane a, untreated cells; Lanes b–g, 15 min, 30 min, 1 hr, 2 hr, 3 hr and 5 hr of incubation in the presence of 100 μM curcumin, respectively. To confirm equal protein loading, the filters were reincubated with a monoclonal b-actin antibody.

Other potential derivatives from natural products like leaf extracts of *Bryophyllum pinnata* as well as fruit pulp of *Phyllanthus emblica* as well as Berberine which is derived from *Berberis asiatica* were also found to possess remarkable anti-HPV and anti- proliferative activities which are being explored currently in *in vitro* cell culture-based experiments in our laboratory.

(b) Elimination of HPV DNA

Praneem: Praneem, a polyherbal formulation based on leaf extracts of *Azadirachta indica* (Neem), a versatile medicinal plant of Indian subcontinent, was originally developed by Talwar and co-workers for treatment of reproductive tract infections and showed virucidal effects against HIV-1 and HSV-2 (Talwar *et al.* 2000) and was found to be pharmacologically safe was put into Phase I clinical trial for testing its ability to eliminate HPV DNA. Neem has been depicted in ancient Ayurvedic literature to possess variety of biological activities and medicinal properties which are being harnessed through traditional and folklore medicine through ages (Satyavati *et al.* 1976, Schmutterer 1995). The phase I study of Praneem for anti-HPV activity on 10 patients each in placebo and treatment arm demonstrated elimination of HPV sequences in upto 80% of the study subjects upon intravaginal application of Praneem for 30 days (exclusive of menstrual period) (**Figure 13.4**). Clearance of HPV infection was accompanied by remission of abnormal cytological and clinical alterations as revealed by Pap smear and colposcopic examination respectively (Unpublished data).

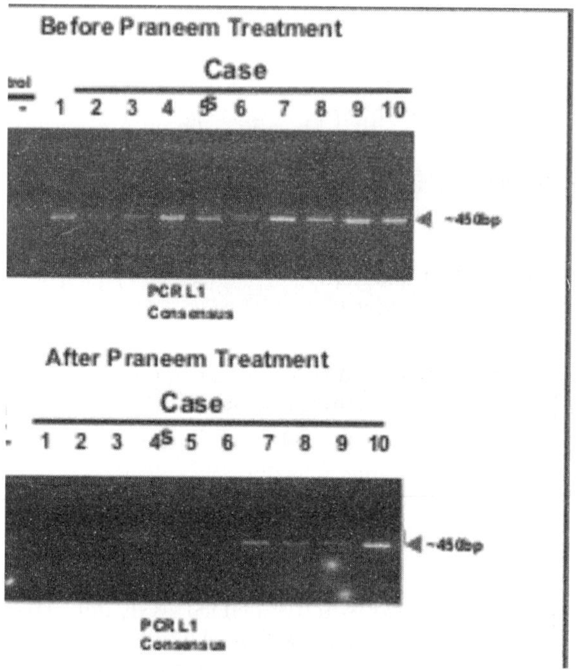

Fig. 13.4 PCR photographs of DNA obtained from cervical scrapes collected before and after Praneem treatment showing clearance of HPV infection in Praneem-treated women.

Basant and Curcumin: Curcumin which showed anti-HPV activity against viral oncogenes are being tested further with Basant which is another potent polyherbal formulation which primarily contain curcumin for elimination of HPV DNA sequences at early pre-cancer stages of cervical lesion. This multi-centric, national trial is in progress and patients are being recruited. The results of this Phase II study will be available by late 2009.

Future Directions

Since herbal derivatives express little or no systemic cytotoxicity, these are most suitable candidates for translation into much awaited anti-cancer and anti-HPV therapeutics. Above mentioned anti-HPV molecules some of which are in phase I/II clinical trials will not only be helpful in preventing as well as treating cancer of the cervix where HPV have a major causative role but will have major therapeutic implications in other HPV-associated malignancies such as oral, esophageal and anogenital precancer, cancer and warts.

REFERENCES

1. Aggarwal B.B., Kumar A. and Bharti A.C. (2003). Anticancer potential of curcumin: preclinical and clinical studies. *Anticancer Res*, **23**:363-98.
2. Bauknecht T., Angel P., Royer H.D. and zur Hausen H. (1992). Identification of a negative regulatory domain in the human papillomavirus type 18 promoter: interaction with the transcriptional repressor YY1. *Embo J*, **11**:4607-17.
3. Bauknecht T., Jundt F., Herr I., Oehler T., Delius H., Shi Y., Angel P. and Zur Hausen H. (1995). A switch region determines the cell type-specific positive or negative action of YY1 on the activity of the human papillomavirus type 18 promoter. *J Virol*, **69**:1-12.
4. Butz K. and Hoppe-Seyler F. (1993). Transcriptional control of human papillomavirus (HPV) oncogene expression: composition of the HPV type 18 upstream regulatory region. *J Virol*, **67**: 6476-86.
5. Chong T., Apt D., Gloss B., Isa M. and Bernard H.U. (1991). The enhancer of human papillomavirus type 16: binding sites for the ubiquitous transcription factors oct-1, NFA, TEF-2, NF1, and AP-1 participate in epithelial cell-specific transcription. *J Virol*, **65**:5933-43.
6. Das B.C., Gopalkrishna V., Hedau S. and Katiyar S. (2000). Cancer of the uterine cervix and human papillomavirus infection. *Curr Science*, **78**:52-63.
7. Das B.C., Hussain S., Nasare V. and Bharadwaj M. (2008). Prospects and prejudices of human papillomavirus vaccines in India. *Vaccine*, **26**:2669-79.
8. Das B.C., Sarin S.K., Kazim S.N. and Bharti A.C. Infections Causing Cancer. In: Shastri S, editor. UICC handbook - Cancer awareness, Prevention and control strategies. Geneva: UICC Press; 2006. p. 119-131.
9. Desaintes C., Hallez S., Van Alphen P. and Burny A. (1992). Transcriptional activation of several heterologous promoters by the E6 protein of human papillomavirus type 16. *J Virol*, **66**:325-33.
10. Dyson N., Howley P.M., Munger K. and Harlow E. (1989). The human papilloma virus-16 E7 oncoprotein is able to bind to the retinoblastoma gene product. *Science*, **243**:934-7.
11. Fontaine V., van der Meijden E., de Graaf J., ter Schegget J. and Struyk L. (2000). A functional NF-kappaB binding site in the human papillomavirus type 16 long control region. *Virology*, **272**: 40-9.
12. Howley P.M. Papillovirinae. Phladelphia: Lippincott-Raven; 1996.
13. Kailash U., Soundararajan C.C., Lakshmy R., Arora R., Vivekanandhan S. and Das B.C. (2006). Telomerase activity as an adjunct to high-risk human papillomavirus types 16 and 18 and cytology screening in cervical cancer. *Br J Cancer*, **95**:1250-7.
14. Mack D.H. and Laimins L.A. (1991). A keratinocyte-specific transcription factor, KRF-1, interacts with AP-1 to activate expression of human papillomavirus type 18 in squamous epithelial cells. *Proc Natl Acad Sci U S A*, **88**:9102-6.
15. Offord E.A. and Beard P. (1990). A member of the activator protein 1 family found in keratinocytes but not in fibroblasts required for transcription from a human papillomavirus type 18 promoter. *J Virol*, **64**:4792-8.
16. Parkin D.M. and Bray F. (2006). Chapter 2: The burden of HPV-related cancers. *Vaccine*, **24 Suppl 3**:S11-25.
17. Parkin D.M., Bray F., Ferlay J. and Pisani P. (2005). Global cancer statistics, 2002. *CA Cancer J Clin*, **55**:74-108.

18. Prusty B.K. and Das B.C. (2005). Constitutive activation of transcription factor AP-1 in cervical cancer and suppression of human papillomavirus (HPV) transcription and AP-1 activity in HeLa cells by curcumin. *Int J Cancer*, **113**:951-60.

19. Prusty B.K., Husain S.A. and Das B.C. (2005). Constitutive activation of nuclear factor -kB: preferntial homodimerization of p50 subunits in cervical carcinoma. *Front Biosci*, **10**:1510-9.

20. Satyavati G.V., Raina M.K. and Sharma M. Azadirachta indica. In: Satyavati GV, Raina MKandSharma M, editors. Medicinal Plants of India. New Delhi: Indian Council of Medical Research; 1976. p. 363.

21. Schmutterer H. The Neem Tree: Source of unique natural products for integrated pest management, medicine, industry and other purposes. Hiedelberg: VCH Weinheim; 1995.

22. Talwar G.P., Raghuvanshi P., Mishra R., Banerjee U., Rattan A., Whaley K.J., Zeitlin L., Achilles S.L., Barre-Sinoussi F., David A., *et al.* (2000). Polyherbal formulations with wide spectrum antimicrobial activity against reproductive tract infections and sexually transmitted pathogens. *Am J Reprod Immunol*, **43**:144-51.

23. Werness B.A., Levine A.J. and Howley P.M. (1990). Association of human papillomavirus types 16 and 18 E6 proteins with p53. *Science*, **248**:76-9.

14

CHAPTER

Optimization of Dendritic Cells and Adenoviral Vectors for Immunotherapy of Cancer

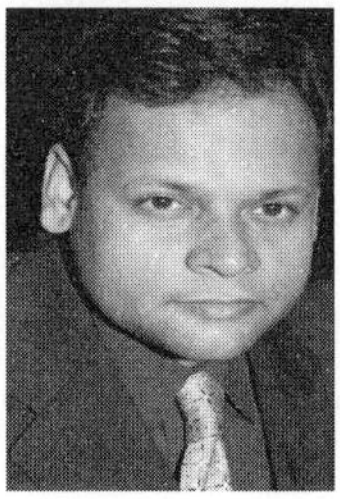

Airi Harui, Sylvia M. Kiertscher, Michael D. Roth and Saroj K. Basak

Pulmonary and Critical Care Medicine, David Geffen School of Medicine at UCLA and the West Los Angeles Veterans Affairs Medical Center, Los Angeles, California

ABSTRACT

Dendritic Cells (DC) are the primary and most potent antigen presenting cells of the immune system. Many different strategies are being evaluated for using DC as cell-based vaccines against diseases such as cancer. The ability to use DC in this manner requires the generation and/or production of a large number of DC, a strategy for efficiently loading them with antigens, and methods to enhance their antigen presentation and stimulation of the most effective immune responses. In this presentation we summarize a number of strategies that have been developed in our laboratory to generate functional and immunocompetent DC *in vitro* and *in situ*, with a particular focus on antigen loading through transduction with modified advenoviral vectors (AdV). These antigen loaded DC have been evaluated for their ability to induce transgene-specific immune responses, the desired outcome, as well as adenoviral vector-specific responses, which may complicate the immunization process as an unwanted side-effect. We have also characterized different subsets of DC for their expression of integrins that mediate adenoviral uptake and the role of these integrin expressing cells in AdV transduction, transgene expression and specific antigen presentation. Collectively, this work has defined several novel strategies for improving and optimizing the combination of DC and AdV vectors for use as cancer immunotherapy reagents.

INTRODUCTION

The goal of cancer immunotherapy is to harness and focus the immune response against antigens that are selectively expressed by cancer cells (tumor antigens). Induction of potent anti-tumor responses depends on efficient antigen delivery and presentation to the immune system. While dendritic cells (DC) are specialized immune cells capable of stimulating potent immune responses, their utility for preparing cancer vaccines is limited by their extremely low numbers *in situ* (1,2). As such, there has been a long-standing interest in methods for generating large numbers of DC so that they can readily be manipulated and used as vaccines against cancer and other diseases.

Dendritic cells can be differentiation from their precursors by stimulating them with a variety of different cytokines including granulocyte macrophage-colony-stimulating factor (GM-CSF), interleukin-3 (IL-3), IL-4, tumor necrosis factor-α (TNF-α) and various receptor ligands (flt-3, CD40-ligand, etc.) (3-10). Of these factors and their combinations, treating DC precursors with GM-CSF alone has been the most extensively studied in mouse models. Our own studies have focused on the generation of DC *in vitro* and *in situ* with GM-CSF alone and in combination with IL-4, which appears to synergize with GM-CSF to produce the most effective DC. The combination of GM-CSF and IL-4 induces the up-regulation of major histocompatibility complex (MHC) expression, costimulatory molecules, antigen processing, cytokine production, and T cell stimulation (11-14). Findings from *in vitro* and preclinical animal models have correlated with studies of the effects of these cytokines when used to treat cancer patients, confirming the potential utility of these cytokines for cancer therapy (15-20).

Purified proteins, peptides and a variety of live and disrupted tumor cell preparations have been loaded into DC as methods for antigen delivery to the immune system. Dendritic cells have been also genetically modified to produce higher and more prolonged cancer antigen expression and increase antigen presentation to the immune system. Genetic modifications of DC have included the delivery of RNA or DNA by a variety of approaches (transfection, electroporation, gene gun delivery etc.) (21,22). One of the most efficient antigen delivery methods employs the use of viral vectors encoding tumor-associated (TAA) or tumor specific antigens (TSA). Viral vectors such as adenoviral vectors (AdV), lentiviral vectors, pox virus, herpesvirus and adeno-associated virus (AAV), etc., have all been tested as approaches for antigen delivery (23). Of the different viral vectors, AdV vectors has been used extensively examined in cancer vaccination studies due to their low pathogenic status, ease of production and capacity to deliver antigen to the immune system (23-25). However, there are also limitations for their use in patient care due to the existence of innate and adaptive host immune responses to AdV, which result in viral neutralization, inflammatory responses and clearance of AdV-transduced cells *in vivo*. The first generation of AdV vectors (FG-AdV), such as E-1 deleted, are replication deficient, but they still express low levels of viral protein after infection, which tend to enhance the stimulation of anti-viral reactions (26,27).

To address this limitation associated with FG-AdV, helper-dependent adenoviral vectors (HD-AdV) were developed that lacks viral coding regions (28). It has been proposed that their lack of viral coding regions should make them less immunogenic to the host. These HD-AdV, when administered *in vivo* in comparison to FG-AdV, result in long term transgene expression consistent with a reduction in host anti-vector responses (29). However, their use as a gene therapy vector has not been extensively evaluated. Our studies in this area focused on the efficiency of HD-AdV for expressing transgene antigens in DC and their impact on the generation of transgene-specific T cells and anti-viral responses in both human and mouse models (30,31).

An important determinant of DC antigen presentation is the efficiency by which they can be loaded with antigen. AdV uptake by target cells depends on two distinct receptors that usually act in collaboration to promote infection. The first step involves the high-affinity coxsackievirus and adenovirus receptors (CAR) that binds to the fiber knob region of AdV capsid. The second step involves lower affinity $\alpha_v\beta_3$ and $\alpha_v\beta_5$ integrin receptors that bind to an Argenine-Glycine-Aspartic acid (RGD) motif expressed on the penton base component of the AdV capsid, resulting in viral internalization (32-35). However, DC do not express CAR receptor and their antigen loading by AdV vectors is entirely dependent on expression of the lower-affinity integrin receptors (32,33). This makes the pattern of integrin expression on DC particularly important in AdV-mediated transgene antigen loading and their antigen presenting capacity. Our studies therefore evaluated the integrin expression pattern of DC and related it to their ability to be transduced by AdV vectors, present transgene antigens and ultimately stimulate antigen specific T cells. We observed that expression of AdV-specific integrin receptors on DC ($\alpha_v\beta_3$ and $\alpha_v\beta_5$ integrins) depends on the differentiation state of the DC and can be modulated by a variety of different growth factors (36-38).

A variety of methods have been used for enhancing the transduction efficiency of AdV vectors including the insertion of additional RGD motifs into the fiber knob region of the AdV capsid to increase affinity to integrin receptors, conjugating other DC receptor ligands to the AdV capsid to redirect binding affinity, etc. (26-29). An even simpler method is to use centrifugation during the transduction process. Interestingly, our studies evaluated the mechanisms by which centrifugation enhances the transduction of DC revealed that this enhances the interaction of AdV vectors with integrins and, similar to other approaches, increases antigen loading and antigen –specific T cell responses (37).

DC Generated by GM-CSF in Combination with IL-4 Result in their Greater Differentiation and Maturation than GM-CSF Alone in Vitro and in Vivo

DC are derived from bone marrow precursors and these precursors are stimulated to differentiate by a variety of cytokines including GM-CSF, IL-3, IL-4, TNF-α, flt-3, CD40-ligand etc. (3-10). In mice, GM-CSF has been proposed as the major growth and differentiation factor for DC. Bone marrow cells from mice, when cultured *in vitro* in presence of GM-CSF alone, result in cells exhibiting dendritic morphology that express increased levels of MHC I, MHC II, CD11c and DEC-205 (39). Similarly, it has been shown that DC can be generated *in situ* by implanting GM-CSF secreting tumors or by administring polyethylene-glycol-modified GM-CSF molecules that produce a sustained exposure to this cytokine (40,41). However, these treatments mainly result in a specific myeloid subpopulation of DC identified by their concurrent expression of the CD11c and CD11b markers.

In contrast, when DC are generated *in vitro* from precursors with GM-CSF in combination with IL-4, the resulting DC express dramatically higher levels of MHC, CD40, CD80, CD86 and DEC-205, produce higher levels of the immunostimulatory cytokine IL-12, and generate higher allo-stimulatory and antigen specific presentation when compared to precursors generated with GM-

CSF alone (8). Furthermore, studies have indicated that DC generated in the presence of GM-CSF/IL-4 are highly immunogenic whereas DC generated in the presence of GM-CSF alone are less immunogenic and can be tolerogenic (41).

To further clarify the role of IL-4 in the generation of DC *in situ*, a mouse model was developed where GM-CSF alone or in combination with IL-4 was delivered by continuous *in vivo* infusion using mini osmotic pumps (10 ?g/day for 7 days) (15). After seven days, spleen and lymph node cells were evaluated for DC subsets, their level of differentiation and their antigen presenting function. The combination of GM-CSF/IL-4 resulted in the generation of both myeloid ($CD11c^+$/$CD11b^+$) and lymphoid DC ($CD11c^+$/$CD8\alpha^+$), whereas GM-CSF only resulted in expansion of only the myeloid DC subset. The DC generated *in situ* with GM-CSF /IL-4 also resulted in greater levels of MHC I and MHC II expression, higher endocytosis, macropinocytosis and allostimulatory activity. Finally, in an immunotherapy model, combining systemic GM-CSF/IL-4 with an adenoviral based vaccination significantly slowed down tumor growth in an antigen specific manner, where as systemic administration of GM-CSF alone (in combination with the same vaccination) failed to regress and inhibit tumor growth.

Importantly, our group also demonstrated that treatment of adherent human peripheral blood leukocytes (PBL) with either GM-CSF or IL-4 alone, each as a single agent, failed to produce functional DC. The generation of human DC only occurred when precursors were treated with the combination of GM-CSF and IL-4, resulting in the differentiation of monocytes ($CD14^{bright}$/$CD83^-$) into to DC ($CD14^{dim}$/CD 83^+) that exhibited the typical function of native human DC including enhanced MHC expression, co-stimulatory molecule expression, antigen processing and T cell stimulatory activity (16). Similar effects were also demonstrated *in vivo* when cancer patients were treated with GM-CSF alone or with the combination of GM-CSF and IL-4 (17,19,20). The treatment of patients with metastatic solid malignancies with GM-CSF (2.5 μg/kg/day) alone resulted in an increased number of circulating monocytes ($CD14^+$) whereas the same treatment in combination with IL-4 (0.5-6.5 μg/kg/day) stimulated these cells to acquire several antigen presenting cell (APC) markers and activity such as increased expression of HLA-DR, CD11c, decreased CD14, increased endocytotic activity and the ability to stimulate T cells in mixed leukocyte reaction (MLR). This combined treatment also resulted in increases in the number of ($CD14^-$/$CD83^+$) cells with APC activity and clinically significant and sustained tumor regression was observed in one patient (17). Further characterization of the cells generated by the systemic treatment of cancer patients with GM-CF and IL-4 demonstrated the expansion and activation of Type-1 DC (DC1). DC1 precursors identified after the *in vivo* therapy were large, more complex and expressed higher levels of HLA-DR, CD11c and CD80 than pre-treatment cells. The MLR activity generated by the DC1 isolated from GM-CSF /IL-4 treated patient were comparable to the MLR activity of monocyte-derived DC generated *in vitro* from the peripheral blood of the same patients (before their *in vivo* exposure). (20).

This combination of human and murine studies performed by our group clearly demonstrate that the systemic administration of GM-CSF in combination with IL-4 provides an optimal, and necessary, stimulus for expanding and differentiating functional DC populations *in vivo*.

Helper Dependent AdV (HD-AdV) Induces Similar Anti-viral Immune Response as That of FG-AdV But Higher Transgene Antigen Expression in DC

Recombinant AdV vectors have been used to present transgene antigens to the immune system

(23-25). However, administration of FG-AdV leads to antiviral immune responses which restrict their use for vaccine purposes. This issue was addressed by developing HD-AdV that lack viral coding regions and thus were proposed to induce less of an anti-viral immune response. However, our study shows that deletion of entire viral coding region and vaccination with HD-AdV (10^6 blue forming unit, BFU) still leads to same high level of antibody response to the AdV vector when compared to vaccination with same amount of FG-AdV. This appears to be explained by the viral capsid, which is highly antigenic and identical in the two vector systems. To reduce viral exposure, DC were first transduced *ex vivo*, allowed to upregulate antigen expression and destroy pre-existing viral capsid, and then used as a vaccination tool. HD-AdV transduced DC expressed higher levels of transgene specific mRNA and protein activity (up to 1,200-fold higher levels of transgene activity) than DC that were transduced with FG-AdV. DC transduced with HD-ADV also stimulated a higher transgene-specific CTL response *in vivo* and the response could be further increased by direct maturation of DC with LPS prior to *in vivo* immunization. Further, in comparison to direct immunization with HD-AdV, the immunization of DC transduced with HD-AdV *ex vivo* was associated with limited antibody response against AdV. Thus, by using this *ex vivo* approach to transduction and antigen loading, vaccination with DC transduced with HD-AdV results in superior vaccination efficiency and reduced anti-viral immune responses (24).

Similar studies were performed with human monocyte-derived DC. Similar to studies with murine DC, these studies revealed that antiviral immune responses to HD-AdV or FG-AdV were similar and are mostly directed towards viral capsid antigens. Transduction of human DC by HD-AdV resulted in higher transgene specific mRNA expression and the transgene activity level was 50 to 275 fold higher than when DC were transduced with FG-AdV (30). Thus, when HD-ADV in combination with DC are used for immunotherapy it results in lower anti-viral immune response and enhanced trangene specific T cell response.

DC Subset Expressing High Levels of $\alpha_v\beta_3$ Integrins Present AdV-encoded Transgene Antigens Most Efficiently

Both human and murine DC lack the primary CAR receptor involved in the first stage of AdV adherence and little is know about the integrin receptor (CD51/CD61or α_v/β_3) patterns on DC that are involved in AdV acquisition and AdV-encoded antigen presentation (32-35). Our studies examined whether there are different DC subsets that exhibit different integrin expression patterns, the role of these different subsets with respect to transgene antigen presentation, and whether the same subsets are present in human DC generated following exposure to GM-CSF and IL-4. Our examination of mouse bone marrow derived DC revealed that less than 10% of DC precursors express α_v (CD51) but the expression of this integrin molecule increases with time in the presence of GM-CSF and IL-4. After 7 days of culture in GM-CSF and IL-4 only 28 % of DC expressed high levels of CD51 ($CD51^{hi}$) and the rest of the DC expressed low levels of ($CD51^{lo}$) (38). Further, studies revealed that these $CD51^{hi}$ DC also express higher MHC I while both subsets express similar levels of MHC II and co-stimulatory molecules. When exposed to AdV, transduction and transgene expression was restricted almost entirely to the $CD51^{hi}$ DC subset. The transduction of $CD51^{hi}$ DC subset can be blocked efficiently with peptide expressing RGD sequence, confirming the role of integrin molecules in viral entry. The $CD51^{hi}$ DC subset also presents transgene-antigen more efficiently to $CD8^+$ T cells than the $CD51^{lo}$ DC subset. Similar to generation of $CD51^{hi}$ DC subset *in vitro* by GM-CSF and IL-4, *in vivo* treatment of mice with GM-CSF and IL-4 resulted in induction of 3 fold more of the $CD11c^{+}/CD51^{+}$ DC subset and rendered these cells susceptible to higher AdV transduction. Our studies with human PBL derived DC with GM-CSF and IL-4 reveal that similar changes are induced in human DC when cultured in presence of GM-CSF and IL-4. Further studies are being conducted to evaluate their antigen presentation ability and how they can be generated in large number to increase and improve DC and AdV mediated vaccination efficiency.

Integrin-dependent AdV Transduction of DC with Centrifugation Results in Higher Transgene Expression and T Cell Activation

DC mediated antigen presentation and T cell activation depends on the level of antigen loading. We have evaluated several different approaches for transducing DC with AdV, comparing them for transgene antigen expression and antigen presentation to T cells (37). Our studies indicate that while conventional Fg-AdV vectors expressing green fluorescent protein (AdV/GFP) produce a concentration dependent expression of GFP, an AdV vector with an additional RGD sequence inserted into its fiber knob (RGD-AdV/GFP) can enhance transgene expression by 9-20 fold at each MOI. Addition of the centrifugation during the transduction period (2000xg) with Ad/GFP resulted in 20- fold higher transduction and transgene expression. However, when the same method of centrifugation was applied with the RGD-AdV/GFP vector it produced almost no effect on transduction and only a 1.5-2 fold increase in GFP expression levels. These results suggested that use of the RGD-AdV vector and the addition of centrifugation were working through the same mechanism – i.e. enhanced interaction of the vector and the DC through integrin receptors. Indeed, we confirmed that the addition of exogenous RGD peptide can block transduction when centrifugation is used to enhance transduction efficiency. Furthermore, transduction by both the RGD-AdV/GFP vectors and by all vectors when combined with centrifugation, was restrictedtothe $CD51^{hi}$ integrin expressing subset of DC. A significant relationship was observed between transgene expression and T cell stimulation regardless of whether transgene expression was increased by using higher MOI, an RGD-modified vector, or by employing centrifugal force.

CONCLUSION

Effective immunotherapy approaches against cancer involve the induction of potent and specific immune responses against cancer antigens. DC can be used in combination with AdV vectors as an approach for cancer immunotherapy. Our studies show that functional DC can be generated in large number and most effectively when precursors are exposed to GM-CSF in combination with IL-4. These cytokines have similar effects in both animal models and in human studies, and are effective both *in vitro* and *in vivo*. The use of HD-AdV vectors in combination with DC can improve antigen presentation to the immune system by their ability to express high transgene expression and by decreasing exposure to adenoviral capsid antiges. DC activating/maturation agents can further improve transgene antigen presentation. A specific subset of DC which expresses high levels of $\alpha_v\beta_3$ and/or $\alpha_v\beta_5$ integrins is highly susceptible to AdV vectors and mediates the majority of the immune response. These integrin expressing DC are optimally expressed following exposure to GM-CSF and IL-4. Finally, a simple method such as centrifugation can improve tarnsgene antigen loading and antigen presentation by integrin expressing DC.

REFERENCES

1. Steinman RM, Banchereau J.Taking dendritic cells into medicine. Nature. 2007 Sep 27;449(7161):419-26.
2. Lin KW, Jacek T, Jacek R. Dendritic cells heterogeneity and its role in cancer immunity. J Cancer Res Ther. 2006 Apr-Jun;2(2):35-40.
3. Rosenzwajg M, Camus S, Guigon M, Gluckman JC. The influence of interleukin (IL)-4, IL-13, and Flt3 ligand on human dendritic cell differentiation from cord blood CD34+ progenitor cells. Exp Hematol. 1998 Jan;26(1):63-72.
4. Morse MA, Zhou LJ, Tedder TF, Lyerly HK, Smith C. Generation of dendritic cells in vitro from peripheral blood mononuclear cells with granulocyte-macrophage-colony-stimulating factor, interleukin-4, and tumor necrosis factor-alpha for use in cancer immunotherapy. Ann Surg. 1997 Jul;226(1):6-16.
5. Daro E, Pulendran B, Brasel K, Teepe M, Pettit D, Lynch DH, Vremec D, Robb L, Shortman K, McKenna HJ, Maliszewski CR, Maraskovsky E. Polyethylene glycol-modified GM-CSF expands CD11b(high)CD11c(high) but notCD11b(low)CD11c(high) murine dendritic cells in vivo: a comparative analysis with Flt3 ligand. J Immunol. 2000 Jul 1;165(1):49-58.
6. Pulendran B, Smith JL, Caspary G, Brasel K, Pettit D, Maraskovsky E, Maliszewski CR. Distinct dendritic cell subsets differentially regulate the class of immune response in vivo. Proc Natl Acad Sci U S A. 1999 Feb 2;96(3):1036-41.
7. Maraskovsky E, Brasel K, Teepe M, Roux ER, Lyman SD, Shortman K, McKenna HJ. Dramatic increase in the numbers of functionally mature dendritic cells in Flt3 ligand-treated mice: multiple dendritic cell subpopulations identified. J Exp Med. 1996 Nov 1;184(5):1953-62.
8. Labeur MS, Roters B, Pers B, Mehling A, Luger TA, Schwarz T, Grabbe S. Generation of tumor immunity by bone marrow-derived dendritic cells correlates with dendritic cell maturation stage. J Immunol. 1999 Jan 1;162(1):168-75.
9. Brossart P, Grünebach F, Stuhler G, Reichardt VL, Möhle R, Kanz L, Brugger W. Generation of functional human dendritic cells from adherent peripheral blood monocytes by CD40 ligation in the absence of granulocyte-macrophage colony-stimulating factor.Blood. 1998 Dec 1;92(11):4238-47.
10. Ureta G, Osorio F, Morales J, Rosemblatt M, Bono MR, Fierro JA. Generation of dendritic cells with regulatory properties. Transplant Proc. 2007 Apr;39(3):633-7.
11. Maroof A, Penny M, Kingston R, Murray C, Islam S, Bedford PA, Knight SC.Interleukin-4 can induce interleukin-4 production in dendritic cells. Immunology. 2006 Feb;117(2):271-9.
12. Menges M, Baumeister T, Rössner S, Stoitzner P, Romani N, Gessner A, Lutz MB. IL-4 supports the generation of a dendritic cell subset from murine bone marrow with altered endocytosis capacity. J Leukoc Biol. 2005 Apr;77(4):535-43. Epub 2004 Dec 23.
13. Lutz MB. IL-3 in dendritic cell development and function: a comparison with GM-CSF and IL-4. Immunobiology. 2004;209(1-2):79-87.
14. Romani N, Gruner S, Brang D, Kämpgen E, Lenz A, Trockenbacher B, Konwalinka G, Fritsch PO, Steinman RM, Schuler G. Proliferating dendritic cell progenitors in human blood. J Exp Med. 1994 Jul 1;180(1):83-93.
15. Basak SK, Harui A, Stolina M, Sharma S, Mitani K, Dubinett SM, Roth MD. Increased dendritic cell number and function following continuous in vivo infusion of granulocyte macrophage-colony-stimulating factor and interleukin-4.Blood. 2002 Apr 15;99(8):2869-79.

16. Kiertscher SM, Roth MD. Human CD14+ leukocytes acquire the phenotype and function of antigen-presenting dendritic cells when cultured in GM-CSF and IL-4. J Leukoc Biol. 1996 Feb;59(2):208-18.

17. Roth MD, Gitlitz BJ, Kiertscher SM, Park AN, Mendenhall M, Moldawer N, Figlin RA.Granulocyte macrophage colony-stimulating factor and interleukin 4 enhance the number and antigen-presenting activity of circulating CD14+ and CD83+ cells in cancer patients. Cancer Res. 2000 Apr 1;60(7):1934-41.

18. Roth MD, Cheng Q, Harui A, Basak SK, Mitani K, Low TA, Kiertscher SM. Helper-dependent adenoviral vectors efficiently express transgenes in human dendritic cells but still stimulate antiviral immune responses. J Immunol. 2002 Oct 15;169(8):4651-6.

19. Gitlitz BJ, Figlin RA, Kiertscher SM, Moldawer N, Rosen F, Roth MD. Phase I trial of granulocyte macrophage-colony stimulating factor and interleukin-4 as a combined immunotherapy for patients with cancer. J Immunother (1997). 2003 Mar-Apr;26(2):171-8.

20. Kiertscher SM, Gitlitz BJ, Figlin RA, Roth MD. Granulocyte/macrophage-colony stimulating factor and interleukin-4 expand and activate type-1 dendritic cells (DC1) when administered in vivo to cancer patients. Int J Cancer. 2003 Nov 1;107(2):256-61.

21. Arthur JF, Butterfield LH, Roth MD, Bui LA, Kiertscher SM, Lau R, Dubinett S, Glaspy J, McBride WH, Economou JS. A comparison of gene transfer methods in human dendritic cells. Cancer Gene Ther. 1997 Jan-Feb;4(1):17-25.

22. Ribas A. Genetically modified dendritic cells for cancer immunotherapy. Curr Gene Ther. 2005 Dec;5(6):619-28.

23. Mossoba ME, Medin JA. Cancer immunotherapy using virally transduced dendritic cells: animal studies and human clinical trials. Expert Rev Vaccines. 2006 Oct;5(5):717-32.

24. Harui A, Roth MD, Kiertscher SM, Mitani K, Basak SK. Vaccination with helper-dependent adenovirus enhances the generation of transgene-specific CTL. Gene Ther. 2004 Nov;11(22):1617-26.

25. Verma IM, Weitzman MD. Gene therapy: twenty-first century medicine. Annu Rev Biochem. 2005;74:711-38.

26. Christ M, Lusky M, Stoeckel F, Dreyer D, Dieterlé A, Michou AI, Pavirani A, Mehtali M. Gene therapy with recombinant adenovirus vectors: evaluation of the host immune response. Immunol Lett. 1997 Jun 1;57(1-3):19-25.

27. Yang Y, Li Q, Ertl HC, Wilson JM. Cellular and humoral immune responses to viral antigens create barriers to lung-directed gene therapy with recombinant adenoviruses. J Virol. 1995 Apr;69(4): 2004-15.

28. Mitani K, Graham FL, Caskey CT, Kochanek S. Rescue, propagation, and partial purification of a helper virus-dependent adenovirus vector. Proc Natl Acad Sci U S A. 1995 Apr 25;92(9):3854-8.

29. Maione D, Wiznerowicz M, Delmastro P, Cortese R, Ciliberto G, La Monica N, Savino R. Prolonged expression and effective readministration of erythropoietin delivered with a fully deleted adenoviral vector. Hum Gene Ther. 2000 Apr 10;11(6):859-68.

30. Roth MD, Cheng Q, Harui A, Basak SK, Mitani K, Low TA, Kiertscher SM. Helper-dependent adenoviral vectors efficiently express transgenes in human dendritic cells but still stimulate antiviral immune responses. J Immunol. 2002 Oct 15;169(8):4651-6.

31. Harui A, Roth MD, Kiertscher SM, Mitani K, Basak SK. Vaccination with helper-dependent adenovirus enhances the generation of transgene-specific CTL. Gene Ther. 2004 Nov;11(22):1617-26.

32. Okada N, Tsukada Y, Nakagawa S, Mizuguchi H, Mori K, Saito T, Fujita T, Yamamoto A, Hayakawa T, Mayumi T. Efficient gene delivery into dendritic cells by fiber-mutant adenovirus vectors. Biochem Biophys Res Commun. 2001 Mar 23;282(1):173-9.

33. Brossart P, Goldrath AW, Butz EA, Martin S, Bevan MJ. Virus-mediated delivery of antigenic epitopes into dendritic cells as a means to induce CTL. J Immunol. 1997 Apr 1;158(7):3270-6.

34. Wickham TJ, Mathias P, Cheresh DA, Nemerow GR. Integrins alpha v beta 3 and alpha v beta 5 promote adenovirus internalization but not virus attachment. Cell. 1993 Apr 23;73(2):309-19.

35. Nemerow GR, Cheresh DA, Wickham TJ. Adenovirus entry into host cells: a role for alpha(v) integrins. Trends Cell Biol. 1994 Feb;4(2):52-5.

36. Basak SK, Kiertscher SM, Harui A, Roth MD. Modifying adenoviral vectors for use as gene-based cancer vaccines. Viral Immunol. 2004;17(2):182-96.

37. Harui A, Roth MD, Sanghvi M, Vira D, Mizuguchi H, Basak SK. Centrifugation enhances integrin-mediated transduction of dendritic cells by conventional and RGD-modified adenoviral vectors. J Immunol Methods. 2006 May 30;312(1-2):94-104.

38. Harui A, Roth MD, Vira D, Sanghvi M, Mizuguchi H, Basak SK. Adenoviral-encoded antigens are presented efficiently by a subset of dendritic cells expressing high levels of alpha(v)beta3 integrins. J Leukoc Biol. 2006 Jun;79(6):1271-8.

39. Inaba K, Inaba M, Romani N, Aya H, Deguchi M, Ikehara S, Muramatsu S, Steinman RM. Generation of large numbers of dendritic cells from mouse bone marrow cultures supplemented with granulocyte/ macrophage colony-stimulating factor. J Exp Med. 1992 Dec 1;176(6):1693-702.

40. Hanada K, Tsunoda R, Hamada H. GM-CSF-induced in vivo expansion of splenic dendritic cells and their strong costimulation activity. J Leukoc Biol. 1996 Aug;60(2):181-90.

41. Daro E, Pulendran B, Brasel K, Teepe M, Pettit D, Lynch DH, Vremec D, Robb L, Shortman K, McKenna HJ, Maliszewski CR, Maraskovsky E. Polyethylene glycol-modified GM-CSF expands CD11b(high)CD11c(high) but notCD11b(low)CD11c(high) murine dendritic cells in vivo: a comparative analysis with Flt3 ligand. J Immunol. 2000 Jul 1;165(1):49-58.

15

CHAPTER

Phase-One Clinical Trial of Dendritic Cell Vaccines for Human Papillomavirus Positive Cervical Cancer

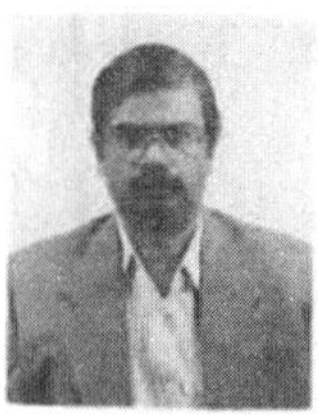

Rajkumar and Priya

Cancer Institute (Wia), Adyar, Chennai

ABSTRACT

Background

Human papillomavirus (HPV) infection is critical for the development of cervical cancer. Cervical cancer cells evade the immune system by down-regulating their major histocompatibility complex (MHC) class I molecules. Since mature dendritic cells (DCs) are potent antigen-presenting cells, expressing both MHC class I and II molecules, they could be primed by autologous tumor lysates and used as vaccines. The objective of the trial was to assess the feasibility and toxicity of DC vaccines.

Materials and Methods

So far ten patients with recurrent or residual cervical cancer have been randomized to a control arm (I) or to receive unprimed mature DCs (II) or mature tumor lysate-primed DCs (III), with three patients in arm I and III and 4 in arm II. Patient-specific DCs were generated in vitro, characterized phenotypically for surface markers and given to the patient in three doses after confirmation of sterility microbiologically. Toxicity was assessed using standard WHO criteria. Immune response was monitored with the delayed-type hypersensitivity (DTH) skin test, proliferation assays, CD3 interferon-???flow cytometric analysis, Cytotoxic T-Lymphocyte (CTL) assay and immunohistochemistry. Autoimmunity was determined by measuring antinuclear antibody levels.

RESULTS

No significant toxicity and no clinical response were observed. A DTH response was seen in two patients in arm III and one in arm II. No autoimmune reaction was observed. One patient in arm III showed increased CD8+ T-cell infiltration after vaccination. This is an ongoing phase one clinical trial.

CONCLUSION

DC vaccination was well tolerated in this study. Further studies are required to assess the clinical efficacy in naïve patients.

16

CHAPTER

Radiation-Enhanced Immunotherapy for Advanced Cancer

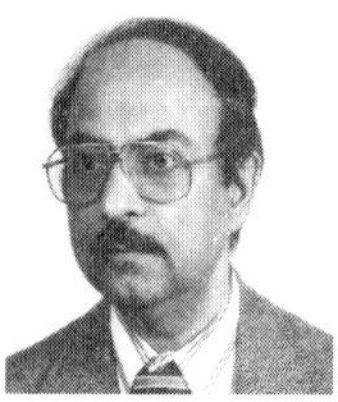

Jayanta Roy-Chowdhury, Chandan Guha, Yujo Kawashita and Namita Roy-Chowdhury

Albert Einstein College of Medicine, Bronx, New York, 10461, USA

Local treatment of primary tumor, such as, surgical resection, treatment with radiofrequency ablation, high intensity focused ultrasound (HIFU), cryotherapy, arterial embolism or radiation therapy often fails to control or eradicate the primary tumor. Recurrence near the location of the original tumor or at distant metastatic sites is a major problem that limits the long-term success of cancer therapy. When patients present with advanced cancer, in most cases, current approaches offer little benefit. For these reasons, many laboratories have focused on immunotherapy of cancer. Cancer cells express unique tumor antigens that include mutated oncoproteins, such as, p53 and ras, unique hybrid proteins expressed from translocated oncogenes, such as, bcr-c-abl and proteins that are expressed during embryogenesis, but are not expressed by normal adult tissues (1). Some of these "oncofetal" proteins serve as epitopes for host humoral and cellular immune response, which could potentially eradicate cancer cells. A brief consideration of the major steps in anti-tumor immune response follows.

A simplified view of natural immune response against tumor cells is presented in Fig. 16.1. Tumor antigens are released from dying tumor cells following treatment with chemotherapy or radiation therapy or from necrotic tumor cells from a growing tumor. The tumor antigens and cellular debris are normally engulfed by macrophages and neutrophils, as well as, by professional antigen presenting cells (APCs), such as, dendritic cells (DC) (2). DCs are normally present as sentinels guarding the entry via skin and mucosal surfaces (3, 4). Although, DCs are derived from hematopoietic stem cells, it is rarely present in circulating blood. However, systemic administration of cytokines, such as, Flt3 ligand (Flt3L) and GMCSF can induce proliferation of immature DCs (5, 6). Following engulfment of the tumor antigens, the DCs process and present the peptide antigens on MHC molecules at the cell surface. Subsequently, if appropriate "danger" signals are present, the DCs are activated and antigen-loaded DCs migrate to draining lymph nodes. In lymph nodes, DCs interact with naive CD4+ T helper cells (Th_0). CD40 ligand (CD40L) expressed at the surface of the helper T cells stimulates the maturation process of the DCs (7). Co-stimulatory interaction between mature DCs and the helper T-cells result in the Th_1 response, which leads to the proliferation of neoantigen-specific CD8+ cytotoxic T-lymphocytes (CTL). Furthermore, mature DCs can cross-present tumor antigenic peptides via Class I MHC molecules to CD8+ naïve CTLs (8-10). The CTLs, in turn, infiltrate the tumors at primary, as well as metastatic sites, inducing death of the tumor cells.

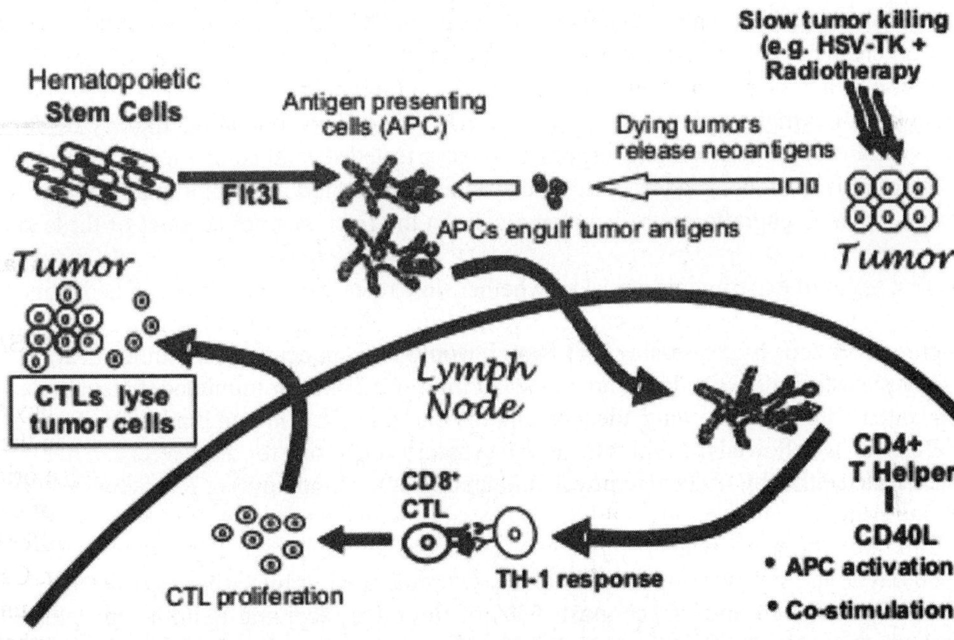

Fig. 16.1 Schematic representation of the envisioned mechanism of radiation-primed immunotherapy of advanced cancer. Cancer neoantigens are released over a long time by cancer cells dying in response to HIR. The antigens are taken up by a large number of APC's derived from bone-marrow cells in response to Flt3L (and other cytokines). Following antigen uptake, APC's migrate to lymph nodes, where they dock with Th0 cells. The APCs stimulate the Th cells, which, in turn, costimulate APC's via CD40L. This interaction results in the "Th1" response, leading to the generation of tumor-specific CTLs that clear tumor cells both at primary and metastatic sites.

Unfortunately, several factors attenuate this natural defense mechanism of the body against cancer. First, cancer neoantigens are not truly foreign proteins, whereby they are often weak antigens. Second, presentation of the neoantigens released from the cancer cells are not presented efficiently to the host immune system because too few uncommitted antigen presenting cells (APC) are present when the neoantigens are released. Third, costimulation of APC's by CD40, expressed by CD4+ helper T-cells (Th_0), occurs in a relatively inefficient manner. Fourth, large tumors secrete immunosuppressive cytokines, such as TGFb and IL10. Fifth, the APC-Th_1 cell costimulation is dampened by signaling by CTLA4 molecules, present on the cell surface of activated lymphocytes. Finally, surgical excision or rapid ablation of the primary tumor by physical means removes the source of the antigen, thereby impeding sustained immune response.

We hypothesize that, potentially, each step of the antitumor immune response can be augmented or modulated by specific therapeutic maneuvers. For example, a slow and prolonged release of tumor antigens could be achieved by tumor irradiation, rather than surgical removal or physical ablation of the cells. Availability of a sufficient number of circulating DCs could be synchronized with the neoantigen release by administration of specific cytokines at appropriate time points during the course of cancer treatment. Maturation of DCs could be assured by administration of CD40L. It is likely that following the initiation of the immune response, the tumor would need to be "debulked" via physical, chemical or molecular approaches, so that the immune response is not attenuated by IL10 secretion by a large primary tumor mass. It is also possible that prevention of CTLA4 expression in activated T-lymphocytes could prolong the APC-Th cell costimulation, thereby resulting in a more intense and sustained immune response. We have tested several components of this comprehensive hypothesis in mouse models of advanced cancer, generated by local implantation of tumor cells or disseminated engraftment of hepatoma cells in the liver. A brief account of these studies follows.

In the first series of experiments we asked whether slow release of putative tumor neoantigens by tumor irradiation (rather than surgical removal), synchronized with increased availability of antigen-presenting cells by expressing Flt3 ligand, would prevent death of the tumor-bearing mice from distant metastasis (11, 12). Immunocompetent mice (C57Bl/6) or immunodeficient nude mice were implanted with a murine lung adenocarcinoma cell line, 3LL in one hind limb. To simulate advanced cancer, we allowed the tumor to grow to a macroscopic size for three weeks. After this the tumor was treated either by surgical removal (amputation of the hind limb) or X-irradiation (60 Gy). The test groups received injections of Flt3L for 10 days, while the control groups received saline. All C57Bl/6 mice that were treated surgically or by X-irradiation, but were not administered Flt3L died by 60 days. The survival was slightly (75 days) prolonged in mice that received Flt3L after surgical ablation of the tumor. In contrast, 55% of the mice receiving radiotherapy plus Flt3L survived long-term. The treatment protocol did not improve the survival in nude mice, indicating that the beneficial effect in the radiotherapy plus Flt3L group was immune mediated. Histological examination showed that the lungs of the mice that died had extensive metastasis, whereas the lungs of surviving mice were clear of metastasis (11). The results supported the first part of our hypothesis that slow release of tumor antigens by tumor irradiation, together with expansion of the number of APC's by Flt3L administration provides immune protection to mice from subsequent distant metastasis.

Next, we wanted to evaluate whether Flt3 ligand-enhanced immune response to tumor antigens can be augmented further by enhancing APC maturation using CD40L, following neoantigen presentation. In this series, mouse 3LL cells were implanted and the tumor implantation and radiation therapy were similar to that in the previous paragraph. In this series, Flt3L was administered daily for 12 days. From day 8-12, one group of mice received 5 daily injections of CD40L. Addition of CD40L in the therapeutic regimen increased the long-term survival of the mice to 70% (13).

Co-incubation of fluorescence-labeled bone marrow-derived, immature DCs and irradiated tumor cells revealed that irradiated tumor cells were engulfed by the DCs, followed by activation of DCs and induction of costimulatory CD86 molecules on their cell surface. Furthermore, dendritic cell maturation after incubation with irradiated HCC was demonstrated by switching of chemokine receptor expression from CCR1 to CCR7, which acts as a "homing" receptor for activated DCs and helps its migration to draining lymph nodes (14, 15).

In the final series of experiments, we asked whether radiation therapy along with Flt3L and CD40L expression could increase the survival of mice with diffuse hepatocellular carcinoma (HCC). Murine BNL1ME HCC cells were transfected with the thymidine kinase gene driven by the radiation-sensitive Egr promoter. The cells were infused into the portal vein of Balb/c mice. Fourteen days later, the mice received X-irradiation to the whole liver (HIR, 25 Gy) in a single dose (control groups did not receive irradiation). Ganciclovir, the prodrug substrate of thymidine kinase, was injected intraperitoneally once on the day of irradiation and once again two weeks later. Mice in various experimental groups received adenoviral vectors expressing Flt3L (Ad-Flet3L, one day after HIR) or CD40L (Ad-CD40L, 8 days after HIR) or both. In control groups, an irrelevant adenoviral vector, expressing *E. coli* b-galactosidase (Ad-LacZ), was injected. All untreated mice died by 35 days. Survival was improved slightly by HIR, combined with ganciclovir administration with or without Ad-LacZ administration, but all mice were dead by 65 days. Combination of ganciclovir, HIR and Ad-CD40L resulted in the long-term survival of 24% of the mice. HIR, ganciclovir and Ad-Flt3 improved the long-term survival to 44%. The best results were obtained when HIR, ganciclovir were combined with both Ad-Flt3 and Ad-CD40L administration, with 84% of the mice exhibiting long-term survival (16). Macroscopic and histological examination of the liver and lungs of the surviving mice did not show evidence of tumor persistence. The treatment regimens did not improve the survival in nude mice, indicating the involvement of the host immune system in the beneficial effect of the treatment protocol. Further evidence for the involvement of the immune system in the protective effect was obtained by measuring the secretion of cytokines characteristic of Th1 cells in response to HCC or CT26, a nonspecific cell line. Splenocytes from Balb/c mice treated with HIR, ganciclovir and Ad-Flt3L secreted higher levels of IL2, IL12 and IFNg in response to HCC than did splenocytes from mice treated with ganciclovir and Ad-Flt3L or ganciclovir and HIR. Such augmented Th1-type cytokine secretion was not found after stimulation of the splenocytes with colon cancer cells. Increased HCC-specific CTL activity was also found by ^{51}Cr release assay in the group treated with HIR, ganciclovir and Ad-Flt3L. Finally, we determined the consequence of ablating CD8+ or CD4+ cells on the protective effect of radioimmunotherapy. Pretreatment of the mice with anti-CD8 or anti-CD4 antibodies nearly abolished the beneficial effect of HIR, ganciclovir and Ad-Flt3L therapy. However, when Ad-CD40L was added to the protocol, the therapeutic benefit of the regimen was maintained despite depletion of CD4+ T cells. The results indicated that, as expected, CD8+ effecter CTLs were essential for the success of the radio-immunotherapy regimen. In this context, the CD4+ cells are necessary mainly for costimulation of mature APC's via CD40L expression. Therefore, when CD40L was overexpressed via the adenoviral vector, the requirement for the CD4+ cells was circumvented. In summary, despite, local treatment (HIR or GCV+RT), mice with diffuse hepatocellular carcinoma died because of hepatic tumor progression, peritoneal carcinomatosis and pulmonary metastasis. Stimulation of dendritic cells by Flt3L and CD40L, following local tumor irradiation cured a high percentage of mice with diffuse HCC. A protective systemic anti-tumor immune response was demonstrated after HIR and immunostimulation by Flt3L and CD40L expression.

RT is conventionally used for local tumor control. Although local control of the primary tumor can prevent development of subsequent systemic metastases, tumor radiation fails to control pre-existing systemic disease. The concept of radiation-enhanced antigen presentation allows us to exploit tumor cell death induced by RT as a potential source of tumor antigens for immunotherapy. *Immunomodulation of RT is a novel strategy of in situ tumor vaccination where primary tumor irradiation can contribute to the control of pre-existing systemic metastatic disease.* Although chemotherapy is the mainstay for the treatment of metastatic cancer, the systemic immunosuppression makes chemotherapy less desirable for immunotherapeutic regimens. The absence of systemic immunosuppression and relatively lesser toxicity makes RT a desirable adjuvant regimen for immunotherapy and tumor vaccination strategies. In conclusion, we have demonstrated an in situ autologous tumor vaccination strategy where the *radiation-enhanced tumor antigen presentation* would be an integral component of immunotherapeutic protocols for solid tumors. Since cancer is a chronic disease, induction of body's own immune system to fight distant microscopic metastatic disease would be highly beneficial in prolonging patient survival and eventual eradication of distant micrometastatic disease in cancer patients.

REFERENCE

1. Urban JL, Schreiber H. Tumor antigens. Annu Rev Immunol 1992;10:617-644.
2. Fonteneau JF, Larsson M, Bhardwaj N. Dendritic cell-dead cell interactions: implications and relevance for immunotherapy. J Immunother 2001;24:294-304.
3. Steinman RM. The dendritic cell system and its role in immunogenicity. Annu Rev Immunol 1991;9:271-296.
4. Banchereau J, Briere F, Caux C, Davoust J, Lebecque S, Liu YJ, Pulendran B, et al. Immunobiology of dendritic cells. Annu Rev Immunol 2000;18:767-811.
5. Bender A, Sapp M, Schuler G, Steinman RM, Bhardwaj N. Improved methods for the generation of dendritic cells from nonproliferating progenitors in human blood. J Immunol Methods 1996;196: 121-135.
6. Maraskovsky E, Brasel K, Teepe M, Roux ER, Lyman SD, Shortman K, McKenna HJ. Dramatic increase in the numbers of functionally mature dendritic cells in Flt3 ligand-treated mice: multiple dendritic cell subpopulations identified. J Exp Med 1996;184:1953-1962.
7. Schoenberger SP, Toes RE, van der Voort EI, Offringa R, Melief CJ. T-cell help for cytotoxic T lymphocytes is mediated by CD40-CD40L interactions [see comments]. Nature 1998;393:480-483.
8. Albert ML, Pearce SF, Francisco LM, Sauter B, Roy P, Silverstein RL, Bhardwaj N. Immature dendritic cells phagocytose apoptotic cells via alphavbeta5 and CD36, and cross-present antigens to cytotoxic T lymphocytes. J Exp Med 1998;188:1359-1368.
9. Harshyne LA, Watkins SC, Gambotto A, Barratt-Boyes SM. Dendritic cells acquire antigens from live cells for cross-presentation to CTL. J Immunol 2001;166:3717-3723.
10. Heath WR, Carbone FR. Cross-presentation, dendritic cells, tolerance and immunity. Annu Rev Immunol 2001;19:47-64.
11. Chakravarty PK, Alfieri A, Thomas EK, Beri V, Tanaka KE, Vikram B, Guha C. Flt3-ligand administration after radiation therapy prolongs survival in a murine model of metastatic lung cancer. Cancer Res 1999;59:6028-6032.

12. Chakravarty PK, Guha C, Alfieri A, Beri V, Niazova Z, Deb NJ, Fan Z, et al. Flt3L Therapy following Localized Tumor Irradiation Generates Long-Term Protective Immune Response in Metastatic Lung Cancer: Its Implication in Designing a Vaccination Strategy. Oncology 2006;70:245-254.

13. Chakravarty PK, Guha C, Alfieri A, Deb NJ, Thomas EK, Vikram B. CD40L alone or in combination with Flt3L following localized radiation therapy increases animal survival in metastatic lung cancer. AACR Proceedings 2002;43:2867A.

14. Sozzani S, Allavena P, D'Amico G, Luini W, Bianchi G, Kataura M, Imai T, et al. Differential regulation of chemokine receptors during dendritic cell maturation: a model for their trafficking properties. J Immunol 1998;161:1083-1086.

15. Sallusto F, Palermo B, Lenig D, Miettinen M, Matikainen S, Julkunen I, Forster R, et al. Distinct patterns and kinetics of chemokine production regulate dendritic cell function. Eur J Immunol 1999;29:1617-1625.

16. Kawashita Y, Deb NJ, Garg M, Fan Z, Alfieri AA, Shah SJ, Chakravarty PK, et al. A novel therapeutic strategy for hepatocellular carcinoma: Immunomodulation by Flt3-Ligand (Flt3L) following whole liver irradiation and radio-inducible HSV-TK gene therapy. Int J Radiat Oncol Biol Phys 2001;51:189A.

17

CHAPTER

Cancer Immunoediting: Professional Editorship by Neem Leaf Glycoprotein

A. Bose, K. Chakraborty, K. Sarkar, S. Goswami, T. Chakrabory, E. Haque, D. Ghosh, I. Mandal-Ghosh, S. Pal[1], S. Laskar[2], U. Chattopadhyay[3] and R. N. Baral

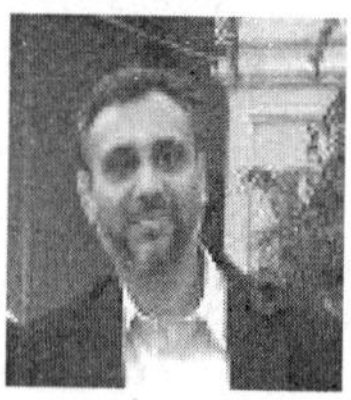

Departmant of Immunoregulation and Immunodiagnostics,
[1]Unit of Clinical Biochemistry,
Chittaranjan National Cancer Institute (CNCI),
37, S. P. Mukherjee Road, Kolkata 700026;
[2]Department of Chemistry, Burdwan University, Burdwan
[3]B. C. Guha Center for Genetic Engineering and Biotechnology,
University of Calcutta, 35 Ballygunge Circular Road, Kolkata- 700019.

INTRODUCTION

The term cancer denotes several types of diseases, having a common property of metastasis. Discovery of several modalities of treatment definitely help in clinical improvement of cancerous diseases, however, complete cure is still dream of oncologists. Multiple etiology, difficulty of selective drug targeting of cancer cells, failure of available treatment to restrict tumor metastasis are few reasons among many. Irrespective of cancer, immune dysfunction is a common experience. Immune system reacts extensively against carcinogenic threat, failure results partial or complete paralysis of it and allows progression of the cancerous diseases. These immune errors are intensified during cancer treatment and make these patients severely immunocompromised. To combat these situations editing of immune errors associated with cancer is very important before treatment, at the time of treatment and after treatment.

In our experience to work with a preparation of neem leaf, we are surprised to see the professional editorship of this neem preparation. In this presentation, some experience with neem in relation to cancer will be shared with eminent immunologists, oncologists and nature lovers with good faith on Indian natural resources. Neem is a plant with versatile bioproperties. It's application in medicine is well recognized in Indian subcontinent from Vedic period and known as 'Sarboroganibarani' (the plant can cure almost all sorts of diseases). Reality behind this myth is experienced by Indian community. Still this plant received comparatively less interest as a subject of scientific research to unreveal the truth behind the common experience. Experience with neem is rightly blended with our everyday's life, as we used it in dental care (commonly known as dantan), in skin care, in maintenance of cloths, in pest control etc. Selection of neem as a professional editor was based on my childhood friendship with this plant and subsequently, my group members extended their faith. Nontoxic nature, availability and cost-effectivenes of this plant is doubtless, however, its bio-action in relation to cancer need to be scientifically established. Our ayurveda gave enough knowledge on this plant, however, modern scientific research was insufficient to prove our faith with scientific evidences. Although eight parts of the plant neem has unique medicinal applications, the leaf was selected based on its easy availability. An aqueous preparation was prepared from these leaves, termed as neem leaf preparation (NLP) and our journey with neem was started with this NLP.

Results and Discussion

NLP is active to restrict the tumor growth

As an initial experiment of our venture with neem, we have taken two groups of mice. One group received NLP, whereas, control group got PBS only. After completion of the treatment protocol, both groups of mice were inoculated with murine carcinoma. Significant restriction of tumor growth was noticed in NLP group. Same observation was obtained when mice were inoculated with melanoma after similar NLP treatment (Baral and Chattopadhyay, 2004).

NLP mediated tumor growth restriction is due to immune activation

Several cancer cell lines in culture were treated with different doses of NLP. However, no cancer cells could be killed by NLP as detected by MTT cytotoxicity assay (Baral and Chattopadhyay, 2004) and AnnexinV-Propidium iodide based apoptosis assay (Bose et al, 2007). Use of NLP in mouse demonstrated few basic changes in their physiological system, prompted us to concentrate on immune system (Baral and Chattopadhyay, 2004). Adoptive transfer of immune cells from NLP treated mice to a group of normal mice resulted significant tumor growth restriction and confirmed the involvement of NLP activated immune system in tumor growth restriction (Haque and Baral, 2006).

A glycoprotein present in NLP may be the active principle

The work with neem was started with an aqueous preparation of neem leaf, termed neem leaf preparation (NLP). We have identified a glycoprotein in this NLP and this neem leaf glycoprotein (NLGP) is responsible for tumor growth restricting and other immunomodulatory functions. Experiments performed with either NLP or NLGP, demonstrated almost similar results. NLGP present within NLP is responsible for NLP induced tumor growth restriction was proved by exposing NLGP into adverse temperature, pH and proteolytic enzymes. In these three conditions tumor growth restricting function of NLP was completely abolished. NLGP is partially characterized and several things need to be further explored on its character.

NLGP and its native form NLP are immunogenic and generated antibody was reactive with NLP as well as carcinoembryonic antigen (Sarkar et al, 2007). Molecular immunology behind this observation is yet to be explored.

NLGP activates various immune cells, except regulatory T cells

Significant upregulation in number of $CD3^+$, $CD8^+$ T cells, $CD56^+$, $CD16^+$ NK cells, $CD14^+$ monocytes/macrophages and $CD3^+CD56^+$ NKT cells from HNSCC patients was noted upon *in vitro* stimulation of PBMC with NLGP. The transformation from naïve to memory phenotype of T cells by NLGP is evidenced by higher expression of the early activation marker CD69, upregulation of CD45RO expression with a simultaneous down regulation of CD45RA and L-selectin (CD62L). NLGP downregulates $CD4^+CD25^+FoxP3^+$ regulatory T cells, having suppressor functions.

NLGP maintains Th1/Th2 balance

NLGP induces higher secretion of Th1 cytokines, IFNg, IL-12 and TNFa, and decreases the release of Th2 cytokines IL-4 and IL-10 from murine and human MNCs. NLGP upregulates the total intracellular glutathione content and nitric oxide release of adherent cells. Moreover, NLGP enhances the total IgG pool with IgG2a as a dominant subclass. NLGP upregulates the expression of T box transcription factor T-bet. These evidences suggest that NLGP may be effective to maintain normal immune homeostasis by upregulating Th1 response in immunosupressed host.

NLGP enhances natural cytotoxicity of immune cells

NLGP helps in the restoration of suppressed killing activity of PBMC from HNSCC patients towards oral (KB), breast (MCF7), colon (COLO-205 & HT-29), leukemia (Jurkat), lymphoma (U937) and erythroleukemia (K562) cell lines. This cytotoxicity is principally associated with perforin-granzyme dependent cytolytic mechinary. Interestingly, NLGP stimulates both T cell and NK cell mediated tumor cell cytotoxicity. However, T cell mediated cytotoxicity is IFNg dependent, whereas, same of NK cell is dependent on IL-12 (Bose and Baral, 2007).

NLP mediated immune stimulation may be used for tumor antigen specific vaccine

In association of the examination of NLP as a nonspecific prophylactic vaccine, we have also tested it as an adjuvant for antigen specific vaccine. In our effort to examine NLP as an adjuvant along with three antigenic systems, namely, carcinoembryonic antigen (CEA), B16melanoma surface antigen (B16MelSAg) (Baral et al, 2005) and breast tumor associated antigen (BTAA) (Mandal-Ghosh et al, 2007), we have observed significant enhancement of the antibody response against specific antigen, when NLP was added with antigen in immunization protocol. These NLP generated antigen specific immunity are active to participate in antitumor immunity as detected by in vitro and in vivo assays. Results showed equal efficacy of NLP with other adjuvants, like, Freunds' oil preparation (Baral et al, 2005) and aluminium hydroxide preparation. First one is toxic for human use and next one can stimulate the humoral immunity only. Thus, NLP might be a better choice as an adjuvant. Comparative studies of NLP with other adjuvants like QS-21 and CpG oligodeoxynucleotide would give better insight on the use of NLP as an adjuvant.

Associated functions of NLP to act as an adjuvant

NLP/NLGP helps in maturation and functioning of professional antigen presenting cells, like, macrophages and dendritic cells. These cells participate in presentation of antigens to either B cells or T cells to achieve antibody production and cytotoxic T lymphocyte (CTL) generating functions. NLP actively participate in CTL generation by stimulating MHC class-I molecules and inducing strong interaction between cytotoxic T cells and APCs by CD28 and CD80/86 crosstalk. We have detected the enhanced secretion of IFNg and IL-12 in this NLP/NLGP linked immunization protocol. This Th1 type immune response definitely has some role in antibody production and induction of antigen specific antitumor immunity.

Other NLGP Induced Immune Mechanisms

For the induction of anti-tumor immunity in optimum level, it is important to move immune cells at the tumor site and reduction of the number as well as functioning of the suppressor regulatory T cells. NLGP is efficient to control this countercurrent, although, mechanism is still unknown. NLP downregulates the $CD4^+CD25^+FoxP3^+$ T Reg cells and by inhibiting CCR4 expression, restricts their movement at tumor site. On the otherhand, NLGP induces the CXC chemokines IP-10/MIG and regulates the balance between two CXCR3 splice variants CXCR3A and CXCR3B (Chakraborty et al, 2008). These immune functions help migration of the NLGP activated immune cells at tumor site to induce cytotoxic reactions either NK mediated or CTL mediated.

CONCLUSION

Above mentioned experiments demonstrated professional editorship by NLP/NLGP to correct errors occasionally found in cancerous diseases. Action of NLP/NLGP in cancer immunoregulation is summarized in figure 17.1. It is effective to combat the both cancer associated and chemotherapy

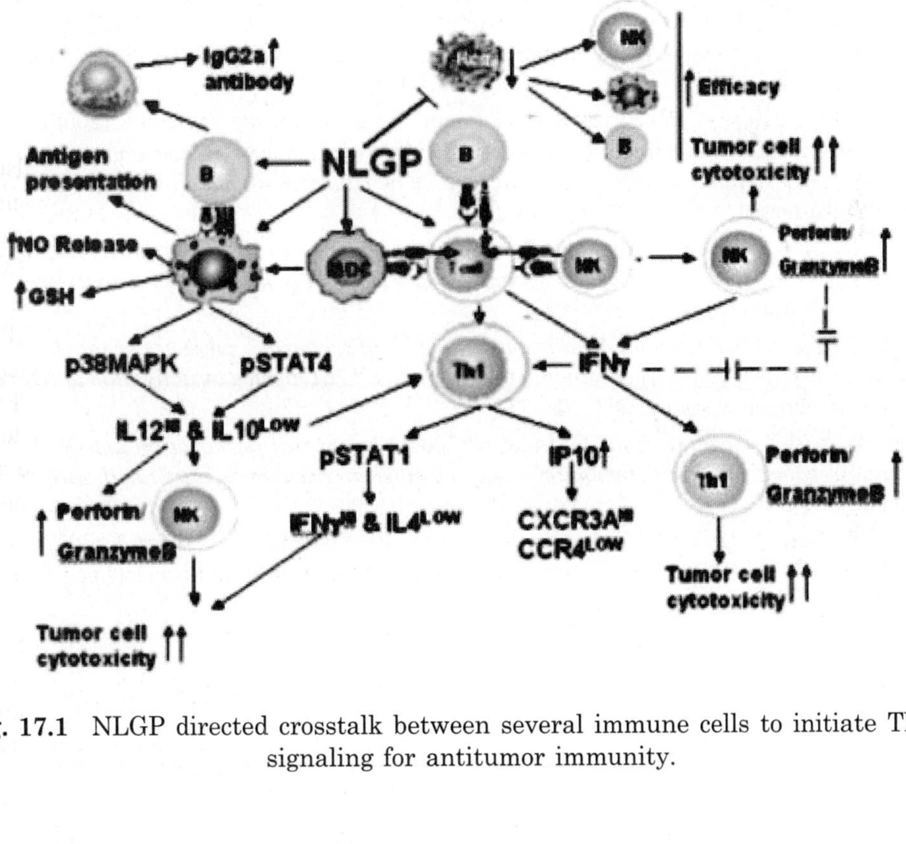

Fig. 17.1 NLGP directed crosstalk between several immune cells to initiate Th1/Tc1 signaling for antitumor immunity.

induced immunosuppression. We have specifically examined the role of NLP in overcoming cyclophosphamide (Ghosh et al, 2006) and cisplatin+5-fluorouracil induced leukepenia in tumor free and tumor bearing mice. These observations have several implications in developing various forms of immunotherapeutic regimens as a prophylactic or therapeutic vaccines of cancer. Again, these vaccines may work in nonspecific and antigen specific manner (Baral RN, 2005) to restrict the tumor growth. Preclinical and clinical studies are required to test possibilities of this vaccine for human neoplastic diseases.

REFERENCES

1. Baral R, Chattopadhyay U (2004) *Neem (Azadirachta indica) leaf mediated immune activation causes prophylactic growth inhibition of murine Ehrlich carcinoma and B16 melanoma*. Int Immunopharmacol, 4, 355-366.
2. Baral RN (2005) *Tumor Vaccine: Current trends in antigen specific immunotherapy*. Ind J Exp Biol, 43, 389-406.
3. Baral R, Mandal I, Chattopadhyay U (2005) *Immunostimulatory neem leaf preparation acts as an adjuvant to enhance the efficacy of poorly immunogenic B16 melanoma surface antigen vaccine*. Int Immunopharmacol, 5, 1343-1352.
4. Bose A, Haque E, Baral R (2007) *Neem leaf preparation induces apoptosis of tumor cells by releasing cytotoxic cytokines from human peripheral blood mononuclear cells*. Phytother Res, 21, 914-920.
5. Bose A, Baral R (2007). *NK cellular cytotoxicity of tumor cells initiated by neem leaf preparation is associated with CD40-CD40L mediated endogenous production of IL-12*. Human Immunol, 68, 823-831.
6. Chakraborty K, Bose A, Pal S, Sarkar K, Goswami S, Chattopadhyay U, Baral R (2008). *Neem leaf glycoprotein restores the impaired chemotactic activity of peripheral blood mononuclear cells from head and neck squamous cell carcinoma patients by maintaining CXCR3/CXCL10 balance*. Int Immunopharmacol, 8, 330-340.
7. Ghosh D, Bose A, Haque E, Baral R (2006). *Pretreatment with neem (Azadirachta indica) leaf preparation in swiss mice diminishes leukopenia and enhances the antitumor activity of cyclophosphamide*. Phytother Res, 20, 814-818.
8. Haque E, Baral R (2006). *Neem (Azadirachta indica) leaf preparation induces prophylactic growth inhibition of murine Ehrlich carcinoma in Swiss and C57BL/6 mice by activation of NK cells and NK-T cells*. Immunobiology, 211, 721-731.
9. Mandal-Ghosh I, Chattopadhyay U, Baral R (2007). *Neem leaf preparation enhances Th1 type immune response and anti-tumor immunity against breast tumor associated antigen*. Cancer Immunity, 7, 8-17.
10. Sarkar K, Bose A, Laskar S, Choudhuri SK, Dey S, Roychowdhury PK, Baral R (2007). *Antibody response against neem leaf preparation recognizes carcinoembryonic antigen*. Int Immunopharmacol, 7, 306-312.

18

CHAPTER

Suppression of Suppressors: Neem Leaf Glycoprotein Guided Crosstalk between Regulatory T Cells and T Cells/Nk Cells/ Macrophages in Cancer

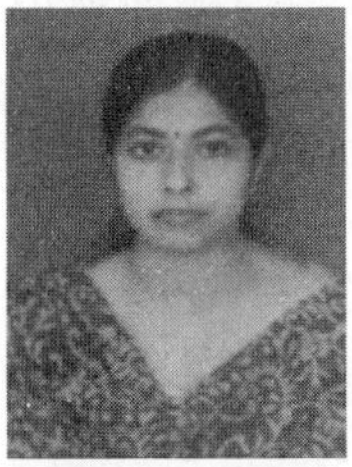

T. Chakrabory, A. Bose, K. Chakraborty, K. Sarkar, S. Goswami, D. Ghosh, S. Pal[1], S. Laskar[2] and R.N. Baral

Departmant of Immunoregulation and Immunodiagnostics, [1]Unit of Clinical Biochemistry, Chittaranjan National Cancer Institute (CNCI), 37, S. P. Mukherjee Road, Kolkata 700026; [2]Department of Chemistry, Burdwan University, Burdwan

INTRODUCTION

Excellent defense system of our body fails sometime and promotes the occurrence of cancer, the phenomena known as tumor escape (Hung *et al*, 2002). The warriors of cancer defense are different immune responsive cells, *viz.*, T cells, NK cells, macrophages, antigen presenting cells (APCs) like dendritic cells etc (Zou, 2006). Often activity of these cells is impaired due to suppressive activity of regulatory T cells (T-Reg), also known as Suppressor T cells (Zou, 2006). The classical T-Reg cells are $CD4^+$ $CD25^+$ and constitutively express CCR4 and CTLA4 on their surface. CCR4 helps T-Reg cells to migrate at the tumor site, where CCL22, the ligand of CCR4, is highly expressed. CTLA4 are responsible for generating negative signaling to other cells like T cells, NK cells and several professional and nonprofessional APCs to suppress, inactivate and also for killing them (Zou, 2006). Another important intracellular marker of T-Reg cells is FoxP3 (Sakaguchi, 2005), which is a transcription factor essential for development, maturation and activation of T-Reg cells.

The normal function of T-Reg is to maintain peripheral tolerance against self antigen reactive T cells (Sakaguchi, 2005). They perform this task by suppressing the activity of T cells and other professional antigen presenting cells that have too high avidity towards self antigens. So their presence and activity in normal body is very much essential. Deficiency in their function in body causes several autoimmune diseases (Sakaguchi, 2005). On the other hand, as some of the tumor antigens are self antigens the over expression and function of T-Reg cells creates serious challenge in efficacy of tumor therapy as they offer a favorable microenvironment for tumor evasion and tumor development by negatively interfering with the immune responses of these anti-tumor cells (Zou, 2006). Maintenance of a balance of their number and function is therefore very important to increase the efficiency of cancer treatment. Finding an immunomodulator that can suppress the suppressive activity of T-Reg cells in cancer condition is therefore very essential.

Our laboratory is working on neem leaf preparation for a couple of years. Immunomodulation (Haque and Baral, 2006; Bose and Baral, 2007) and cancer immunoprophylaxis (Baral and Chattopadhyay, 2004) by nontoxic preparation of neem leaf (Haque et al, 2006), which is recently characterized as a glycoprotein (Chakraborty et al, 2008), was previously reported from our laboratory. It was also clearly suggested by studies utilizing adoptive cell transfer technology and several in vitro assays that neem leaf component(s) may be responsible for activation of various immunocompetent cells, including T, NK/NK-T cells, macrophages, dendritic cells, those are occasionally suppressed in cancer condition (Haque and Baral, 2006; Bose and Baral, 2007). Moreover, it optimally regulates the secretion of an array of cytokines (Bose and Baral, 2007) and chemokines (Chakraborty et al, 2008). In the context of these reported findings, here, we have attempted to elucidate the role of neem leaf glycoprotein (NLGP) in regulation of the homeostasis of T-Reg cells in cancer.

Results and Discussion

Enhanced T-Reg Population in Cancer Can be Downregulated by NLGP

$CD4^+CD25^+FoxP3^+$ T-Reg cells are upregulated in cancer, specifically at the site of tumor and seriously interferes with the normal functions of several immunocompetent cells. Using head and neck squamous cell carcinoma (HNSCC) as a model, we have also found that these T-Reg cells are increased in the circulation of patients. Creation of a tumor microenvironment in vitro generates T-Reg cells too with significant upregulation in the transcription factor FoxP3. FoxP3 negatively interacts with nuclear factor for activation of T cells (NFAT), which is responsible for the T cell activation (Tone *et al.*, 2007). Accordingly, T cell activation and function is seriously hampered. NLGP significantly downregulates T-Reg cells, especially expression of FoxP3 as detected in protein and mRNA level. This downregulation withdraws the inhibitory effect of FoxP3 on NFAT to enhance the T cell functions, including cytotoxicity and cytokine secretion.

T-Reg Mediated Suppression of Immune Cellular Function is Reversed by NLGP

We have observed earlier that NLGP can activate T cells, macrophages and NK cells, principally monitored by expression of early activation marker CD69 and secretion of IFN?. NLGP stimulated

T cells, macrophages and NK cells are able to kill more number of tumor cells as tested in vitro. Magnetic bead separated T-Reg cells inhibit these functions of immune cells, including diminished tumor cell cytotoxicity. Supplementation of NLGP in these cultures withdraws suppressive activities of T-Reg cells on various immune cells. These cells become more cytotoxic to tumor cells and secretes optimum amount of IFN?. NLGP may regulate other immune functions in presence of T-Reg cells, which is yet to be disclosed. Mechanism of NLGP action on T-Reg cells is not known yet, however, we may propose a hypothesis in light of the antigen presentation. NLGP activates APCs (macrophages and dendritic cells) and upregulates expression of co-stimulatory molecules, like, CD80, CD86 and enhances CD28 expression on T cells. At the sametime NLGP downregulates the upregulated intracellular expression of CTLA4. These NLGP regulated events promote cytotoxicity and other functions of T cells. These T cell functions again assisted by antigen presenting functions of NLGP matured dendritic cells. This maturation process is hampered in tumor microenvironment and dendritic cells release IDO (Indoleamine 2, 3-dioxygenase) and PDLs (programmed death ligands) to promote T-Reg functions and causes T cell anergy.

T-Reg Mediated Suppression of Cytokine Secretion is Reversed by NLGP

Our experience with HNSCC suggests the suppression in secretion of IFNg/IL-12 and enhancement of IL-10. In the creation of this situation, T-Reg cells have prominent role, as we observed addition of these suppressor cells in normal immune cell culture causes creation of same situation producing low IFN?/IL-12 and high IL-10. Interestingly, this abnormal situation could be controlled NLGP to create cytokine homeostasis. This effect become prominent due to removal of T-Reg cells from the system, proving the prominent role of T-Reg in cancer associated immunosuppression. TGFβ is another important cytokine in this scenario (Zou, 2006). Unfortunately, TGFβ is yet to be included in our experimental protocol. NLGP may initiate suppression of the T-Reg functions by creating physiological cytokine homeostasis.

NLGP Restricts the Movement of T-Reg Cells at Tumor site

Leukocyte infiltration at tumor site is very common experience of cancer histopathologists. Recent studies indicated that T-Reg cells are predominant within this tumor infiltrating leukocytes/lymphocytes. This traffic by principally guided by CCL22, which transduce its signal through the receptor CCR4. Upregulated expression of CCR4 was noticed in cancer (Zou, 2006), which could be downregulated by NLGP. Data obtained from chemotaxis assay suggests that tumor condition inhibits the movement of leucocytes in Boyden's chamber and this restricted movement is propagated by NLGP. This propogation is possibly by NLGP mediated inhibition of CCL22/CCR4. However, this hypothesis is yet to be confirmed.

CONCLUSION

Results of our preliminary study suggests that T-Reg might hold the central position of cancer associated immunosuppression. Downregulation of the number of T-Reg cells in circulation and tumor site by NLGP might be a good effort for cancer immunotherapy. Inhibition of their function and migration at tumor site by NLGP utilizing different mechanisms would enhance the efficacy of various immunocompetent cells to destruct tumor cells.

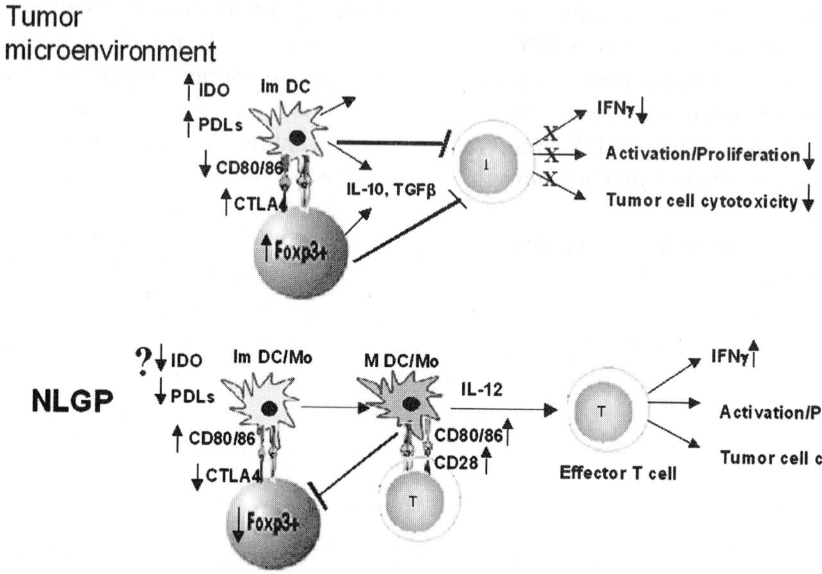

Fig. 18.1 FoxP3+ T-Reg cell mediated dysfunction of T cell activities in tumor microenvironment and possible role of NLGP in rectification of these dysfunctions. Im DC, immature DC; M DC, mature DC; Mo, macrophages; IDO, Indoleamine 2, 3-dioxygenase; PDLs, programmed death ligands

REFERENCES

1. Baral R, Chattopadhyay U (2004) *Neem (Azadirachta indica) leaf mediated immune activation causes prophylactic growth inhibition of murine Ehrlich carcinoma and B16 melanoma.* Int Immunopharmacol, **4**, 355-366.
2. Bose A, Baral R (2007). *NK cellular cytotoxicity of tumor cells initiated by neem leaf preparation is associated with CD40-CD40L mediated endogenous production of IL-12.* Human Immunol, **68**, 823-831.
3. Chakraborty K, Bose A, Pal S, Sarkar K, Goswami S, Chattopadhyay U, Baral R (2008). *Neem leaf glycoprotein restores the impaired chemotactic activity of peripheral blood mononuclear cells from head and neck squamous cell carcinoma patients by maintaining CXCR3/CXCL10 balance.* Int Immunopharmacol, **8**, 330-340.
4. Haque E, Mandal I, Pal S, Baral R (2006). *Prophylactic dose of neem (Azadirachta indica) leaf preparation restricting murine tumor growth is nontoxic, hematostimulatory and immunostimulatory.* Immunopharmacol Immunotoxicol, **28**, 1-18.
5. Haque E, Baral R (2006). *Neem (Azadirachta indica) leaf preparation induces prophylactic growth inhibition of murine Ehrlich carcinoma in Swiss and C57BL/6 mice by activation of NK cells and NK-T cells.* Immunobiology, **211**, 721-731.

6. Hung TK , Nicholas PR (2002). *Natural selection of tumor variants in the generation of "tumor escape" phenotypes.* Nat Immunol, **3**, 999–1005.

7. Sakaguchi S (2005).*Naturally arising Foxp3-expressing CD25+CD4+ regulatory T cells in immunological tolerance to self and non-self.* Nat Immunol, **6**, 345-352.

8. Tone Y, Furuuchi K, Kojima Y, Tykocinski ML, Greene MI Tone M (2007) *Smad3 and NFAT cooperate to induce Foxp3 expression through its enhancer*, Nat Immunol. (Epub ahead of print, December 23).

9. Zou W (2006). *Regulatory T cells, tumor immunity and immunotherapy*. Nature Reviews/Immunology, **6**, 295-360.

19

CHAPTER

Mycobacterium Indicus Pranii Vaccine (Mw) in Cancers

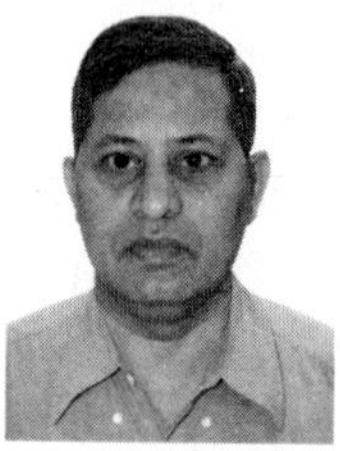

Bakulesh Khamar

Director Research, Cadila Pharmaceuticals Ltd., Ahmedabad

INTRODUCTION

Immuvac is a novel therapeutic agent available commercially in India since 1998. It contains heat killed (autoclaved) Mycobacterium Indicus pranii.(Mycobacterium w, Mw). It shares antigens with *M. tuberculosis* and *M. leprae*[1-3]

Mw has following unique feature.

(a) It elicits Th1 response and does not elicit Th2 response.

(b) It elicits increased Th1 response on increase of the dose but does not elicit Th2 response even on higher dosage as well as on repeated administration.

(c) It is a potent activator of macrophages. This can be demonstrated even in normal healthy individuals.

(d) Its action seems to be universal and not limited by-to species or strain. i.e. it provides protection against tuberculosis in animals where inof different genetic strains. Whereas BCG is effective in (BALB/C BYJ and C57BC/6N strains6N strains of mice,) Mw protects all the 4 strains against H37Rv, C3H/He and CBA/N strain of the mice (16).

(e) The major part of its effect comes from CD4 cells. CD8 (Cytotoxic T) cells also participate. Elimination of CD4 as well as CD8 cells results in elimination of the effects.

(f) It is possible to transfer the induced effect by transfer of immune cells to syngenic animals.

(g) Systemic side effects typically seen with other products are not seen even with significantly higher dose of Mw.

(h) It induces immune responses:

Immune mechanisms play an important role in maintenance of health. They are divided into humoral mechanisms & cell mediated mechanisms. Humoral mechanisms are responsible for protection against majority of acute infectious diseases. They provide protection by generating antibodies against antigens from pathogens. Administration of prophylactic vaccines raises antibody titers and provides protection. Disease like Cancer, Tuberculosis, Leprosy, HIV etc are associated with poor cell mediated immunity and have immune deviation with decreased Th1 type response and increased Th2 type response. Restoration and invigoration of Th1 response seems to be responsible for therapeutic effects with Mw seen in diseases like Cancer, Tuberculosis and Leprosy.

IN VITRO STUDIES (NON IMMUNOLOGICAL)

Mw kills cancer cells at a significantly lower concentration. The effect begins around 4 hours and is over by 12 hours. The death is through apoptosis. The effect is demonstrated against varieties of cell lines, e.g. breast cancer, leukemia, pancreatic cancer, prostrate cancer et al. (Figure 19.1)

Mw is also synergistic to chemotherapy agents. The cytotoxic drugs like Gemcitabine and 5-Fluorouracil when used along with Mw demonstrate synergistic activity. (Fig.19.2)

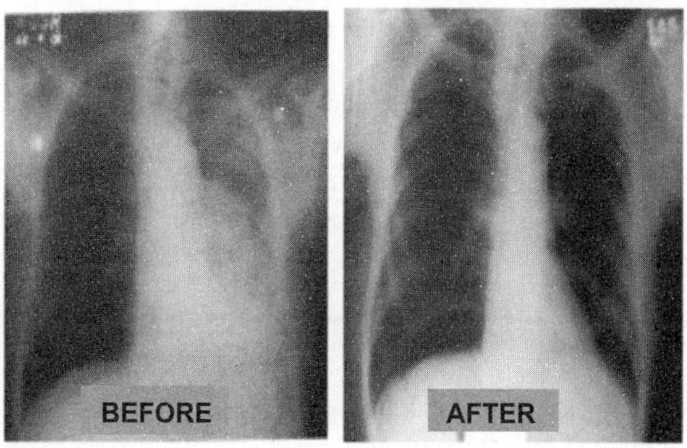

Fig. 19.1

IN VIVO - ANIMAL STUDIES

Immunization with Mw protects animals from developing myeloma. It is also effective when used as a therapy following induction of tumor. The protection is seen only when Mw is given intradermally and is not seen when it is given intraperitoneally. (Personal communication from Dr. Dipankar Nandi, Indian Institute of Science Bangalore).

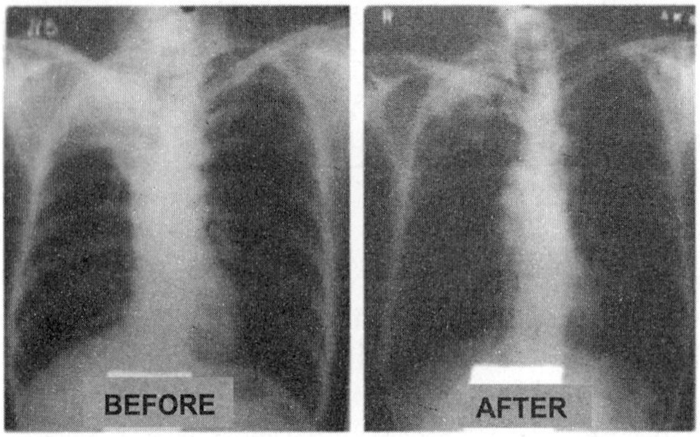

Fig. 19.2

Similarly it delays metastasis to lungs in aggressive mouse melanoma model (Intravenous injection). There is also significant improvemet of survival. (Personal communication from Dr. Gavin P.Robertson, PennState College of Medicine, USA).

HUMAN CLINICAL STUDIES

(a) Mw alone: Monotherapy

(i) Improvement in quality of life and symptoms in Head and Neck cancers [9]

In a prospective single arm study, Mw was evaluated for its effects on quality of life and symptomsas a palliative therapy. Mw (0.1 ml containing $0.5X10^9$ autoclaved bacilli each) was injected intradermally with all aseptic precautions. Four injections, weekly and later on four injections monthly (0.1 ml each) were given. Patients were followed up for 6 months. There was no major side effect. 27% patients had pain relief. Symptom control was seen in 15% patients. Improvement in quality of life was observed in 82% of patients. 4% of patients had no effect. The beneficial effect lasted for three months in 27% patients and more than six months in 13% patients. The effect was more marked in dysphagia, ulcer and fistula. Effect was insignificant in strider, change in voice and metastatic nodes. Four patients are alive and symptom free for more than one year.

CONCLUSIONS

Immunotherapy with Mw can safely be used to improve quality of life and control of symptoms in terminally ill patients with Head & Neck cancer.

(ii) Use of Immunomodulater Mw vaccine for Palliative Treatment in advanced & incurable cancer patients [10]

In another study Mw was evaluated for its effect on tumor size, symptoms, and quality of life in 100 patients of advanced cases of carcinoma. The inclusion criteria were positive biopsy of malignancy, measurable disease, and patients at an advanced stage,where all available established treatments had been given, and cancer has been confirmed to be incurable by a team of oncologists with life expectancy of more than two months. Intradermal 0.1ml Mw was

7. Fotedar A, Mehra NK, Mustafa AS, Talwar GP.Local reactions to intradermal instillation of *Mw* and ICRC bacilli in mice.Lepr India. 1978; 50(4):520-33.

8. Prasad HK, Singh AK, Talwar GP.Ability of M. leprae, *Mw* and ICRC bacillus to produce macrophage activating factors from lymphocytes of leprosy patients. Lepr India. 1978; 50(4):539-49.

9. R. I. Dave, U. B. Tripathi, B. J. Parikh, K. M. Patel, H. K. Shukla_Improvement in quality of life and symptom control with Mw (CADI-05) in head and neck cancer. *Journal of Clinical Oncology*, 2007 ASCO Annual Meeting Proceedings Part I. Vol 25, No. 18S, 2007: 21186

10. R. I. Dave, S. V. Shah, K. M. Patel, U. B. Tripathi, A. S. Kapadia, H. P. Panchal.Use of Immunomodulater Mw vaccine for Palliative Treatment in advanced & incurable cancer patients *Journal of Clinical Oncology*, 2005 ASCO Annual Meeting Proceedings. Vol 23, No. 16S, Part I of II, 2005: 2592

11. R. I. Dave, U. Tripathi, S. Shah, K. M. Patel. Poly TLR agonist polyantigenic vaccine (Mw) in palliative therapy of head and neck cancer. *Journal of Clinical Oncology*, 2006 ASCO Annual Meeting Proceedings Part I. Vol 24, No. 18S, 2006: 12512

12. Chaudhuri P, Mukhopadhyay S .Bladder preserving approach for muscle invasive bladder cancer—role of Mw. J Indian Med Assoc. 2003;101(9):559-60.

13. M. C. Pant, R. Hadi, R. Prasad, D. Dalela, R. Pant, D. Parmar, M. Srivastava, S. Parikh. Role of immuno-therapy as a adjuvant treatment in advance head & neck cancer, patient receiving chemo radiotherapy. *Journal of Clinical Oncology*, 2005 ASCO Annual Meeting Proceedings. Vol 23, No. 16S, Part I of II, 2005: 2598

14. S. K. Sarkar, C. Dasgupta. Role of Mw as an adjuvant treatment of Head & Neck Cancer—A Randomized trial *Journal of Clinical Oncology*, 2005 ASCO Annual Meeting Proceedings. Vol 23, No. 16S, Part I of II, 2005: 5588

15. Sur PK, Dastidar AG.Role of Mw as adjuvant treatment of lung cancer (non-small cell lung cancer).J Indian Med Assoc. 2003; 101(2):118, 120

16. Singh IG, Mukherjee R, Talwar GP. Resistance to intravenous innoculation of *Mycobacterium tuberculosis* H37Rv in mice of different inbred strains following immunization with a leprosy vaccine based on Mycobacterium w. Vaccine 1991;9,10-14.

17. G.P. Talwar et al. Leprosy in India, 1978, 50; 492-598.

18. G.P.Talwar. An immunotherapeutic vaccine for multibacillary Leprosy. Intern. Rev. Immunol. 1999; 18;229-249.

20
CHAPTER

Biology of Head and Neck Cancer Metastasis

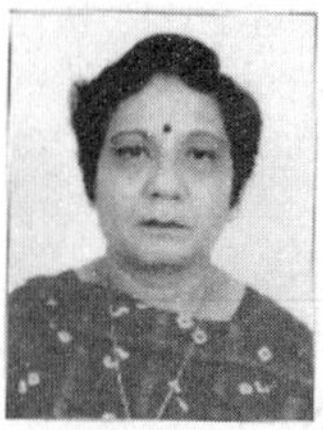

Ranju Ralhan and Jatinder Kaur

Department of Biochemistry, All India Institute of Medical Sciences, Ansari Nagar, New Delhi 110016

ABSTRACT

Advances in treatment of head and neck/oral squamous cell carcinoma (HNOSCC) have not been successful in significantly improving its prognosis over the past three decades. There is an urgent need for novel, more effective therapies to prevent relapse, control metastases and improve overall survival of HNOSCC patients. Recent investigations have provided insights into the mechanisms of cellular adhesion, invasion, and angiogenesis-key processes involved in metatstasis. The detection of metastatic signatures in primary tumors by genomic and proteomic analyses has facilitated understanding of the biology of HNOSCC metastasis and opened new avenues toward their molecular diagnosis and prognosis. Current trials looking at sentinel node mapping may allow evaluation of the nodal status of early HNOSCC and identify a subset of patients at risk for distant metastasis. Improved understanding of HNOSCC biology will also lead to introduction of molecularly targeted treatment strategies for more effective management of these cancers.

INTRODUCTION

Head and neck/oral squamous cell carcinoma (HNOSCC) accounts for over 600,000 cases worldwide annually and is the sixth most common cause of cancer deaths (1). Often more than 50% of all HNOSCC patients have advanced disease at the time of diagnosis. Despite multimodality therapy including surgery, radiation, and chemotherapy, the five-year survival rate of HNOSCC patients is poor, less than 50% (2). This is primarily because patients continue to die from metastatic disease at regional and distant sites, though loco-regional recurrence and second primary tumors are also causes of death in these patients. The treatment of late stage HNOSCC can be very devastating, associated with disfigurement, psychosomatic problems and poor quality of life in survivors. The most reliable prognostic indicator of regional and distant treatment failure for HNOSCC patients is the presence of metastasis in cervical lymph nodes (3-7), though a high rate of occult nodal metastasis (20-40%) is observed in patients with squamous cell carcinoma of tongue (SCCOT) with no evidence of regional spread on clinical or radiological evaluation (reviewed in 7). Recent developments in DNA microarray and proteomic technologies have led to the identification of metastatic signatures in primary HNOSCCs and facilitated understanding of the functions of metastasis-related proteins involved in adhesion, invasion, dissemination, and survival, and defining the appropriate biomarkers and targets for the treatment of this disease.

HEAD AND NECK CARCINOGENESIS

The development of head and neck cancer is a tobacco related multistep and multifocal process involving field cancerization and intraepithelial clonal spread (Figure 20.1). Several epigenetic, genetic and metabolic alterations resulting from exposure to tobacco carcinogens, alcohol or human papilloma virus have been identified in the multistep process of head and neck carcinogenesis. These have been extensively reviewed by us and others and thus will not be described here (8-12).

BIOLOGY OF METASTASIS

Metastasis, the spread of cancer from the site of primary tumor growth to distant organs, is a leading cause of cancer morbidity and mortality. The metastastic process is very complex and it's genetic and biochemical determinants remain incompletely understood in most cancers, including head and neck cancer. The process of metastasis requires generation of new blood and lymph vessels (lymphangiogenesis), invasion from the primary tumor involving breakdown of the extra-cellular matrix (ECM), escape from immune surveillance, intravasation, survival, arrest and extravasation of the circulatory system, transport to other sites with adhesion, subsequent invasion of the organ that hosts the metastasis, and tumor proliferation at the secondary site (Figure 20.2). In addition, autonomy in growth signaling, evasion of apoptosis, unresponsiveness to growth inhibitory signaling, limitless replication, and angiogenesis are also needed for successful invasion and metastasis (13). The organ-specific metastasis may result from (i) tumor cell arrest based on the pattern of blood flow from the primary tumor to the first capillary bed and the ability of the tumor cells to form aggregates; (ii) tumor cell adhesion—specific adhesive interactions between tumor cells and the endothelia of certain organs; or (iii) tumor cell niches—the microenvironment of a distant organ creating a permissive site for metastatic colonization. However, the molecular factors that may contribute to organ-specific metastasis of HNOSCC remain largely obscure.

HEAD AND NECK CANCER METASTASIS

The development of local-regional and distant metastases begins with the initiation of the primary tumor and ends with the establishment of metastatic clones through-out the host. Several processes including the differential expression of cell adhesion molecules, release of metalloproteinases, and

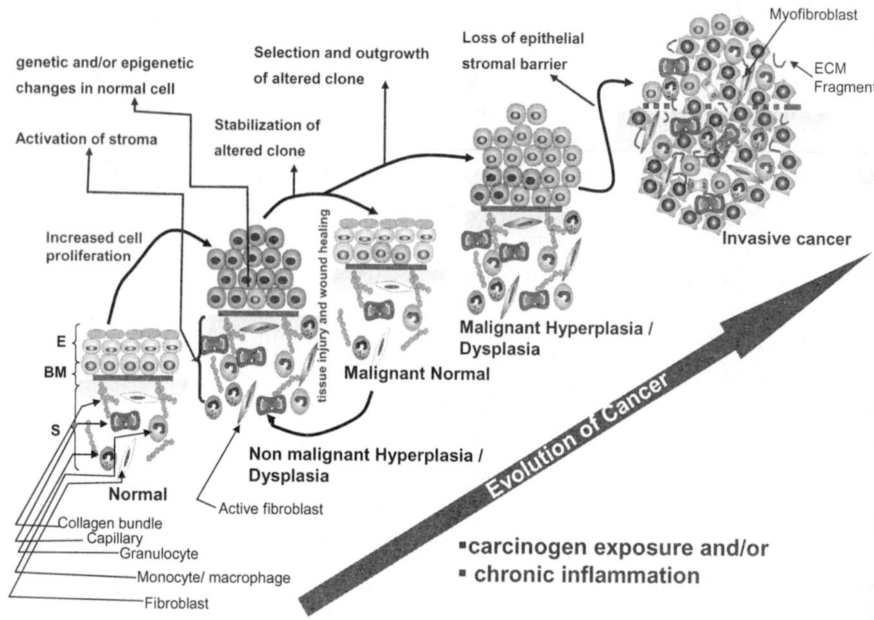

Fig. 20.1 Proposed Multistep process of development of head and neck cancer. A normal well-differentiated stratified epithelium, made up of cells such as keratinocytes in the epidermis (E), is separated by a well-delineated basement membrane (BM) from the stromal compartment(S). This stromal compartment normally contains collagen bundles that surround resting fibroblasts, mature blood vessels encircled by an uninterrupted basement membrane (capillary), and a few resident leukocytes (monocytes and macrophages). During the course of tumorigenesis carcinogen exposure and/or chronic inflammation likely involves a chronic process of tissue injury and wound healing which helps in the accumulation of genetic and/or epigenetic changes and stabilization of cell population harboring these changes. It also causes continuous change in tissue microenvironment in the form of activated stroma which applies a selection pressure on the cells of the particular niche. In this changing tissue microenvironment, certain genetically and/or epigenetically altered cells gain selective advantage over normal unaltered cells and out growth of these altered cells leads to evolution of cancer phenotype.

angiogenesis occur at multiple points in the metastatic cascade. The loss of normal cell–cell and cell–ECM contacts are amongst the earliest events in the process of metastasis. E-cadherin is a calcium-dependent protein that maintains epithelial cell adhesion and polarity and plays a key role in junctional adherence through the binding of the extracelluar domains of E-cadherin molecules in neighboring cells (14). This adhesion depends on an association with the cytoplasmic catenins. β-Catenin plays a key role in Wnt-mediated signal transduction and cell adhesion (15,16). The loss of E-cadherin/β-catenin-mediated adherens junctions is one of the most important hallmarks of the epithelial–mesenchymal transition (EMT) and tumor progression. Loss or reduction of E-cadherin expression occurs early in epithelial carcinogenesis, and correlates with the development of lymph node metastasis, aggressive tumor behavior and poor prognosis (17-19). Mechanistically, cadherins

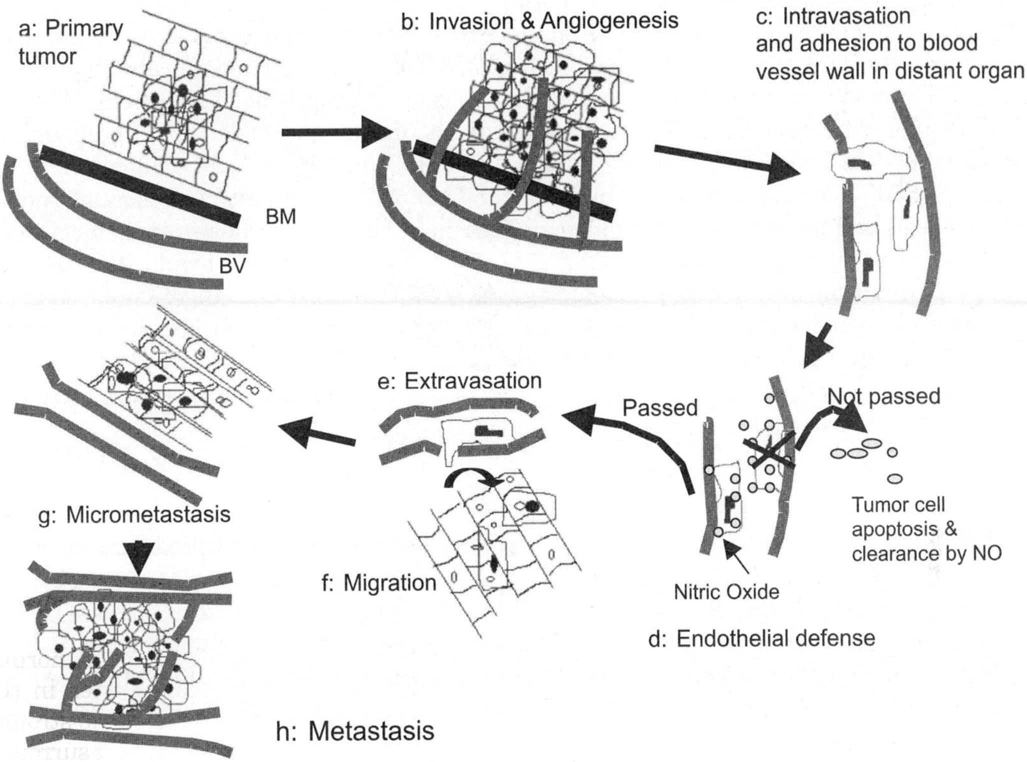

Fig. 20.2 Schematic depiction of metastasis. The process of metastasis begins with invasion from the primary tumor (a,b) involving breakdown of the extra-cellular matrix (ECM); (b) requires generation of new blood and lymph vessels (lymphangiogenesis), (c) intravasation and adhesion to the walls of the blood vessels in distant organ, survival, arrest, (d) escape from immune surveillance and (e) extravasation of the circulatory system and transport to other sites with (g) adhesion, (h) subsequent invasion of the organ that hosts the metastasis, and tumor proliferation at the secondary site. Abbreviations: BM: Basement membrane, BV: Blood vessel, NO: Nitric Oxide.

initiate a program of signal transduction that suppresses growth, proliferation, and migration (20). The reduction of E-cadherin and β-catenin expression is associated with regional metastasis of oral squamous cell carcinoma (OSCC) (21,22).

Angiogenesis

The second step in establishment of distant metastases is the development of an intratumor vascular system. Angiogenesis, the generation of new blood vessels, plays an important role in the growth of primary tumors by maintaining a supply of oxygen and nutrients that supports tumor spread and metastasis (23). In addition, it provides tumor microemboli access to the host vascular system. Quantita-tion of tumor angiogenesis can predict the likelihood of nodal metastases in many solid tumor systems, including carcinoma of the tongue, floor of mouth and nasopharynx (24-29).

Several cytokines produced by HNOSCC stimulate endothelial cell proliferation, migration, assembly and alter the expression of cell surface receptors. These cytokines include basic fibroblast growth factor (b-FGF), vascular endothelial cell growth factor (VEGF) and transforming growth factor-β (TGF-β). While many factors have been implicated in promoting angiogenesis, VEGF is one of the most potent mediators of tumor angiogenesis, inducing endothelial cell proliferation, migration, survival and capillary tube formation (30-33). The VEGF family comprises of six proteins: VEGF-A-E and placenta growth factor (34). VEGF-A plays an essential role in vasculogenesis and angiogenesis. Lymphangiogenesis is also important in tumor metastasis, although its role is still not clearly understood (35). The lymphatic system is involved in the metastatic spread of several human cancers, including HNOSCC (36-38). VEGF-C, VEGF-D, and their receptor on the lymphatic endothelium, VEGFR3, are proposed to control lymphangiogenesis. Overexpression of VEGF is associated with poor prognosis and metastases in SCCOT (39-41). VEGF-A and/or VEGF-C expression have been reported to correlate with regional lymph node metastases in SCCOT (42-44).

Invasion

In addition to cytokines active on the host endothelial cells, tumor cells also produce a variety of proteinases that act on the ECM components. These proteinases play critical roles at two points in the metastatic cascade during (i) intravasation into blood vessels and lymphatic channels at the site of the primary tumor, and (ii) extravasation of tumor cells at the site of the distant metastasis. The first step of tumor invasion involves attachment to components in the subdermal ECM, particularly laminin which serves as the binding site for other laminin molecules and for collagen, enctatin and the epithelial cell surface.

Integrins are a class of high-molecular-weight transmembrane glycoproteins composed of two noncovalently bound subunits (α and β), which attach to ECM and cytoskeletal components. The integrin α6β4 is uniquely expressed in HNOSCCs and shown to correlate with early recurrence and reduced disease free survival (45). Both the α6 and β4 integrin subunits can function as laminin receptor and bind laminin. Soluble factors derived from endothelial cells transiently increase adherence of HNOSCC to fibronectin and vitronectin and increase surface expression of the β-integrins 1 and 4, but not 3 (46). Alterations in tumor cell adherence and the expression of these cell surface ligands may facilitate invasion, metastasis and neovascularization. Following attachment to laminin molecules in the base-ment membrane, invasion of malignant cells is facilitated by the secretion of several classes of enzymes that degrade particular components of the ECM. In order to limit the activity of tumor-derived proteinases, tumors also produce proteinase inhibitors. Tissue-derived metalloproteinase inhibitors (TIMP-1 and TIMP-2) have been identified that bind to specific activated MMPs and prevent ECM degradation. Specific HNOSCC-derived MMPs responsible for the degradation of fibrillar collagen (collagens I, II, III, V), laminins and other basement membrane components (collagen IV, gelatin) have been identified (47-52).

Another family of metalloproteinases, Stromelysins 2 and 3 have also been identified in both HNOSCC and chemically induced SCC, and up-regulation of their mRNA is positively correlated with increased stromal invasion (53,54). Plasminogen activators (PAs) catalyze the synthesis of plasmin from plasminogen; plasmin is a fibrinolytic enzyme that degrades type IV collagen and laminin. Although two forms of PA exist, the urokinase type (u-PA) has been shown to be important in HNOSCC invasion and metastasis (55). Although u-PA is produced by several primary HNOSCC cultures, its levels are significantly reduced with time (56). The transcription factor ets-1 is implicated in regulation of ST3 and correlates with nodal invasion in HNOSCC (57,58). Migration of tumor cells through the degraded base-ment membrane into the stroma is the final step in the sequence of tumor invasion. This process is also observed as tumors invade vascular or lymphatic channels (intravasation) or exit these channels at distant sites (extravasation).

Lower levels of cytoskeletal organization are associated with higher levels of invasiveness and increased frequency of metastasis. The polymerization and depolymerization of the cytoskeletal components and hence cellular motility, is regulated in part by the binding of microtubule associated proteins (MAPs). The phosphorylation of MAP-2 by protein kinase A (PKA) depolymerizes microtubules and destabilizes the cytoskeleton. Manipulation of PP-2A activity in HNOSCC has also been shown to affect migration and invasion in HNOSCC *in vitro*. Inhibition of PP-2A with okadaic acid reduced the invasion of HNOSCC lines through laminin and vitronectin. Increasing PP-2A activity with either ceramide or dihydroxyvitamin D_3 decreased invasion through these matrix components (59,60).

In summary, the process of tumor invasion involves attachment of the tumor to the basement membrane, degradation of ECM components, and migration of the malignant cells into the surrounding stroma.

Invasion into Local Stroma and Vascular System

MMPs are a large family of zinc-dependent enzymes that catalyze the disassembly of ECM and facilitate tumor cell invasion and metastasis by at least three distinct mechanisms: ECM degradation; attachment to ECM components; and cellular motility. Aberrant expression of MMP-9 is an early event in epithelial carcinogenesis and correlates with aggressive tumor behavior (61,62). EMT explains certain features of cancer progression, including tumor cell invasion and metastasis (63,64). In EMT, epithelial cells lose their apical-basal polarity, cell–cell adhesion, and cytoskeletal structure (65). These cells begin to express surface proteins that characterize mesenchymal cells, and become capable of migrating through the basement membrane and basal lamina into the extracellular space. Induction of EMT in HNOSCC drives tumor progression (66). Understanding the mechanisms of EMT has provided insight into the molecular mechanisms of metastasis and led to the development of novel targets for prevention of metastasis.

Tumor proliferation at the secondary site is a prerequisite for metastasis. Various growth factors and their receptors, including interleukin (IL)-8, transforming growth factor (TGF)-α, epidermal growth factor (EGF), and epidermal growth factor receptor (EGFR) regulate tumor proliferation. EGFR is a transmembrane tyrosine kinase receptor. Signaling through this receptor leads to the activation of multiple signaling proteins that initiate a cascade of several signal pathways including, (i) Ras-Raf-mitogen-activated protein kinase (MAPK) pathway, (ii) phosphatidylinositol 3-kinase (PI3K)-Akt pathway, and (iii) signal transducer and activators of transcription (STAT) pathway, which convey the signals to promote cellular responses, such as proliferation and survival (67). EGFR overexpression is a prognostic marker in HNOSCC (68-73).

The Wnt/β-catenin signaling pathway plays a crucial role in the development and progression of cancer (74,75). Wnt proteins are a large family of secreted glycoproteins with at least 19 known human family members that bind to the Frizzeled receptors (76-78) and LRP5/6 co-receptors (79,80).

Wnt/β-catenin signaling, which is only activated when both Frizzeled and LRP5/6 receptors are complexed with Wnt ligands, plays an important role in regulating cell proliferation and differentiation (81). β-catenin, a key downstream component of the Wnt/β-catenin signaling pathway, also plays an important role in cell–cell adhesion, and a switch between these two processes is associated with EMT and cancer development and progression. Extracellular Wnt proteins bind to Frizzeled receptors, which in turn mediates phosphorylation of the Dishevelled protein through binding to Axin. Dishevelled inhibits phosphorylation of β-catenin by disrupting a complex consisting of adenomatous polyposis coli (APC), Axin, and glycogen synthase kinase 3-β (GSK3β). Unphosphorylated β-catenin then translocates into the nucleus and associates with the T-cell factor/lymphoid-enhancer factor (Tcf/Lef) family to form a functional transcription factor that mediates the transactivation of target genes involved in the promotion of tumor progression, invasion, and metastasis, such as c-Myc, cyclin D1, MMP7, gastrin, and ITF-2 (82-89).

In cancer cells, Wnt/β-catenin signaling initiates proliferation, de-differentiation, EMT and directly up-regulates MMP expression (90-92). Thus, activation of the Wnt/β-catenin signaling pathway can have a significant impact on tumor progression. Uraguchi *et al.* (93) demonstrated that oral squamous cell carcinomas express Wnt proteins and activate the signaling pathway suggesting that enhanced Wnt expression and signaling accelerate the progression of carcinomas by activating EMT and local invasiveness. Thus, the Wnt/β-catenin signaling pathway could play a central role in the progression and metastasis of SCCOT. Although our understanding of this signaling pathway has significantly improved with the identification of key regulator proteins over the past decade, little is known about the role of the Wnt/β-catenin signaling pathway and its principal mediator, β-catenin, in HNOSCC. Further work is required to understand the detailed biology of HNOSCC metastasis and to evaluate the potential for targeted therapies.

Nodal Metastasis

Lymph node metastasis is the single most reliable independent prognostic factor for HNOSCC, hence it is critical to identify patients who have cervical lymph node metastases even though they have no clinical evidence of nodal spread. As the sensitivity of preoperative imaging by CT or MRI and clinical examination is only ~70% (94) and there are no imaging techniques capable of detecting micrometastasis in cervical lymph nodes, predictive markers that indicate a high risk of cervical lymph node metastasis will have a major role in determining the optimal therapeutic strategy for these patients.

Tumor thickness is a powerful predictive factor for occult lymph node metastasis in oral cancer (18,95). Lim et al. (18) reported that patients with SCCOT tumors >4 mm thickness should be considered at high risk for late cervical metastasis. Although tumor thickness has gained recognition as an important feature that is predictive of nodal metastasis, the tumor thickness cut-off value has not been definitively determined and ranges from 2 to 10 mm in different series (18,95).

Intense efforts are directed towards investigation of molecular markers that will predict cervical lymph node metastasis. Many molecular markers, including EGFR, VEGF, and β-catenin, have been suggested to be predictive factors for cervical lymph node metastases. *p53* is a tumor suppressor gene that negatively regulates the cell cycle and serves to protect the integrity of the genome. Approximately 50% of cancers of the head and neck studied harbor a *p53* mutation (96). Studies evaluating the utility of *p53* as a predictor of regional nodal disease in SCCOT have shown mixed results (97-99). Cyclin D1 is a proto-oncogene located on chromosome 11q13 that is elevated in response to extracellular mitogens and is a rate-limiting regulator of G_1-phase progression through the cell cycle (100). Cyclin D1 has been shown to bc associated with increased lymph node involvement in anterior tongue cancer (101-103). Ki-67 is a proliferation marker, and the Ki-67 index is correlated with poor prognosis in SCCOT (104). With regards to angiogenesis-related factors, tumor microvessel density has been found to be correlated with regional recurrence in $T_{1-3}N_0$ SCCOT (105). Podoplanin, a mucin-like glycoprotein important in lymphangiogenesis (106) , is expressed in oral cancer and correlates with lymph node metastasis and poor clinical outcomes (107). However, none of these markers has been validated in larger, prospectively acquired, clinically annotated specimen sets, and warrant further investigations for translation into clinical practice.

DNA microarray analysis has been used to identify distinct gene expression profiles of HNOSCC and a comprehensive database has been created (108,109). Over 20 studies of cDNA microarray analysis of HNOSCC have been reported (110). Molecular profiling of 82 primary HNOSCC tumors for determining the potential of predicting the presence of lymph node metastasis at the time of diagnosis, led to identification of 102 predictor genes that correctly predicted local lymph node metastases, suggesting that gene expression of the primary tumor could decipher the metastatic state (111). O'Donnell et al. (112) also reported a metastatic gene expression signature from 18 primary tumors of patients with SCCOT. Comparative genomic hybridization (CGH) first developed by Kallioniemi *et al.* (113) is used for detecting individual gains, losses, and amplifications in genes. Several genetic analyses of HNOSCC based on CGH have been reported (114-117). Recently, using proteomics, Lin-C/VELI3/MALS-3 (Lin-7C) has been shown to mediate OSCC metastasis with beta-catenin signaling and decrease in Lin-7C expression level in primary tumors is clinically linked to the development of cervical lymph node metastasis (118). It is hypothesized that Lin-7C might suppress metastasis in oral carcinogenesis and that Lin-7C up-regulation, possibly by demethylation in primary OSCC and probably other types of human cancers may suppress tumor invasion and metastasis. Further development of these biological investigations may provide the means for screening HNOSCC patients for the presence of large numbers of genes or proteins simultaneously and should be helpful as biomarkers to predict regional metastasis of HNOSCC through revealing the gene expression signatures.

Distant Metastasis

A significant percentage of malignant tumors may gain access to the vascular system yet few develop distant metastases. It is estimated that only 0.1 % of all circulating tumor cells eventually develop into secondary tumors. Tumors will exist in the circulation as single cells, small tumor microemboli with a fibrin 'cocoon', or tumor cells in aggregates with host lymphocytes and platelets. Tumors can circumvent detection by circulating host immune surveillance by forming a fibrin shell around tumor microemboli. While the vast majority of circulating tumor cells will either not survive host immune defense mechanisms, or be destroyed by mechanical trauma of the circulatory system, or carried to an unfavorable secondary site, some will survive to establish metastases.

Many tumors in the head and neck have predictable anatomic patterns of metastases. HNOSCC and thyroid malignan-cies most commonly metastasize to the lung which is the first capillary bed to be encountered by circulating tumor cells. Only rarely will metastases appear in the liver or bone. In contrast, Adenoid cystic carcinomas will spread along nerve sheaths (perineural extension) and will present with proximal lesion along cranial nerves. The use of orthotopic transplantation models of

HNOSCC has shown that cervical lymph node and pulmonary metastases are seen with greater frequency when compared to tumor growth in the flank (119-121). The extravasation of tumors at the secondary site leads to the development of micrometastases and eventually fatal macrometastases. The proliferation of these tumors within the substance of the target organ duplicates the events seen at the primary including attachment to ma-trix, production of proteinases, and angiogenesis.

Biological Predictors of Metastasis

The identification of particular genes/proteins, which can consistently predict the aggressiveness, metastatic potential or occurrence of distant metastases, would be of great clinical importance in HNOSCCs. There are two categories of potential tumors markers: those obtained from a histological assessment of the primary tumor and/or regional nodes and serum tumor markers. Histological data obtained from the primary tumor and regional nodes is most useful in the prognosis of distant metastases. Serum markers can be effective in screening for metastasis in asymptomatic patients. In HNOSCC, the strongest histopathologic predictor of distant metastases is the presence of extracapsular exten-sion in the cervical lymph nodes (122-126).

With the increased availability of molecular diagnostic techniques, surgical pathologists have shifted the focus away from the relationship between the tumor and the surrounding tissue to more precisely examining the tumor itself to provide accurate prognostic information. Mutations in key cell cycle regulating genes including *p53, cyclin D1* and *p27* have shown consistently strong correlations with the development of distant metastases, while alterations in Ki-67, retinoblastoma (Rb), Bcl-2, Bax and Bak proteins were less predictive (123-127). However, not all head and neck malignancies harbor these mutations. Therefore, the variable expression of these mutations limits their usefulness as routine prognostic indicators of metastasis.

Serum tumor markers have shown great utility as screening tools for the development of local recurrences and distant metastases in a variety of tumor systems. The overproduction of thyroglobulin by differentiated thyroid carcinoma is an example of how a particular gene product can be effectively used to monitor tumor recurrence. Yearly, thyroglobulin determination in conjunction with ^{131}1 scan has increased the sensitivity and specificity in detection of recurrent and metastatic carcinoma (127,128). Unfortunately, a sensitive and specific serum marker for HNOSCC has yet to be identified (129,130). One potentially exciting new area for tumor surveillance in HNOSCC is in the area of immunological markers. The immune suppressive effects of HNOSCC are well known and are due to the production of immunosuppressive cytokines and the induction of a population of CD34+ natural suppressor cells (131). High intramural $CD34^+$ content and synthesis of high levels of granulocyte-macrophage colony-stimulating factor correlate significantly with local recurrence and distant metastasis (132).

In summary, we have focused on the clinical significance and mechanisms of metastasis of HNOSCC. Cervical lymph node metastasis is a critical event and is the most reliable predictor of poor treatment outcomes. Therefore, patients with node-positive tumors, especially with ECS, need treatment intensification to improve prognosis. cDNA microarrays, array-based CGH, integrative genomics and proteomic approaches will be useful, and prospective multi-institutional validation of markers of metastasis will lead to important progress and novel potential targets for therapy will emerge, which could improve survival and quality of life for HNOSCC patients.

REFERENCES

1. Jemal, A., Siegel, R., Ward, E., Murray, T., Xu, J., and Thun, M. J. 2007. Cancer statistics, 2007. *CA Cancer J Clin* 57:43-66.
2. Silverman, S., Jr. 2001. Demographics and occurrence of oral and pharyngeal cancers. The outcomes, the trends, the challenge. *J Am Dent Assoc* 132 Suppl:7S-11S.
3. Veness, M. J., Porceddu, S., Palme, C. E., and Morgan, G. J. 2007. Cutaneous head and neck squamous cell carcinoma metastatic to parotid and cervical lymph nodes. *Head Neck* 29:621-31.
4. Lim, Y. C., Koo, B. S., Lee, J. S., Lim, J. Y., and Choi, E. C. 2006. Distributions of cervical lymph node metastases in oropharyngeal carcinoma: therapeutic implications for the N0 neck. *Laryngoscope* 116:1148-52.
5. Ferlito, A., Rinaldo, A., Robbins, K. T., and Silver, C. E. 2006. Neck dissection: past, present and future? *J Laryngol Otol* 120:87-92.
6. Goto, M., Hasegawa, Y., Terada, A., Hyodo, I., Hanai, N., Ijichi, K., Yamada, H., Fujimoto, Y., and Ogawa, T. 2005. Prognostic significance of late cervical metastasis and distant failure in patients with stage I and II oral tongue cancers. *Oral Oncol* 41:62-9.
7. Sano, D. and Myers, J. N. 2007. Metastasis of squamous cell carcinoma of the oral tongue. *Cancer Metastasis Rev* 26:645-62.
8. Chimenos-Kustner, E., Font-Costa, I., and Lopez-Lopez, J. 2004. Oral cancer risk and molecular markers. *Med Oral Patol Oral Cir Bucal* 9:381-4; 377-80.
9. Warnakulasuriya, K. A. and Ralhan, R. 2007. Clinical, pathological, cellular and molecular lesions caused by oral smokeless tobacco—a review. *J Oral Pathol Med* 36:63-77.
10. Mithani, S. K., Mydlarz, W. K., Grumbine, F. L., Smith, I. M., and Califano, J. A. 2007. Molecular genetics of premalignant oral lesions. *Oral Dis* 13:126-33.
11. Ralhan, R. 2007. Genomic and proteomics signature in oral cancer. *Int J human Genet* 7:57-66.
12. Ralhan, R. and Kaur, J. 2003. Tobacco Associated Molecular Changes. In M., P., M.K., N., and P., S., eds., *Advances in Oncology*, p. pp 128-154. Jaypee Brothers Med Publ (P) Ltd., New Delhi.
13. Hanahan, D. and Weinberg, R. A. 2000. The hallmarks of cancer. *Cell* 100:57-70.
14. Vasioukhin, V., Bauer, C., Degenstein, L., Wise, B., and Fuchs, E. 2001. Hyperproliferation and defects in epithelial polarity upon conditional ablation of alpha-catenin in skin. *Cell* 104:605-17.
15. Beavon, I. R. 2000. The E-cadherin-catenin complex in tumour metastasis: structure, function and regulation. *Eur J Cancer* 36:1607-20.
16. Polakis, P. 2001. More than one way to skin a catenin. *Cell* 105:563-6.
17. Diniz-Freitas, M., Garcia-Caballero, T., Antunez-Lopez, J., Gandara-Rey, J. M., and Garcia-Garcia, A. 2006. Reduced E-cadherin expression is an indicator of unfavourable prognosis in oral squamous cell carcinoma. *Oral Oncol* 42:190-200.
18. Lim, S. C., Zhang, S., Ishii, G., Endoh, Y., Kodama, K., Miyamoto, S., Hayashi, R., Ebihara, S., Cho, J. S., and Ochiai, A. 2004. Predictive markers for late cervical metastasis in stage I and II invasive squamous cell carcinoma of the oral tongue. *Clin Cancer Res* 10:166-72.
19. Margulis, A., Zhang, W., Alt-Holland, A., Crawford, H. C., Fusenig, N. E., and Garlick, J. A. 2005. E-cadherin suppression accelerates squamous cell carcinoma progression in three-dimensional, human tissue constructs. *Cancer Res* 65:1783-91.
20. Christofori, G. and Semb, H. 1999. The role of the cell-adhesion molecule E-cadherin as a tumour-suppressor gene. *Trends Biochem Sci* 24:73-6.

21. Chow, V., Yuen, A. P., Lam, K. Y., Tsao, G. S., Ho, W. K., and Wei, W. I. 2001. A comparative study of the clinicopathological significance of E-cadherin and catenins (alpha, beta, gamma) expression in the surgical management of oral tongue carcinoma. *J Cancer Res Clin Oncol* 127:59-63.
22. Tanaka, N., Odajima, T., Ogi, K., Ikeda, T., and Satoh, M. 2003. Expression of E-cadherin, alpha-catenin, and beta-catenin in the process of lymph node metastasis in oral squamous cell carcinoma. *Br J Cancer* 89:557-63.
23. Kerbel, R. S. 2000. Tumor angiogenesis: past, present and the near future. *Carcinogenesis* 21:505-15.
24. Albo, D., Granick, M. S., Jhala, N., Atkinson, B., and Solomon, M. P. 1994. The relationship of angiogenesis to biological activity in human squamous cell carcinomas of the head and neck. *Ann Plast Surg* 32:588-94.
25. Dray, T. G., Hardin, N. J., and Sofferman, R. A. 1995. Angiogenesis as a prognostic marker in early head and neck cancer. *Ann Otol Rhinol Laryngol* 104:724-9.
26. Hegde, P. U., Brenski, A. C., Caldarelli, D. D., Hutchinson, J., Panje, W. R., Wood, N. B., Leurgans, S., Preisler, H. D., Taylor, S. G. t., Caldarelli, L., and Coon, J. S. 1998. Tumor angiogenesis and p53 mutations: prognosis in head and neck cancer. *Arch Otolaryngol Head Neck Surg* 124:80-5.
27. Klijanienko, J., el-Naggar, A. K., de Braud, F., Rodriguez-Peralto, J. L., Rodriguez, R., Itzhaki, M., Russo, A., Janot, F., Luboinski, B., and Cvitkovic, E. 1995. Tumor vascularization, mitotic index, histopathologic grade, and DNA ploidy in the assessment of 114 head and neck squamous cell carcinomas. *Cancer* 75:1649-56.
28. Roychowdhury, D. F., Tseng, A., Jr., Fu, K. K., Weinburg, V., and Weidner, N. 1996. New prognostic factors in nasopharyngeal carcinoma. Tumor angiogenesis and C-erbB2 expression. *Cancer* 77:1419-26.
29. Zatterstrom, U. K., Brun, E., Willen, R., Kjellen, E., and Wennerberg, J. 1995. Tumor angiogenesis and prognosis in squamous cell carcinoma of the head and neck. *Head Neck* 17:312-8.
30. Yancopoulos, G. D., Davis, S., Gale, N. W., Rudge, J. S., Wiegand, S. J., and Holash, J. 2000. Vascular-specific growth factors and blood vessel formation. *Nature* 407:242-8.
31. Jain, R. K. 2003. Molecular regulation of vessel maturation. *Nat Med* 9:685-93.
32. Folkman, J. 1985. Tumor angiogenesis. *Adv Cancer Res* 43:175-203.
33. Denhart, B. C., Guidi, A. J., Tognazzi, K., Dvorak, H. F., and Brown, L. F. 1997. Vascular permeability factor/vascular endothelial growth factor and its receptors in oral and laryngeal squamous cell carcinoma and dysplasia. *Lab Invest* 77:659-64.
34. Neufeld, G., Cohen, T., Gitay-Goren, H., Poltorak, Z., Tessler, S., Sharon, R., Gengrinovitch, S., and Levi, B. Z. 1996. Similarities and differences between the vascular endothelial growth factor (VEGF) splice variants. *Cancer Metastasis Rev* 15:153-8.
35. Clarijs, R., Ruiter, D. J., and de Waal, R. M. 2001. Lymphangiogenesis in malignant tumours: Does it occur? *J Pathol* 193:143-6.
36. Beasley, N. J., Prevo, R., Banerji, S., Leek, R. D., Moore, J., van Trappen, P., Cox, G., Harris, A. L., and Jackson, D. G. 2002. Intratumoral lymphangiogenesis and lymph node metastasis in head and neck cancer. *Cancer Res* 62:1315-20.
37. Maula, S. M., Luukkaa, M., Grenman, R., Jackson, D., Jalkanen, S., and Ristamaki, R. 2003. Intratumoral lymphatics are essential for the metastatic spread and prognosis in squamous cell carcinomas of the head and neck region. *Cancer Res* 63:1920-6.
38. Hall, F. T., Freeman, J. L., Asa, S. L., Jackson, D. G., and Beasley, N. J. 2003. Intratumoral lymphatics and lymph node metastases in papillary thyroid carcinoma. *Arch Otolaryngol Head Neck Surg* 129:716-9.

39. Maeda, T., Matsumura, S., Hiranuma, H., Jikko, A., Furukawa, S., Ishida, T., and Fuchihata, H. 1998. Expression of vascular endothelial growth factor in human oral squamous cell carcinoma: its association with tumour progression and p53 gene status. *J Clin Pathol* 51:771-5.

40. Smith, B. D., Smith, G. L., Carter, D., Sasaki, C. T., and Haffty, B. G. 2000. Prognostic significance of vascular endothelial growth factor protein levels in oral and oropharyngeal squamous cell carcinoma. *J Clin Oncol* 18:2046-52.

41. Uehara, M., Sano, K., Ikeda, H., Sekine, J., Irie, A., Yokota, T., Tobita, T., Ohba, S., and Inokuchi, T. 2004. Expression of vascular endothelial growth factor and prognosis of oral squamous cell carcinoma. *Oral Oncol* 40:321-5.

42. Tanigaki, Y., Nagashima, Y., Kitamura, Y., Matsuda, H., Mikami, Y., and Tsukuda, M. 2004. The expression of vascular endothelial growth factor-A and -C, and receptors 1 and 3: correlation with lymph node metastasis and prognosis in tongue squamous cell carcinoma. *Int J Mol Med* 14:389-95.

43. Kishimoto, K., Sasaki, A., Yoshihama, Y., Mese, H., Tsukamoto, G., and Matsumura, T. 2003. Expression of vascular endothelial growth factor-C predicts regional lymph node metastasis in early oral squamous cell carcinoma. *Oral Oncol* 39:391-6.

44. Shintani, S., Li, C., Ishikawa, T., Mihara, M., Nakashiro, K., and Hamakawa, H. 2004. Expression of vascular endothelial growth factor A, B, C, and D in oral squamous cell carcinoma. *Oral Oncol* 40:13-20.

45. Van Waes, C. and Carey, T. E. 1992. Overexpression of the A9 antigen/alpha 6 beta 4 integrin in head and neck cancer. *Otolaryngol Clin North Am* 25:1117-39.

46. Taitz, A., Petruzzelli, G. J., Lozano, Y., Shankar, R., and Young, M. R. 1995. Bi-directional stimulation of adherence to extracellular matrix components by human head and neck squamous carcinoma cells and endothelial cells. *Cancer Lett* 96:253-60.

47. Rosenthal, E. L. and Matrisian, L. M. 2006. Matrix metalloproteases in head and neck cancer. *Head Neck* 28:639-48.

48. Ruokolainen, H., Paakko, P., and Turpeenniemi-Hujanen, T. 2006. Tissue and circulating immunoreactive protein for MMP-2 and TIMP-2 in head and neck squamous cell carcinoma—tissue immunoreactivity predicts aggressive clinical course. *Mod Pathol* 19:208-17.

49. Basile, J. R., Holmbeck, K., Bugge, T. H., and Gutkind, J. S. 2007. MT1-MMP controls tumor-induced angiogenesis through the release of semaphorin 4D. *J Biol Chem* 282:6899-905.

50. Gorogh, T., Beier, U. H., Baumken, J., Meyer, J. E., Hoffmann, M., Gottschlich, S., and Maune, S. 2006. Metalloproteinases and their inhibitors: influence on tumor invasiveness and metastasis formation in head and neck squamous cell carcinomas. *Head Neck* 28:31-9.

51. Yoshizaki, T., Sato, H., Maruyama, Y., Murono, S., Furukawa, M., Park, C. S., and Seiki, M. 1997. Increased expression of membrane type 1-matrix metalloproteinase in head and neck carcinoma. *Cancer* 79:139-44.

52. Charous, S. J., Stricklin, G. P., Nanney, L. B., Netterville, J. L., and Burkey, B. B. 1997. Expression of matrix metalloproteinases and tissue inhibitor of metalloproteinases in head and neck squamous cell carcinoma. *Ann Otol Rhinol Laryngol* 106:271-8.

53. Soni, S., Mathur, M., Shukla, N. K., Deo, S. V., and Ralhan, R. 2003. Stromelysin-3 expression is an early event in human oral tumorigenesis. *Int J Cancer* 107:309-16.

54. Arora, S., Kaur, J., Sharma, C., Mathur, M., Bahadur, S., Shukla, N. K., Deo, S. V., and Ralhan, R. 2005. Stromelysin 3, Ets-1, and vascular endothelial growth factor expression in oral precancerous and cancerous lesions: correlation with microvessel density, progression, and prognosis. *Clin Cancer Res* 11:2272-84.

55. Ossowski, L., Russo-Payne, H., and Wilson, E. L. 1991. Inhibition of urokinase-type plasminogen activator by antibodies: the effect on dissemination of a human tumor in the nude mouse. *Cancer Res* 51:274-81.

56. Petruzzelli, G. J., Snyderman, C. H., and Johnson, J. T. 1994. In vitro urokinase type plasminogen activator levels and total plasminogen activator activity in squamous cell carcinomas of the head and neck. *Arch Otolaryngol Head Neck Surg* 120:989-92.

57. Pande, P., Soni, S., Chakravarti, N., Mathur, M., Shukla, N. K., and Ralhan, R. 2001. Prognostic impact of Ets-1 overexpression in betel and tobacco related oral cancer. *Cancer Detect Prev* 25: 496-501.

58. Pande, P., Mathur, M., Shukla, N. K., and Ralhan, R. 1999. Ets-1: a plausible marker of invasive potential and lymph node metastasis in human oral squamous cell carcinomas. *J Pathol* 189:40-5.

59. Lozano, Y., Taitz, A., Petruzzelli, G. J., Djordjevic, A., and Young, M. R. 1996. Prostaglandin E2-protein kinase A signaling and protein phosphatases-1 and -2A regulate human head and neck squamous cell carcinoma motility, adherence, and cytoskeletal organization. *Prostaglandins* 51:35-48.

60. Meisinger, J., Patel, S., Vellody, K., Bergstrom, R., Benefield, J., Lozano, Y., and Young, M. R. 1997. Protein phosphatase-2A association with microtubules and its role in restricting the invasiveness of human head and neck squamous cell carcinoma cells. *Cancer Lett* 111:87-95.

61. Kupferman, M. E., Fini, M. E., Muller, W. J., Weber, R., Cheng, Y., and Muschel, R. J. 2000. Matrix metalloproteinase 9 promoter activity is induced coincident with invasion during tumor progression. *Am J Pathol* 157:1777-83.

62. Katayama, A., Bandoh, N., Kishibe, K., Takahara, M., Ogino, T., Nonaka, S., and Harabuchi, Y. 2004. Expressions of matrix metalloproteinases in early-stage oral squamous cell carcinoma as predictive indicators for tumor metastases and prognosis. *Clin Cancer Res* 10:634-40.

63. Birchmeier, C., Birchmeier, W., and Brand-Saberi, B. 1996. Epithelial-mesenchymal transitions in cancer progression. *Acta Anat (Basel)* 156:217-26.

64. Thiery, J. P. 2002. Epithelial-mesenchymal transitions in tumour progression. *Nat Rev Cancer* 2: 442-54.

65. Kang, Y. and Massague, J. 2004. Epithelial-mesenchymal transitions: twist in development and metastasis. *Cell* 118:277-9.

66. Grille, S. J., Bellacosa, A., Upson, J., Klein-Szanto, A. J., van Roy, F., Lee-Kwon, W., Donowitz, M., Tsichlis, P. N., and Larue, L. 2003. The protein kinase Akt induces epithelial mesenchymal transition and promotes enhanced motility and invasiveness of squamous cell carcinoma lines. *Cancer Res* 63:2172-8.

67. Ullrich, A. and Schlessinger, J. 1990. Signal transduction by receptors with tyrosine kinase activity. *Cell* 61:203-12.

68. Rubin Grandis, J., Melhem, M. F., Gooding, W. E., Day, R., Holst, V. A., Wagener, M. M., Drenning, S. D., and Tweardy, D. J. 1998. Levels of TGF-alpha and EGFR protein in head and neck squamous cell carcinoma and patient survival. *J Natl Cancer Inst* 90:824-32.

69. Xia, W., Lau, Y. K., Zhang, H. Z., Xiao, F. Y., Johnston, D. A., Liu, A. R., Li, L., Katz, R. L., and Hung, M. C. 1999. Combination of EGFR, HER-2/neu, and HER-3 is a stronger predictor for the outcome of oral squamous cell carcinoma than any individual family members. *Clin Cancer Res* 5:4164-74.

70. Forastiere, A. A. 1999. Induction and adjuvant chemotherapy for head and neck cancer: future perspectives. *Acta Otorhinolaryngol Belg* 53:277-80.

71. Ang, K. K., Berkey, B. A., Tu, X., Zhang, H. Z., Katz, R., Hammond, E. H., Fu, K. K., and Milas, L. 2002. Impact of epidermal growth factor receptor expression on survival and pattern of relapse in patients with advanced head and neck carcinoma. *Cancer Res* 62:7350-6.

72. Bei, R., Budillon, A., Masuelli, L., Cereda, V., Vitolo, D., Di Gennaro, E., Ripavecchia, V., Palumbo, C., Ionna, F., Losito, S., Modesti, A., Kraus, M. H., and Muraro, R. 2004. Frequent overexpression of multiple ErbB receptors by head and neck squamous cell carcinoma contrasts with rare antibody immunity in patients. *J Pathol* 204:317-25.

73. Ulanovski, D., Stern, Y., Roizman, P., Shpitzer, T., Popovtzer, A., and Feinmesser, R. 2004. Expression of EGFR and Cerb-B2 as prognostic factors in cancer of the tongue. *Oral Oncol* 40:532-7.

74. Waltzer, L. and Bienz, M. 1999. The control of beta-catenin and TCF during embryonic development and cancer. *Cancer Metastasis Rev* 18:231-46.

75. Behrens, J. 2000. Control of beta-catenin signaling in tumor development. *Ann N Y Acad Sci* 910:21-33; discussion 33-5.

76. Yang-Snyder, J., Miller, J. R., Brown, J. D., Lai, C. J., and Moon, R. T. 1996. A frizzled homolog functions in a vertebrate Wnt signaling pathway. *Curr Biol* 6:1302-6.

77. Bhanot, P., Brink, M., Samos, C. H., Hsieh, J. C., Wang, Y., Macke, J. P., Andrew, D., Nathans, J., and Nusse, R. 1996. A new member of the frizzled family from Drosophila functions as a Wingless receptor. *Nature* 382:225-30.

78. He, X., Saint-Jeannet, J. P., Wang, Y., Nathans, J., Dawid, I., and Varmus, H. 1997. A member of the Frizzled protein family mediating axis induction by Wnt-5A. *Science* 275:1652-4.

79. Pinson, K. I., Brennan, J., Monkley, S., Avery, B. J., and Skarnes, W. C. 2000. An LDL-receptor-related protein mediates Wnt signalling in mice. *Nature* 407:535-8.

80. Tamai, K., Semenov, M., Kato, Y., Spokony, R., Liu, C., Katsuyama, Y., Hess, F., Saint-Jeannet, J. P., and He, X. 2000. LDL-receptor-related proteins in Wnt signal transduction. *Nature* 407:530-5.

81. Seidensticker, M. J. and Behrens, J. 2000. Biochemical interactions in the wnt pathway. *Biochim Biophys Acta* 1495:168-82.

82. Luu, H. H., Zhang, R., Haydon, R. C., Rayburn, E., Kang, Q., Si, W., Park, J. K., Wang, H., Peng, Y., Jiang, W., and He, T. C. 2004. Wnt/beta-catenin signaling pathway as a novel cancer drug target. *Curr Cancer Drug Targets* 4:653-71.

83. Shtutman, M., Zhurinsky, J., Simcha, I., Albanese, C., D'Amico, M., Pestell, R., and Ben-Ze'ev, A. 1999. The cyclin D1 gene is a target of the beta-catenin/LEF-1 pathway. *Proc Natl Acad Sci U S A* 96:5522-7.

84. Tetsu, O. and McCormick, F. 1999. Beta-catenin regulates expression of cyclin D1 in colon carcinoma cells. *Nature* 398:422-6.

85. Crawford, H. C., Fingleton, B. M., Rudolph-Owen, L. A., Goss, K. J., Rubinfeld, B., Polakis, P., and Matrisian, L. M. 1999. The metalloproteinase matrilysin is a target of beta-catenin transactivation in intestinal tumors. *Oncogene* 18:2883-91.

86. Koh, T. J., Bulitta, C. J., Fleming, J. V., Dockray, G. J., Varro, A., and Wang, T. C. 2000. Gastrin is a target of the beta-catenin/TCF-4 growth-signaling pathway in a model of intestinal polyposis. *J Clin Invest* 106:533-9.

87. Kolligs, F. T., Nieman, M. T., Winer, I., Hu, G., Van Mater, D., Feng, Y., Smith, I. M., Wu, R., Zhai, Y., Cho, K. R., and Fearon, E. R. 2002. ITF-2, a downstream target of the Wnt/TCF pathway, is activated in human cancers with beta-catenin defects and promotes neoplastic transformation. *Cancer Cell* 1:145-55.

88. Kolligs, F. T., Bommer, G., and Goke, B. 2002. Wnt/beta-catenin/tcf signaling: a critical pathway in gastrointestinal tumorigenesis. *Digestion* 66:131-44.

89. He, T. C., Sparks, A. B., Rago, C., Hermeking, H., Zawel, L., da Costa, L. T., Morin, P. J., Vogelstein, B., and Kinzler, K. W. 1998. Identification of c-MYC as a target of the APC pathway. *Science* 281:1509-12.

90. Eger, A., Stockinger, A., Schaffhauser, B., Beug, H., and Foisner, R. 2000. Epithelial mesenchymal transition by c-Fos estrogen receptor activation involves nuclear translocation of beta-catenin and upregulation of beta-catenin/lymphoid enhancer binding factor-1 transcriptional activity. *J Cell Biol* 148:173-88.

91. Lo Muzio, L. 2001. A possible role for the WNT-1 pathway in oral carcinogenesis. *Crit Rev Oral Biol Med* 12:152-65.

92. Takahashi, M., Tsunoda, T., Seiki, M., Nakamura, Y., and Furukawa, Y. 2002. Identification of membrane-type matrix metalloproteinase-1 as a target of the beta-catenin/Tcf4 complex in human colorectal cancers. *Oncogene* 21:5861-7.

93. Uraguchi, M., Morikawa, M., Shirakawa, M., Sanada, K., and Imai, K. 2004. Activation of WNT family expression and signaling in squamous cell carcinomas of the oral cavity. *J Dent Res* 83: 327-32.

94. Woolgar, J. A. 1999. Pathology of the N0 neck. *Br J Oral Maxillofac Surg* 37:205-9.

95. Yuen, A. P., Ng, R. W., Lam, P. K., and Ho, A. 2007. Preoperative measurement of tumor thickness of oral tongue carcinoma with intraoral ultrasonography. *Head Neck.*

96. Ford, A. C. and Grandis, J. R. 2003. Targeting epidermal growth factor receptor in head and neck cancer. *Head Neck* 25:67-73.

97. Keum, K. C., Chung, E. J., Koom, W. S., Cho, J. H., Cho, S. H., Choi, E. C., Lee, C. G., Suh, C. O., and Kim, G. E. 2006. Predictive value of p53 and PCNA expression for occult neck metastases in patients with clinically node-negative oral tongue cancer. *Otolaryngol Head Neck Surg* 135:858-64.

98. Hogmo, A., Kuylenstierna, R., Lindholm, J., and Munck-Wikland, E. 1999. Predictive value of malignancy grading systems, DNA content, p53, and angiogenesis for stage I tongue carcinomas. *J Clin Pathol* 52:35-40.

99. Ahomadegbe, J. C., Barrois, M., Fogel, S., Le Bihan, M. L., Douc-Rasy, S., Duvillard, P., Armand, J. P., and Riou, G. 1995. High incidence of p53 alterations (mutation, deletion, overexpression) in head and neck primary tumors and metastases; absence of correlation with clinical outcome. Frequent protein overexpression in normal epithelium and in early non-invasive lesions. *Oncogene* 10:1217-27.

100. Sherr, C. J. 1995. D-type cyclins. *Trends Biochem Sci* 20:187-90.

101. Soni, S., Kaur, J., Kumar, A., Chakravarti, N., Mathur, M., Bahadur, S., Shukla, N. K., Deo, S. V., and Ralhan, R. 2005. Alterations of rb pathway components are frequent events in patients with oral epithelial dysplasia and predict clinical outcome in patients with squamous cell carcinoma. *Oncology* 68:314-25.

102. Bova, R. J., Quinn, D. I., Nankervis, J. S., Cole, I. E., Sheridan, B. F., Jensen, M. J., Morgan, G. J., Hughes, C. J., and Sutherland, R. L. 1999. Cyclin D1 and p16INK4A expression predict reduced survival in carcinoma of the anterior tongue. *Clin Cancer Res* 5:2810-9.

103. Carlos de Vicente, J., Herrero-Zapatero, A., Fresno, M. F., and Lopez-Arranz, J. S. 2002. Expression of cyclin D1 and Ki-67 in squamous cell carcinoma of the oral cavity: clinicopathological and prognostic significance. *Oral Oncol* 38:301-8.

104. Xie, X., De Angelis, P., Clausen, O. P., and Boysen, M. 1999. Prognostic significance of proliferative and apoptotic markers in oral tongue squamous cell carcinomas. *Oral Oncol* 35:502-9.

105. Williams, J. K., Carlson, G. W., Cohen, C., Derose, P. B., Hunter, S., and Jurkiewicz, M. J. 1994. Tumor angiogenesis as a prognostic factor in oral cavity tumors. *Am J Surg* 168:373-80.

106. Kahn, H. J. and Marks, A. 2002. A new monoclonal antibody, D2-40, for detection of lymphatic invasion in primary tumors. *Lab Invest* 82:1255-7.

107. Yuan, P., Temam, S., El-Naggar, A., Zhou, X., Liu, D. D., Lee, J. J., and Mao, L. 2006. Overexpression of podoplanin in oral cancer and its association with poor clinical outcome. *Cancer* 107:563-9.

108. El-Naggar, A. K., Kim, H. W., Clayman, G. L., Coombes, M. M., Le, B., Lai, S., Zhan, F., Luna, M. A., Hong, W. K., and Lee, J. J. 2002. Differential expression profiling of head and neck squamous carcinoma: significance in their phenotypic and biological classification. *Oncogene* 21:8206-19.

109. Sok, J. C., Kuriakose, M. A., Mahajan, V. B., Pearlman, A. N., DeLacure, M. D., and Chen, F. A. 2003. Tissue-specific gene expression of head and neck squamous cell carcinoma in vivo by complementary DNA microarray analysis. *Arch Otolaryngol Head Neck Surg* 129:760-70.

110. Choi, P. and Chen, C. 2005. Genetic expression profiles and biologic pathway alterations in head and neck squamous cell carcinoma. *Cancer* 104:1113-28.

111. Roepman, P., Wessels, L. F., Kettelarij, N., Kemmeren, P., Miles, A. J., Lijnzaad, P., Tilanus, M. G., Koole, R., Hordijk, G. J., van der Vliet, P. C., Reinders, M. J., Slootweg, P. J., and Holstege, F. C. 2005. An expression profile for diagnosis of lymph node metastases from primary head and neck squamous cell carcinomas. *Nat Genet* 37:182-6.

112. O'Donnell, R. K., Kupferman, M., Wei, S. J., Singhal, S., Weber, R., O'Malley, B., Cheng, Y., Putt, M., Feldman, M., Ziober, B., and Muschel, R. J. 2005. Gene expression signature predicts lymphatic metastasis in squamous cell carcinoma of the oral cavity. *Oncogene* 24:1244-51.

113. Kallioniemi, A., Kallioniemi, O. P., Sudar, D., Rutovitz, D., Gray, J. W., Waldman, F., and Pinkel, D. 1992. Comparative genomic hybridization for molecular cytogenetic analysis of solid tumors. *Science* 258:818-21.

114. Squire, J. A., Bayani, J., Luk, C., Unwin, L., Tokunaga, J., MacMillan, C., Irish, J., Brown, D., Gullane, P., and Kamel-Reid, S. 2002. Molecular cytogenetic analysis of head and neck squamous cell carcinoma: By comparative genomic hybridization, spectral karyotyping, and expression array analysis. *Head Neck* 24:874-87.

115. Huang, Q., Yu, G. P., McCormick, S. A., Mo, J., Datta, B., Mahimkar, M., Lazarus, P., Schaffer, A. A., Desper, R., and Schantz, S. P. 2002. Genetic differences detected by comparative genomic hybridization in head and neck squamous cell carcinomas from different tumor sites: construction of oncogenetic trees for tumor progression. *Genes Chromosomes Cancer* 34:224-33.

116. Dahlgren, L., Mellin, H., Wangsa, D., Heselmeyer-Haddad, K., Bjornestal, L., Lindholm, J., Munck-Wikland, E., Auer, G., Ried, T., and Dalianis, T. 2003. Comparative genomic hybridization analysis of tonsillar cancer reveals a different pattern of genomic imbalances in human papillomavirus-positive and -negative tumors. *Int J Cancer* 107:244-9.

117. Garnis, C., Campbell, J., Zhang, L., Rosin, M. P., and Lam, W. L. 2004. OCGR array: an oral cancer genomic regional array for comparative genomic hybridization analysis. *Oral Oncol* 40:511-9.

118. Onda, T., Uzawa, K., Nakashima, D., Saito, K., Iwadate, Y., Seki, N., Shibahara, T., and Tanzawa, H. 2007. Lin-7C/VELI3/MALS-3: an essential component in metastasis of human squamous cell carcinoma. *Cancer Res* 67:9643-8.

119. Manzotti, C., Audisio, R. A., and Pratesi, G. 1993. Importance of orthotopic implantation for human tumors as model systems: relevance to metastasis and invasion. *Clin Exp Metastasis* 11:5-14.

120. Dinesman, A., Haughey, B., Gates, G. A., Aufdemorte, T., and Von Hoff, D. D. 1990. Development of a new in vivo model for head and neck cancer. *Otolaryngol Head Neck Surg* 103:766-74.

121. Sales, E. W., Fitch, K. A., Sudetic, P. A., Schechter, G. L., Faulconer, R. J., and Somers, K. D. 1991. Growth and histopathology of human head and neck squamous cell carcinoma implanted intraorally in nude mice. *Otolaryngol Head Neck Surg* 104:351-7.

122. Alvi, A. and Johnson, J. T. 1997. Development of distant metastasis after treatment of advanced-stage head and neck cancer. *Head Neck* 19:500-5.

123. Zoller, M., Goodman, M. L., and Cummings, C. W. 1978. Guidelines for prognosis in head and neck cancer with nodal metastasis. *Laryngoscope* 88:135-40.

124. Calhoun, K. H., Fulmer, P., Weiss, R., and Hokanson, J. A. 1994. Distant metastases from head and neck squamous cell carcinomas. *Laryngoscope* 104:1199-205.

125. Johnson, J. T., Barnes, E. L., Myers, E. N., Schramm, V. L., Jr., Borochovitz, D., and Sigler, B. A. 1981. The extracapsular spread of tumors in cervical node metastasis. *Arch Otolaryngol* 107:725-9.

126. Myers, E. N. and Fagan, J. F. 1999. Management of the neck in cancer of the larynx. *Ann Otol Rhinol Laryngol* 108:828-32.

127. Bradford, C. R., Wolf, G. T., Carey, T. E., Zhu, S., Beals, T. F., Truelson, J. M., McClatchey, K. D., and Fisher, S. G. 1999. Predictive markers for response to chemotherapy, organ preservation, and survival in patients with advanced laryngeal carcinoma. *Otolaryngol Head Neck Surg* 121:534-8.

128. Shaha, A. R., Shah, J. P., and Loree, T. R. 1998. Patterns of failure in differentiated carcinoma of the thyroid based on risk groups. *Head Neck* 20:26-30.

129. Rassekh, C. H., Johnson, J. T., and Eibling, D. E. 1994. Circulating markers in squamous cell carcinoma of the head and neck: a review. *Eur J Cancer B Oral Oncol* 30B:23-8.

130. Straka, M. B., Wagner, R. L., Johnson, J. T., Kachman, K. K., and Eibling, D. E. 1992. The lack of utility of a tumor marker panel in head and neck carcinoma. Squamous cell carcinoma antigen, carcinoembryonic antigen, lipid-associated sialic acid, and CA-125. *Arch Otolaryngol Head Neck Surg* 118:802-5.

131. Taitz, A., Petruzzelli, G., Pak, A. S., Wright, M. A., Matthews, J. P., Raslan, W. F., Lozano, Y., and Young, M. R. 1995. Immune parameters of mice bearing human head and neck cancer. *Cancer Immunol Immunother* 40:283-91.

132. Young, M. R., Wright, M. A., Lozano, Y., Prechel, M. M., Benefield, J., Leonetti, J. P., Collins, S. L., and Petruzzelli, G. J. 1997. Increased recurrence and metastasis in patients whose primary head and neck squamous cell carcinomas secreted granulocyte-macrophage colony-stimulating factor and contained CD34+ natural suppressor cells. *Int J Cancer* 74:69-74.

21

CHAPTER

MTA Family of Master Co-regulators in Invasion and Metastasis

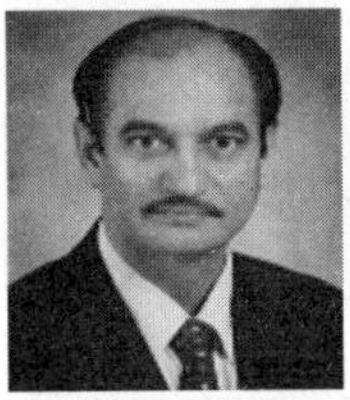

Poonam Molli[1] and Rakesh Kumar[1, 2]

[1]Molecular and Cellular Oncology, The University of Texas M. D. Anderson Cancer Center, Houston, Texas, USA; [1]Molecular and Cellular Biology, Baylor College of Medicine, Houston, Texas, USA.

ABSTRACT

Nuclear receptors (NRs) by interacting with nucleosome remodeling complexes modulate the transcription of target genes. NRs rely on coregulators like coactivators to potentiate transcription and on corepressors to inhibit transcription of the target genes. Metastasis-associated proteins (MTA) family of novel NR coregulator that form independent nucleosome remodeling and deacetylation (NuRD) complexes and either repress the transcription of genes by recruiting histone deacetylases onto their target genes or activate genes through recruitment of RNA polymerase II onto the gene promoter. Over expression of MTA1 in cancer and metastasis and subsequent identification of additional gene family members, namely MTA1s, MTA2, and MTA3, and their role in breast cancer has establishment significance of the MTA family in pathophysiological conditions. Interestingly, repression of estrogen receptor transactivation functions by MTA1, MTA1s, and MTA2 and regulation of MTA3 by estrogen signaling have revealed a role for these proteins in modulating hormonal responses in normal mammary glands and in breast cancer. Here, we highlight the action of MTA proteins on NR signaling, invasion, and metastasis.

Introduction to the MTA Family

MTA1, the founding member of the MTA family, was discovered in a differential screen conducted to identify the candidate genes selectively expressed between highly metastatic and nonmetastatic rat mammary adenocarcinoma cell lines and cloned as the metastasis-associated tumor gene (*mta1*) (Toh et al 1994). Metastasis is a complex disease involving several series of events that includes stimulation or repression of numerous gene products, resulting in the detachment of neoplastic cells from the primary site, angiogenesis, extravasation and arrest at secondary sites (Nicolson et al 1988). In addition to metastatic cells, MTA1 is expressed in almost all organs of the rat, including the liver, lung, heart, and kidneys, but the highest levels is found in the testes, which indicates that MTA1 is also functional in normal tissues. Despite widespread expression of the MTA1 protein, the molecular functions of the MTA family remained a mystery until the proteomic analysis of the nucleosome remodeling and deacetylation (NuRD) complex identified MTA1 and MTA2 as integral to the histone deacetylase (HDAC) complexes, suggesting that MTA1 might be involved in nucleosomal remodeling and transcriptional regulation of genes thus providing first clue about the role of the MTA family of proteins in chromatin remodeling (Singh et al 2007). Subsequently, MTA3, the third member of the MTA family, was identified by a search of genomic and EST sequences. Two RNA species were transcribed, one encoding a protein of 515 amino acids (MTA3) and the other encoding a protein of 595 amino acids named MTA3 long form (MTA3L). MTA3 was identified to be a part of the Mi2–NuRD complex by co-immunoprecipitation with Mi2, MBD3, and HDAC1 (Fujita et al 2003). MTA1s, a naturally occurring variant of MTA1, was accidentally discovered in our laboratory while pursuing the role of MTA1 in transcriptional regulation of estrogen receptor-a (ER) (Kumar et al 2002). MTA1s is an alternative spliced form of MTA1 mRNA. The resulting MTA1s gene product lacks the C-terminal region of other MTA family members. In addition, using a polyclonal antibody against purified zymogen granule membrane components from rat pancreas, researchers identified ZG29p, a cDNA coding for the 29-kDa protein. ZG29p is an N-terminal truncated form of MTA1, coded by the last seven exons of MTA1 and present in the zymogen granules of the pancreas. ZG29p mediates interaction with amylase and is involved in condensation-sorting in the exocrine rat pancreas (Kleene et al 2000).

All three primary members of the MTA family share a high degree of sequence similarity. Analysis of the primary structure of MTA proteins shows that MTA2 and MTA3 are 68% and 80% identical to MTA1, respectively, with the highest homology in the N-terminal half of the proteins (Fig. 21.1). In contrast, the C-terminal half of MTA family members are divergent. In general, the MTA proteins (with the exception of the ZG29p variant) contain one BAH domain, one ELM domain, and one SANT domain that is similar to the DNA binding domain of Myb-related proteins. Toward the C-terminal end, the members of the MTA family share a highly conserved GATA-type zinc finger motif that indicates the capability of direct interaction with DNA. In addition to these protein domains, the C-terminal region of MTA1 has two src-homology (SH) domain-binding motifs. An SH3 binding motif is situated between amino acid residues 545 and 552, and an SH2 binding motif between residues 697 and 705. Both MTA2 and MTA3 also contain SH2 and SH3 binding domains. The SH domains are known to be involved in signal transduction, such as kinases (src-family, btk, Fps, and zap-70), adaptors and scaffolding proteins (NCk1, NCK2, GRB2, and Shc). Thus, MTA1 has a unique protein primary structure that suggests that it might function in signal transduction and DNA-binding. MTA1 and MTA2 contain nuclear localization signals and are nuclear in localization. MTA3 does not contain a predicted nuclear localization signal, but localizes to both the cytoplasmic and nuclear compartments. MTA1s – the C terminal truncated form of MTA1, is predominantly localized in the cytoplasm due to the loss of the nuclear localization signal (Manavathi et al. 2007).

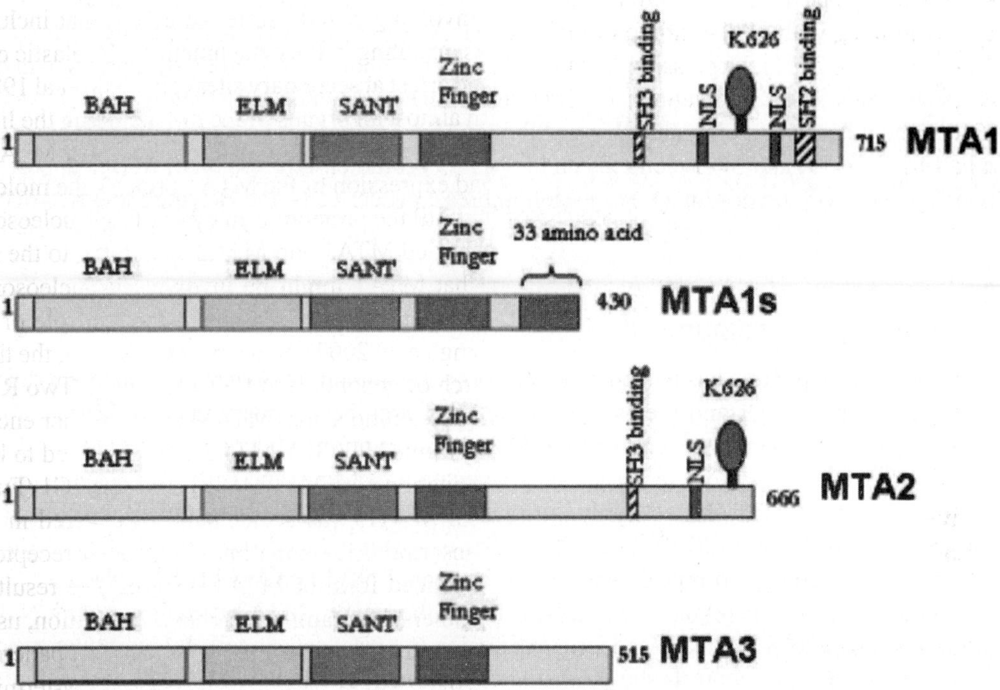

Fig. 21.1 Structural domains of MTA family members. Comparison of physical structures of the MTA family proteins. BAH, ELM and SANT domains located at the N-terminus are highly conserved whereas C-terminal region of MTA proteins is divergent. NLS-nuclear localization signal.

Expression and Regulators of the MTA Genes

MTA1 is expressed in almost all organs, including the lung, liver, kidney, heart, and testes, suggesting that MTA1 is essential for the normal functioning of these organs. MTA1 is over expressed in a variety of cancer cell lines, including ovarian, lung, gastric, and colorectal cancers, but not in melanoma or sarcoma. MTA1 over expression and a concomitant enhancement of invasiveness have been observed in several cancers, including breast, colorectal, gastric, lung, and prostrate cancers. Similarly, MTA1 over expression is correlated with increased tumor grade, angiogenesis and relapse chances in breast cancers. Over expression of MTA1 also correlate with invasiveness or lymph node metastasis in gastric, colorectal, and esophageal carcinomas (Singh et al 2007).

Recent findings provide some clues about the regulation of MTA1 protein expression (Singh et al 2007). Heregulin-beta1, a ligand for human epidermal growth factor receptors HER3 and HER4, has been shown to induce the expression of MTA1 in breast cancer cells. A recent study in the normal diploid human fibroblasts identified MTA1 a mechanistic mediator of c-MYC-regulated transformation thus linking MTA1 promoter as a C-MYC target (Zhang et al 2005). Further, MTA1 is also transcriptionally up regulated under hypoxia through a poorly understood mechanism (Yoo et al 2006). Although MTA1 and MTA2 share a great degree of structural similarity, regulation of

MTA2 promoter appears to be different than that of MTA1. MTA2 promoter contains ETS-1 binding elements along with SP-1-binding motifs, and MTA2 transcription is regulated by both ETS-1 and SP-1 (Xia et al 2001). Expression of MTA3 has been demonstrated to be estrogen regulated in breast cancer cells. MTA3 contains half estrogen response elements (ERE) along with AP-1 and SP-1 sites, and it has been shown that ER-α, AP-1, and SP-1 transcription factors directly bind onto these half ERE, AP-1, and SP-1 elements on the MTA3 promoter. Expression of MTA3 appears to be tissue-specific with predominant expression in breast cancer cells and B-lymphocytes, whereas MTA1 and MTA2 are ubiquitously expressed. At present, regulation of ZP29 gene transcription is not known.

MTA Family and Hormone Action

MTA family of co-regulators has gained importance, owing to their involvement in mammary gland development, breast cancer and metastasis. Of all three members, a great deal of information is available regarding the hormonal regulation of MTA3 transcription. Abundant expression of MTA3 in ERα-positive cell lines and its absence in ER-negative cell lines indicated the dependency of MTA3 transcription on ERα. Interestingly, estrogen and a functional ERα pathway were found to be indispensable for the transcription of MTA3. The estrogen induced stimulation of MTA3 transcription was abrogated by co-repressors of ERα function, MTA1 and MTA1s thus placing MTA1 and MTAs as an upstream regulator of MTA3. In another study, MTA3-containing Mi-2/NuRD complex was shown to influence E-cadherin expression in breast cancer cells by inhibiting expression Snail, which in turn controls the epithelial-to-mesenchymal transition (EMT) (Mishra et al 2004). In all, these studies indicate a role for MTA1 and MTA1s in the EMT and metastasis of breast cancer cells. In accordance, constitutive over expression of MTA1 in MCF-7 cells resulted in the onset of aggressive phenotypes like invasion and anchorage-independent growth. Later, MTA1–NuRD complex was shown to associate with a Lim domain only 4 (LMO4) a transcriptional co-regulator that is found to be over expressed in breast cancers, and cooperatively repress the transcription functions of ERα and transcription of E2 responsive genes (Singh et al 2005). Recent studies associated MTA1 with ERα dependent repression of BRCA1 gene and centrosomal amplification and thereby linking MTA1 to genomic instability and tumorigenesis (Molli et al 2007). Similar to MTA1, over expression of MTA1s efficiently suppressed estrogen-stimulated ERα transactivation functions. Mechanistic studies showed that the repression was due to cytoplasmic sequestration of ERα by MTA1s (kumar et al 2002). Recently, MTA2 was also shown to interact physically with ERα and repress its transcriptional functions. MTA2-associated HDAC activity was shown to be involved in deacetylation of ERα at lysine 303. Over expression of MTA2 was found to render cells unresponsive to estrogen and suppress estrogen-induced colony formation in breast cancer cells (Cui et al 2006).

Majority of the studies conducted in the past identified MTA1 as a co-repressor, where it associated with HDACs and brought about transcriptional repression of the target genes or was involved in direct deacetylation of its binding proteins. A recent study showed that MTA1 can also function as a transcriptional activator (Fig 21.2). Study of the mechanism behind the transcription activation functions of MTA1 led to the identification of an acetylation site on Lys626. Acetylation at this site by acetyl transferase-like p300 allowed MTA1 to recruit RNA polymerase II (pol II) on the breast cancer-amplified sequence 3 (BCAS3) enhancer region (Gururaj et al (2006). In addition, our laboratory has identified co-existence of two transcriptional co-activators, MICoA and NRIF3 with

MTA1, both of which were found to co-activate ERα transactivation functions. The co-activator role of MTA1 was identified in yet another study that linked MTA1 with mammary gland development. Over expression of the mammary tumor-like virus (MMTV)-MTA1 transgene in the mouse mammary gland resulted in increased ductal extension, enhanced ductal branching, and proliferation. The noted increase in ductal growth and ductal branching in MTA1-transgenic mice was attributed to the alteration in the ratios of progesterone receptor isoforms. This phenotype was accompanied by increased expression of β-casein and β-catenin, a central component of the cadherin cell-adhesion complex and the canonical Wnt pathway (Bagheri Yarmand et al (2004). In addition, the transgenic mice also showed a high incidence of spontaneous B cell lymphomas including diffuse large B cell lymphomas (DLBCL). Lymphocytes and lymphoma cells from MTA1-TG mice were hyper-proliferative. Lymphomas from MTA1-TG mice showed up-regulation of paired box gene 5 (Pax5), a molecule previously implicated in B-cell lymphogenesis. Interestingly, once again acetylated MTA1 was found to get recruited onto the Pax5 promoter to stimulate Pax5 transcription (Balasenthil et al 2007a and 2007b).

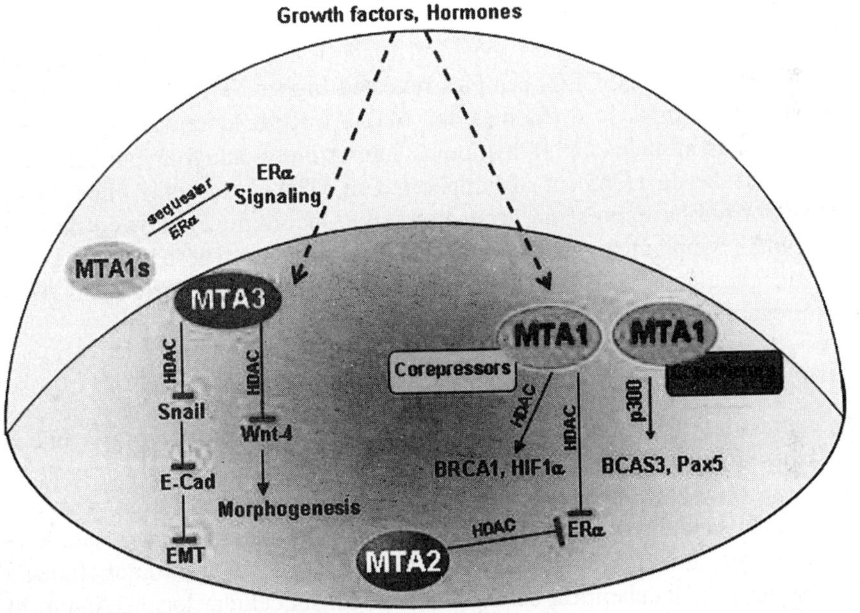

Fig. 21.2 Schematic diagram showing role of MTA family members in nuclear receptor signaling pathway. MTA1s sequesters ERa in the cytoplasm. MTA1 and MTA2 associates with HDACs and repress the E2-ERa transactivation at EREs. MTA1 also interacts with p300 and activate BCAS3 and Pax5 transcription. MTA3 associates with NuRD complex and repress Snail an inhibitor of E-cadherin and thereby promotes EMT.

In contrast to the hyper-branching and tumor formation in MTA1-transgenic mice, MTA3-transgenic mice exhibit hypo-branching. The mammary gland hypo-branching phenotype observed in MTA3-TG mice was remarkably similar to the defective branching in Wnt4 knockout mice. The study established that MTA3 repressed Wnt4- mediated morphogenesis of murine mammary glands (Zhang et al 2006).

MTA Proteins in Human Diseases

Large body of evidence from cell-based model systems and mouse models has firmly established the significance of MTA1 in cancer metastasis (Manavathi et al 2007b). MTA1 over expression in mouse mammary gland epithelium leads to the formation of mammary gland adenocarcinomas. In addition, tumors formed in MMTV-PyV-mT-transgenic mice- a reliable model for multistage tumorigenesis of human breast cancer show elevated levels of MTA1. In addition to breast cancer, MTA1 over expression was also found in a tissue microarray analysis of 102 gastrointestinal carcinoids. In an independent study, 13 of 34 patients with gastric carcinoma exhibited over expression of MTA1 mRNA. In a microarray study containing 70 endometrial adenocarcinomas of various grades, MTA1 was over expressed in 53 tumors. Increased expression of MTA1 mRNA was also observed in human colorectal carcinoma and HCC cells compared to normal tissue. Furthermore, in esophageal squamous cell carcinoma, 30 of 70 samples displayed over expression of the MTA1 protein compared to normal and these patients showed a higher degree of lymph node metastasis and poorer prognosis. A DNA microarray analysis combined with immuno-histochemistry analysis showed that MTA1 is also selectively over expressed in metastatic prostate cancer compared with clinically localized prostate cancer and benign prostate tissue. In yet another study involving 74 non-small cell lung cancer (NSCLC) samples revealed higher MTA1 mRNA levels in NSCLC samples compared to normal. In thymomas, the MTA1 mRNA level was significantly higher in stage IV thymoma than in stage I and II thymomas. Interestingly, data from our lab clearly indicated a role for MTA1 in the development of lymphomas in MTA1 transgenic mice. In support, data mining analysis of public expression array datasets (Oncomine 2) showed that 75 out of 76 specimens of human lymphomas (98.6%) show MTA1 expression. These findings together suggest a strong positive correlation between MTA1 over expression and tumorigenesis. However, very little is known regarding the roles of MTA2 and MTA3 in human cancers.

Outstanding Issues

Because the expression of MTA family members is not restricted to cancer cells, one of the major outstanding issues is the lack of our understanding of role for MTA1 family of proteins in normal cells. In this context, we have recently generated a mice deficient of MTA1, and on-goings studies are directed to understand the contribution of MTA1 in the normal physiology and tumor progression, and whether one could target selective functions of MTA1 to anti-tumor strategies. Another intriguing question is the biochemical basis of differential subcellular localization of MTA family members and whether it is further affected by the extracellular signals. In addition, there is a clear need to define specific cellular function for various domains of MTA1 (or other family members). Furthermore, to fully appreciate the master regulatory function of MTA1 (or other MTA family members), it is vital to understand the nature of the biochemical switch responsible for co-repressor versus co-activator activity of MTA1. Although it is possible that both co-activators and co-repressors exist in common transcriptional complexes and the final consequence on gene expression is the balance between their activities. And finally, it will be important to start defining the cellular pathways which in-turn regulates the expression of MTA1, and consequently, its function in physiologically relevant setting.

REFERENCES

1. Bagheri-Yarmand, R., Talukder, A. H., Wang, R. A., Vadlamudi, R. K., and Kumar, R. Metastasis-associated protein 1 deregulation causes inappropriate mammary gland development and tumorigenesis. *Development* (2004) **131,** 3469-79.
2. Balasenthil, S., Bhageri-Yarnand, R., Gururaj, A. E., Talukder, A. H. and Kumar, R. Overexpression of MTA1 causes diffuse large B-cell lymphoma (DLBCL). *Cancer Res* (2007a) **67,** 7062-67.
3. Balasenthil S., Gururaj A. E., Talukder A. H., Bagheri-Yarmand R., et al. Identification of Pax5 as a Target of MTA1 in B-Cell Lymphomas. *Cancer Res* (2007b) **67,** 7132-38.
4. Cui, Y., Niu, A., Pestell, R., Kumar, R., Curran, E. M., Liu, Y., and Fuqua, S. A. Metastasis-associated protein 2 is a repressor of estrogen receptor alpha whose overexpression leads to estrogen-independent growth of human breast cancer cells. *Mol Endocrinol* (2006) **20,** 2020-35.
5. Fujita, N., Jaye, D. L., Kajita, M., Geigerman, C., Moreno, C. S., and Wade, P. A. MTA3, a Mi-2/NuRD complex subunit, regulates an invasive growth pathway in breast cancer. *Cell* (2003) **113,** 207-19.
6. Gururaj, A. E., Singh, R. R., Rayala, S. K., Holm, C., den Hollander, P., Zhang, H., Balasenthil, S., Talukder, A. H., Landberg, G., and Kumar, R. MTA1, a transcriptional activator of breast cancer amplified sequence 3. *Proc Natl Acad Sci USA* (2006) **103,** 6670-5.
7. Kleene, R., Classes, B., Zdzieblo, J and Schrader, M. SH3 binding sites of ZG29p mediate an interaction with amylase and are involved in condensation-sorting in the exocrine rat pancreas. *Biochemistry* (2000) **39,** 9893-900.
8. Kumar, R., Wang, R. A., Mazumdar, A., Talukder, A. H., Mandal, M., Yang, Z., Bagheri-Yarmand, R., Sahin, A., Hortobagyi, G., Adam, L., Barnes, C. J., and Vadlamudi, R. K. A naturally occurring MTA1 variant sequesters oestrogen receptor-alpha in the cytoplasm. *Nature* (2002) **418,** 654-57.
9. Manavathi, B. and Kumar, R. Metastasis associated antigens, an emerging family of multifaceted master coregulators. *J Biol Chem* (2007) **282,** 1529-533.
10. Manavathi, B., Singh K and Kumar, R. MTA family of coregulators in nuclear receptor biology and pathology *NRS* (2007) **5,** 1-8.
11. Mishra, S. K., Talukder, A. H., Gururaj, A. E., Yang, Z., Singh, R. R., Mahoney, M. G., Franci, C., Vadlamudi, R. K., and Kumar, R. Upstream determinants of estrogen receptor-alpha regulation of metastatic tumor antigen 3 pathway. *J Biol Chem* (2004) **279,** 32709-15.
12. Nicolson, G. L. Cancer metastasis: tumor cell and host organ properties important in metastasis to specific secondary sites. *Biochim Biophys Acta* (1988) **948,** 175-24.
13. Molli P.R., Singh R. R., Lee S. W., and Kumar R. MTA1-mediated transcriptional repression of BRCA1 tumor suppressor gene. *Onocogene – In Press* (2007).
14. Singh, R.R, Barnes, C. J., Talukder, A. H., Fuqua, S. A., and Kumar, R. Negative regulation of estrogen receptor alpha transactivation functions by LIM domain only 4 protein. *Cancer Res* (2005) **65,** 10594-601.
15. Singh R.R., and Kumar R. MTA Family of Transcriptional Metaregulators in Mammary Gland Morphogenesis and Breast Cancer. *J Mammary Gland Biol Neoplasia* (2007) **12,** 115– 125.
16. Toh, Y., Pensil, S. D., Nicolson G. L. A novel candidate metastasis-associated gene, mta1, differentially expressed in highly metastatic mammary adenocarcinoma cell lines. cDNA cloning, expression, and protein analyses. *J Biol Chem* (1994) **269,** 22958-963.

17. Xia, L. and Zhang, Y. Sp1 and ETS family transcription factors regulate the mouse Mta2 gene expression. *Gene* (2001) **268,** 77-85.

18. Yoo, Y. G., Kong, G., and Lee, M. O. Metastasis-associated protein 1 enhances stability of hypoxia-inducible factor-1alpha protein by recruiting histone deacetylase 1. *EMBO J* (2006) **25,** 1231-41.

19. Zhang, X. Y., DeSalle, L. M., Patel, J. H., Capobianco, A. J., Yu, D., Thomas-Tikhonenko, A., and McMahon, S. B. Metastasis-associated protein 1 (MTA1) is an essential downstream effector of the c-MYC oncoprotein. *Proc Natl Acad Sci USA* (2005) **102,** 13968-73.

20. Zhang, H., Singh, R.R., Talukder, A.H., and Kumar, R. Metastatic tumor antigen 3 is a direct corepressor of the Wnt4 pathway. *Genes Dev* (2006), **20,** 2943-48.

22

CHAPTER

Role of Hormonal and Cytokine Environment of Tumor-bearing Host in Manifestation of Gender-Dependent Differential Induction of Apoptosis of Tumor Cells: Implication in Gender Dimorphism of Tumor Growth

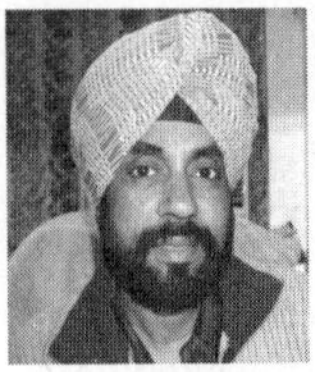

Vivekanand Gupta and Sukh Mahendra Singh

School of Biotechnology, Banaras Hindu University, Varanasi–221005

ABSTRACT

Although a sizeable number of clinical tumors have a spontaneous origin, adequate knowledge of their relationship with the host's immune system is still lacking. In view of this our laboratory has been engaged in studying the immunosuppressive effects of a transplantable T cell lymphoma of spontaneous origin, designated as Dalton's Lymphoma (DL), in a murine model. It was demonstrated in one of our previous studies that gender hormones could modulate tumor growth through direct or indirect actions. Thus the present investigation was initiated to study if a gender-dependent differential induction of tumor cell apoptosis is responsible for the manifestation of gender dimorphism observed in the growth of a transplantable murine T cell lymphoma. Tumor cell samples obtained from male tumor-bearing mice showed a higher number of cells with apoptotic morphology compared to that observed in female tumor-bearing mice. In this report we demonstrate that male hormone androgen and female hormone estrogen can differentially modulate tumor cell proliferation and apoptosis through alteration in the expression pattern of cell death regulating genes: p53 and CAD. Tumor cells cells were shown to express mRNA for androgen and estrogen receptors. Further these gonadal hormones also induced tumor cells to produce tumor growth regulating proteins: VEGF, TGF-β, IL-2, IL-2R, SOCS, Hsp-70 and IFN-γ which in turn either through autocrine action on tumor cells or via TAM-derived NO were observed to regulate tumor cell apoptosis leading to gender dimorphism of tumor growth. In addition we also observed gender dimorphism with respect to myeloid differentiation of bone marrow precursor cells; gender-dependent differential action of anti-tumor drugs and efficacy of adoptive immunotherapy using macrophage-derived dendritic cells. The study has clinical significance as these results will helps in understanding the mechanism of gender dimorphism with respect to the progression of T-cells tumors.

INTRODUCTION

Tumor growth has a complex relationship with the host's immune and endocrine systems (1-3). Hormones and cytokines, of both host and tumor origin have been shown to be involved in the regulation of tumor progression in either directions (4,5). Nevertheless, the mechanism(s) of hormone-dependent differential regulation of tumor progression varies with the etiology of individual tumor clones as well as on the profile of hormones and cytokines of the tumor-bearing host (6-8). However, existence of gender dimorphism and the associated mechanisms in the progressive growth of several types of tumors remains unclear. Nearly 18 % of total human malignancies are of lymphocytic origin (9), and are considered as one of the most complicated neoplasm for clinical management (10,11). However, very little information is found in literature regarding the effect of gender-specific hormones in the regulation of such lymphocytic tumors. Moreover, existence of receptors for gender-specific hormones has also been demonstrated on lymphocytes (12).

Using a murine model of a transplantable T-cell lymphoma of spontaneous origin designated as Dalton's lymphoma (DL), we have been investigating several aspects of host-tumor relationship. DL is a T-cell tumor that originates in thymus of DBA strain (H-2^d) of mice (13,14). DL can grow in the form of either an ascitic or a solid tumor (15) and has been reported to possess chromosomal aberrations (16). Like some lymphoma and leukemia of human origin, DL cells do not metastasize to other lymphoid organs (17). During the course of our previous investigation, we observed that the progression of the ascitic DL growth is rapid in syngenic BALB/c (H-2^d) mice, causing death of the host in a relatively short time. Further we have reported that DL growth is associated with thymus regression, modulation of macrophage activation, humoral and T cell-mediated immune responses associated with an alteration of T_{H1}/T_{H2} cytokine balance (18-28).

Using this tumor model we recently reported that growth of this tumor showed gender dimorphism, which was found to be dependent on gender specific hormones: testosterone, progesterone, prolactin and cytokines: IL-4, IL-10, and TNF-α leading to a differential proliferation of tumor cells (29,30). Reports indicate that in addition to cell proliferation, rate of the induction of apoptosis also play an indispensable role in determining the rate of tumor progression and its outcome (31,32). To the best of our knowledge this is the first report of its kind to show that there exists gender dimorphism of tumor cell death, which in turn may influence tumor growth in gender specific-manner.

MATERIALS AND METHODS

Mice and Tumor System

Pathogen-free inbred adult male and female mice of BALB/c (H-2^d) strain were used at 8-12 weeks of age. Dalton's lymphoma (DL) is maintained in ascitic form by serial transplantation in BALB/c mice or in an *in vitro* cell culture system by serial passage as described earlier (33). Tumor cells (1.5×10^5) were transplanted to age and weight matched male and female mice (6 mice per group) in 0.5 ml phosphate buffered saline (PBS) intraperitoneally (21). Tumor cells were obtained from the tumor-bearing host on indicated days post-DL transplantation.

Reagents

Tissue culture medium RPMI 1640 and fetal calf serum (FCS) were purchased from Hyclone (Logan, Utah, USA). MTT [3-(4,5-dimethylthiazol-2yl)-2, 5-diphenyl tetrazolium bromide] and most of the other chemicals were purchased from the Sigma Chemical Co. (St. Louis, MO, USA). Antibodies against Interleukin-2 (IL-2), Interleukin-2 receptor (IL-2R), Interferon-gamma (IFN-γ), Tumor growth factor-beta (TGF-β), Suppressor of cytokine signaling-5 (SOCS-5), Heat shock protein 70 (Hsp70), Vascular endothelial growth factor (VEGF), p53, Caspase-activated DNase (CAD) and actin were purchased from Imgenex (San Diego, CA, USA) and Chemicon (Hampshire, NF, UK). Secondary antibodies conjugated to alkaline phosphatase were obtained from Bangalore Genie (Bangalore, India). BCIP/NBT was purchased from Amresco (Solon, Ohio, USA). All the cell cultures were carried out at 37 ^{0}C in a CO_2 incubator (Sheldon, Oregon, USA) having 5% CO_2 in air in a humidified atmosphere in culture medium supplement with 20 mg ml^{-1} gentamycin, 100 ìg ml^{-1} Streptomycin and 100 IU Penicillin (Himedia, Mumbai, India).

Estimation of Tumor Cell Survival in Vitro by MTT Assay

Tumor cell survival was assayed according to a method described earlier (29). DL cells were seeded (1.5×10^5 viable cells $well^{-1}$), in a 96 well tissue culture plate in culture conditions mentioned in the materials and for 72 hours. Cell survival was measured by MTT assay following a method described by Mosmann (34) with slight modifications as described earlier (29).

Morphological Evaluation of Apoptotic DL Cells

Apoptotic tumor cell population was enumerated by a method described earlier (22). Apoptotic cells were identified on the basis of morphological features that included contracted cell bodies, condensed, uniformly circumscribed, and densely stained chromatin; or membrane-bound apoptotic bodies containing one or more nuclear fragments.

Percent DNA Fragmentation

Induction of apoptosis in tumor cells was also confirmed by a quantitative determination of DNA fragmentation following a method given by Sellins and Cohen (35) with slight modifications using diphenyl amine method (30).

Tumor-associated Macrophages (TAM)

TAM were isolated and the monolayers prepared following a method described earlier by lavage of the peritoneal cavity (25) after 10 days of tumor transplantation. TAM were finally plated in a 96 well flat bottom tissue culture plate at a cell density of 1×10^5 cells well^{-1} in the presence or absence of LPS (10 μg ml^{-1}) + IFN-γ (10 U ml^{-1}) for 24 hours to activate the TAM. The culture supernatant was then harvested and assayed for nitrite content by a method described in the following section.

Nitrite Assay

The concentration of stable nitrite (NO_2^-), the end product from NO generation in the ascitic fluid and in the culture supernant of tumor-associated macrophage (TAM) was determined by method of Ding et.al. (36) based on Griess reaction as described earlier (24).

Preparation of DL-cell-free Ascitic Fluid

DL cell-free ascitic fluid (DLAF) was prepared according to the method described previously (37).

Estimation of DL cell Multiplication Rate (MR) and Population Doubling Time (PDT)

Multiplication rate (MR) and population doubling time (PDT) of DL cells under conditions as indicated in results (Table I) was carried out following a standard method (38). The MR and PDT were calculated with following formula.

$$\text{Multiplication rate (MR)} = 3.32\,(\log N_h - \log N_1)/ t_1 - t_2$$

Where N_h = Number of cells harvested, N_1 = Number of cells seeded, t_1 = time zero, t_2 = time of cell harvesting at 96 hours.

Population doubling time was taken as the time (hours) taken for cell number to double and this was the reciprocal of multiplication rate i.e. 1 / MR.

ELISA for Detection of Cytokines in Ascitic Fluid and Tumor Culture Supernatant

A standard ELISA was performed to detect the presence of indicated proteins in the ascitic fluid, and culture supernatant following a method described earlier (Singh et al., 2006).

Western Immunoblot Analysis

Samples of cell lysate were processed for Western blotting following a method described earlier (30).

RT-PCR for Espression of mRNA for Androgen and Estrogen Receptors

RT-PCR analysis for the expression of mRNA for estrogen and androgen receptors was carried out according to a method described earlier (30).using a one step RT-PCR cell to cDNA kit (Ambion, Texas, USA). The primer sequence for estrogen receptor (alpha) 5'-AATTCTGACAATCGA CGCCAG-3(forward); 5'-GTGCTTCAACATTCTCCCTCCTC -3 (reverse). The primer sequence for androgen rcccptor; 5'-GGAGAACTCTTCAGAGCAAG -3(forward); 5'-AGCTGAGTCAT CCTGATCTG -3 (reverse). The primer sequence for ²-actin 5'-GGCACAGTGTGGGTGAC-3(forward);5'CTGGCACCACACCTTCTAC-3' 0(reverse). (Hysel India, New Delhi,.India).

RESULTS

Effect of Androgen, Estrogen and Their Antagonists on in Vitro Survival of Tumor Cells

The effect of androgen and estrogen on the in vitro survival of tumor cells was estimated by MTT assay. Results are shown in Fig 22.1. Although both androgen and estrogen showed an augmentory effect on tumor cell proliferation in a dose-dependent manner, estrogen was found to be better in augmentation of tumor cell survival compared to androgen. Optimum augmentory effect of both the hormones on cell survival was observed at a dose of 1 μM. Therefore, in all subsequent experiments cells were treated in vitro with these hormones at a dose of 1μM. In same set of experiment tumor cells were also incubated in medium alone or containing androgen and estrogen in the presence of antagonists against the respective hormones as indicated in Fig 22.1. Presence of flutamide, an antagonist of androgen or tamoxifen, an antagonist of estrogen, in the presence of androgen or estrogen respectively, significantly reversed the modulatory effect of the respective hormones on tumor cell proliferation.

Gender Dimorphism of Tumor Growth Kinetics in Vitro

Tumor cells (1×10^5) obtained.from male and female mice were cultured in vitro up to 96 hours followed by estimation of multiplication rate and population-doubling time as described in materials and methods by counting the number of viable tumor cells by trypan blue dye exclusion test. Results are shown in Table 22.1. DL cells obtained from female mice showed a higher growth kinetics compared to those obtained from male mice.

Effect of in Vivo Administration of Hormone Antagonists on The Survival of DL Cells in Vitro and Life Span of DL-bearing Mice

DL was transplanted to male and female mice in groups of 10 mice flowed by daily i.p. administration of flutamide (10 mg/kg body weight) to male mice and tamoxifen (10 mg/kg body weight) to female mice for 10 days in 0.5 ml volme of PBS. The control mice received only PBS administration. On the 11th day the tumor cells were harvested and plated in wells of 96 well culture plate for 72 h followed by estimation of cell viability by MTT assay. Results are shown in Table 22.2a. In vivo administration of flutamide to male mice resulted in an augmentation of cell survival compared

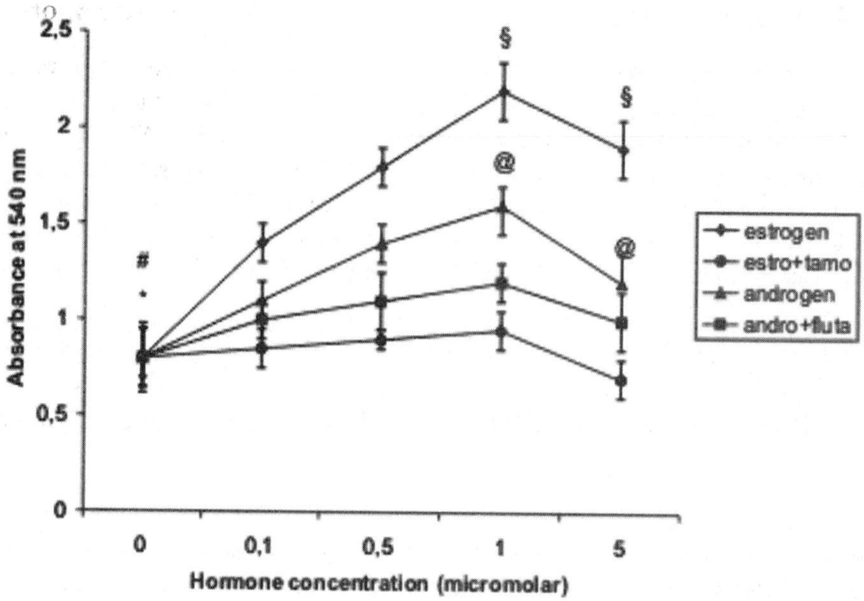

Fig. 22.1 Effect of androgen, estrogen, and their antagonists on proliferation of tumor cells in vitro. Values are mean ± SD. *p<0.05 vs values for DL cells incubated in medium containing androgen #p<0.05 vs values for DL cells incubated in medium containing estrogen § p<0.05 vs values for DL cells incubated in medium containing androgen with their respective antagonists at the respective concentration of the hormone. @ p<0.05 vs values for DL cells incubated in medium containing estrogen with their respective antagonists at the respective concentration of the hormone.

Table 22.1 Gender differences and differentially regulate tumor-growth

Source of tumor cells and in vitro incubation culture conditions	Multiplication rate / 24 h ± S.D.	Population doubling time (h) ± S.D.
Male (Incubation: Medium alone without hormones)	0.43 ± 0.02	55.6 ± 0.7
Female (Incubation: Medium alone without hormones)	0.58 ± 0.01 *	41.4 ± 0.9 *

The values are mean ± SD of three independent experiments conducted in triplicate. * $p < 0.05$ compared to values for cell samples of male tumor-bearing mice.

to male DL-bearing mice without drug administration. On the other hand the survival of the DL cells obtained from female DL-bearing mice administered with tamoxifen showed an inhibition in the survival ability in vitro compared to the DL cells of female mice without administration of tamoxifen. Mice similarly treated with hormone antagonists were monitored for the survival time.

Table 22.2a Effect of in vivo administration of androgen antagonist flutamide and estrogen antagonist tamoxifen to male and female tumor-bearing mice respectively on thesurvival of DL cells in vitro.

Treatment of tumor-bearing mice	Absorbance at 540 nm±SD
Female without tamoxifen	2.47±0.04
Female with tamoxifen (10 mg/kg body weight/day)	1.26±0.01*
Male without flutamide	1.15±0.02
Male with flutamide (mg/kg body weight)	1.76±0.03**

*p<0.05 vs values for DL cells obtained from male tumor-bearing mice without flutamide administration
**p< vs values for DL cells obtained from female tumor-bearing mice without tamoxifen administration

The results are shown in Table 22.2b. In vivo administration of flutamide resulted in an inhibitionj of the survival time of male DL-bearing mice compared to the mice administered with PBS alone. In vivo administration of tamoxifen to female tumor-bearing mice resulted in an augmentation of the survival time compared to the respective controls.d

Table 22.2b Survival of DL-bearing male and female mice following in vivo administra tion of flutamide and tamoxifen respectively.

Days following DL transplantation	% of surviving mice			
	Male tumor-bearing mice		Female tumor-bearing mice	
	Without treatment	Flutamide 10mg/kg body weight/day for 10 days)	Without treatment	Tamoxifen (10 mg/kg body weight/day for 10 days)
15	100	100	100	100
20	100	80	60	80
22	60	40	30	50
25	10	05	0	20
30	0	0	0	0

PBS alone or Flutamide or tamoxifen in 0.5 ml of PBS were administered i.p. to male or female mice (in groups of 10 mice each) respectively at a dose of 10 mg/kg body weight for 10 days on daily basis. The mean survival of mice was recorded and the values shown in the table indicate the % of mice surviving on the respective days indicated on the left side of the table.

Gender Dimorphism in the Induction of Apoptosis in Tumor Cells

To check if the existence of gender dimorphism of tumor cell death, DL cells obtained from male and female tumor bearing host 10 days-post tumor transplantation were enumerated under microscope for percentage of cells exhibiting typical feature of apoptotic morphology (Fig 22.2a) or processed for quantitative estimation of percent specific DNA fragmentation (Fig 22.2b). The percentage of apoptotic tumor cells was significantly higher in the tumor cell population obtained from male tumor-bearing mice compared to those obtained from the female tumor-bearing mice. Similarly DNA fragmentation was also found to be significantly higher in the tumor cell samples obtained from male mice compared to those from female tumor-bearing mice.

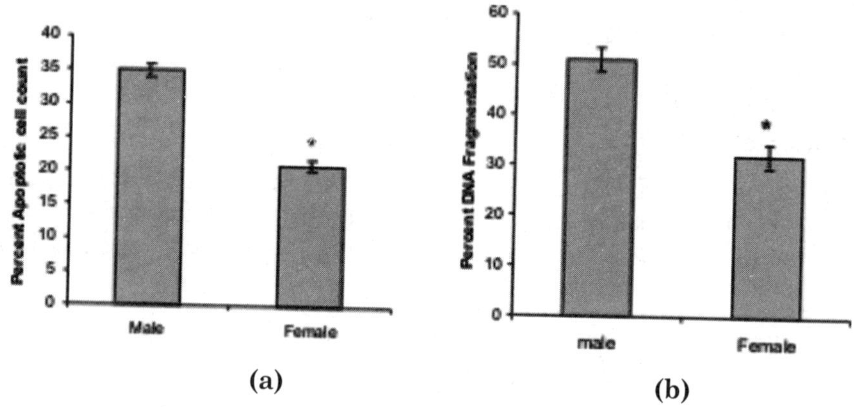

Fig. 22.2 Gender-specific difference in tumor cell apoptosis. Percent apoptotic cell count (a) and percent specific DNA fragmentation (b) of DL cells obtained from male and female tumor-bearing mice 10 days after tumor transplantation. Values are mean ± SD. * $p < 0.05$ vs values for DL cell samples obtained from male tumor-bearing mice.

Effect of Androgen, Estrogen and their Antagonists on Induction of Apoptosis in Tumor Cells in Vitro

In the next set of experiment we checked the effect of androgen, estrogen and their respective antagonists: flutamide and tamoxifen, on the induction of apoptosis in tumor cells. In vitro serially passaged DL cells (1×10^5) were incubated in medium alone or containing androgen (1 μM) or estrogen (1 μM) in the absence or presence of flutamide (1 μM) or tamoxifen (1 μM) respectively for 72 hours followed by estimation of apoptosis by enumerating percentage apoptotic cells. Results are shown in Fig. 22.3. Percent of tumor cells with apoptotic morphology was found to significantly increase following incubation in vitro in medium containing androgen while the percentage of apoptotic cells remained significantly lower in samples of tumor cells in medium alone or containing estrogen. Presence of androgen and estrogen antagonists did not alter the percentage of apoptotic cells incubated in medium without any hormone. However, presence of flutamide along with androgen caused a significant decrease in the count of apoptotic tumor cells compared to those incubated in medium containing androgen alone. On the other hand presence of tamoxifen along with estrogen caused an increase in the apoptotic count of tumor cells compared to that in tumor cells incubated in medium containing only estrogen.

Nitric Oxide Content in Ascitic Fluid of Male and Female Tumor-bearing Host

Ascitic fluid of male and female tumor-bearing host obtained from 10 days-post tumor transplantation was analyzed for NO content as described in materials and methods. Results are shown in

Fig 22.4. NO content in the ascitic fluid of female tumor-bearing mice was found to be significantly lower than that in the ascitic fluid of male tumor-bearing mice.

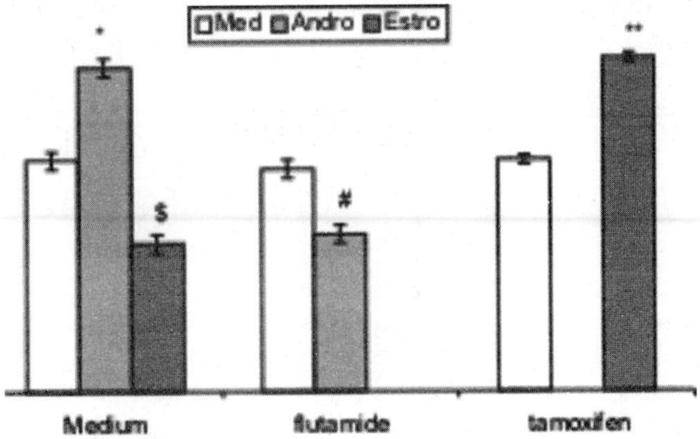

Fig. 22.3 Effect of androgen, estrogen, and their antagonists on the induction of apoptosis in tumor cells in vitro. Values are mean ± S.D. *$ p < 0.05 vs. values of cells incubated in medium alone. # p < 0.05 vs. values for DL cells incubated in medium containing androgen without flutamide. **p < 0.05 vs. values for DL cells incubated in medium containing estrogen without tamoxifane.

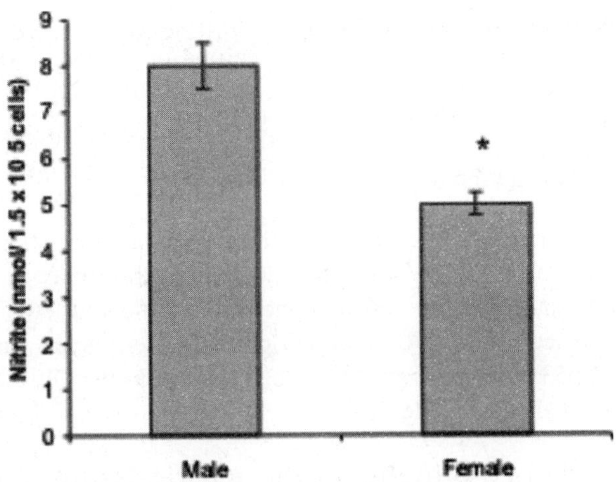

Fig 22.4 Effect of gender dimorphism on the content of NO in the ascitic fluid of male and female tumor-bearing mice. Values shown are mean ± S.D. * $p < 0.05$ vs. values for ascitic fluid of male tumor-bearing mice.

Gender Dimorphism of NO Production by TAM

Next we checked if TAM obtained from male and female tumor-bearing mice showed a differential production of NO. TAM ($1x10^5$) obtained from male and female mice were incubated in presence or absence of LPS (10 μg ml $^{-1}$) plus IFN-γ (10 U ml $^{-1}$) for 24 hours followed by assaying of NO content in the culture supernatant. Results are shown in Fig. 22.5. TAM treated with LPS+IFN-γ of both male and female mice produce higher amount of NO compare to untreated TAM. However, the level of NO in the culture supernatant of TAM obtained from male mice was significantly higher than that of female mice.

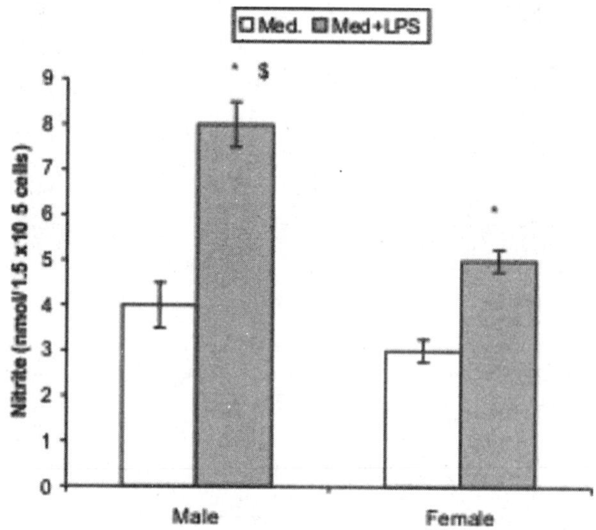

Fig. 22.5 Production of NO by TAM obtained from male and female tumor-bearing mice. Values shown are mean ± S.D. * $p < 0.05$ vs. values of corresponding TAM incubated in medium alone. \$ $p < 0.05$ vs. values for LPS + IFN-g treated TAM obtained from female tumor-bearing mice.

Expression of p53 and CAD Proteins in DL Cells is Gender-Dependent

We also checked if the tumor cells obtained from male and female mice showed a difference in the level of CAD and p53 proteins, which have been demonstrated to play an important role in the induction of apoptosis. Lysate of tumor cells obtained from male and female tumor-bearing mice was immunoblotted for detection of CAD and p53 proteins. Results are shown in Fig. 22.6 a, b. Expression of CAD and p53 proteins were found to be higher in the DL cell lysate of male mice compare to that in the DL cells of female mice.

Tumor Growth Regulatory Proteins in the Ascitic Fluid of Male and Female Tumor-bearing Mice

Ascitic fluid collected from male and female tumor-bearing mice was check by ELISA for the presence of IL-2, TGF-β and IFN-γ. Results are shown in Fig. 22.7. The level of IFN-γ was found to be significantly less in the DLAF of female tumor-bearing mice, whereas the levels of IL-2 and TGF-β were significantly higher in the DLAF of the female tumor-bearing mice compared to the DLAF of male mice.

Immunoblotting of DL Cell Lysate for Detection of IL-2R, VEGF, Hsp70 and SOCS-5

Lysate of DL cells (1×10^8 cells) obtained from male and female tumor-bearing mice, 10 days post tumor transplantation, was immunoblotted for detection of IL-2R, VEGF, Hsp70 and SOCS-5 as described in materials and methods. Results are shown in Fig. 22.8 a, b. Expression of SOCS-5, IL-2R, VEGF and Hsp70 was found to increase in the DL cells obtained from female mice compared to those from male tumor-bearing mice.

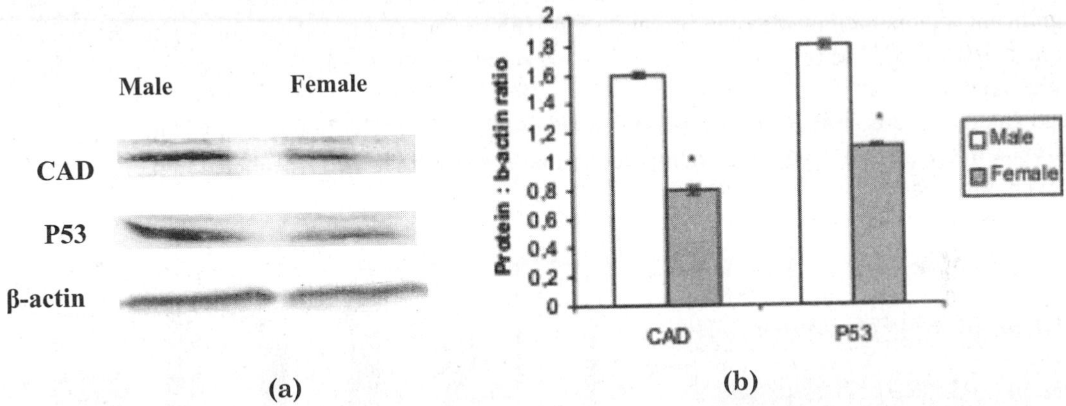

Fig. 22.6 Expression of CAD and p53 proteins in DL cells obtained from male and female tumor-bearing mice. (a) Western blot showing expression of CAD, p53 and β–actin: Lane 1 DL cells of male mice, Lane 2 DL cells of female mice: (b) Blot shown in Fig. 22.6a was scanned by a gel dumentation system and the band size was analyzed by Quantity One software as described in the materials and methods. Values shown are ratio of CAD or p53 vs. β–actin.

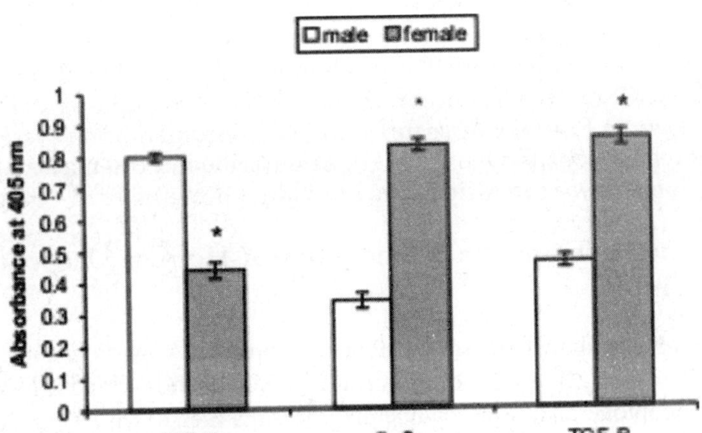

Fig. 22.7 Immuno-detection of IFN–γ, IL-2 and TGF–β in the ascitic fluid of male and female tumor-bearing mice by ELISA. The values shown are mean ± SD. *$p < 0.05$ vs values for DLAF obtained from male tumor-bearing mice.

Detection of Tumor Growth Regulatory Factors in the Culture Supernant of DL Cells Treated With Androgen and Estrogen in Vitro

DL cells (1×10^7 ml $^{-1}$) from the serially passaged stock were treated in vitro in medium alone or containing androgen (1μM) or estrogen (1μM) for 72 hours and cell free culture supernatant was harvested and checked for presence of IL-2, IL-2R, VEGF, TGF-β and IFN-γ by ELISA as described in materials and methods. Results are shown in Fig. 22.9. Treatment of DL cells in vitro with androgen had little effect on the production of IL-2, IL-2R, and TGF-β as compared to DL cells incubated in medium alone. On the other hand treatment of DL cells with androgen resulted in a significant augmentation of in the production of IFN-γ compared to those incubated in medium alone or estrogen. Treatment of DL cells with estrogen in vitro resulted in a comparatively much higher augmentation in the production of IL-2, IL-2R, VEGF, and TGF-β compared to that in androgen treated DL cells. However estrogen treatment of DL cells resulted in a decline in the expression of IFN-γ in the culture supernatant compared to that in case of DL cells incubated in medium alone or with androgen.

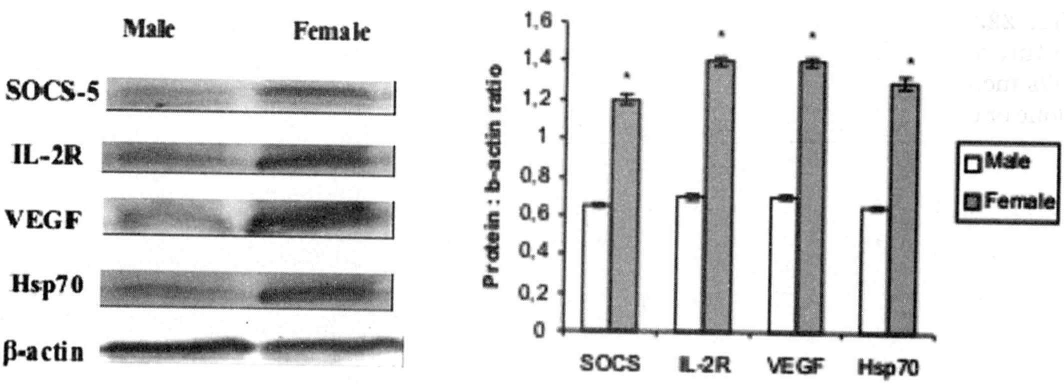

(a) (b)

Fig. 22.8 Western blot analysis of DL cells obtained male and female mice for expression of IL–2R, VEGF, SOCS-5, Hsp70. Lane 1: DL cells of male mice; Lane: 2: DL cells of female mice. The blot shown in Fig. 8a was scanned by a gel documentation system and the band size was analyzed by Quantity One software as described in the materials and methods. Values shown are ratio of the individual proteins vs. β – actin.

Effect of Cytokine Antibodies on the Induction of Hormone Dependent Apoptosis of DL Cells in Vitro

DL cells (1×10^7) were incubated in medium alone or in presence of androgen or estrogen (1μM) in with or without antibodies (250 × dilution) against IL-2, VEGF, TGF-β and IFN-γ for 72 hours and the percentage of apoptotic cells were enumerated. Results are shown in Fig. 22.10. Presence of antibodies significantly altered the level of hormone induced modulation of the count of apoptotic cells.

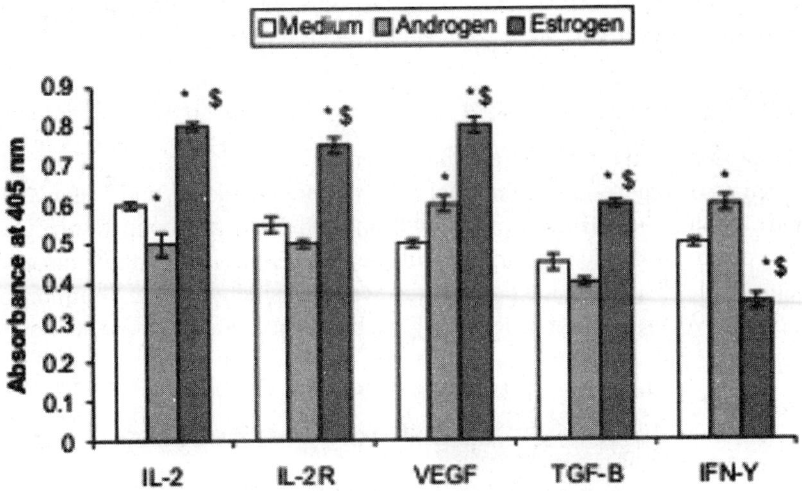

Fig. 22.9 Immuno-detection of IL-2, IL-2R, VEGF, TGF-β and IFN-γ in the DL cell culture supernatant. Values shown are mean ± S.D. * $p < 0.05$ vs. values for samples of DL cells incubated in medium alone. \$ $p < 0.05$ vs. values for DL cells incubated in medium alone or containing androgen. Range of inter-assay coefficient of variation: 1.6 to 7.1; Range of intra-assay coefficient of variation: 1.25 to 6.0.

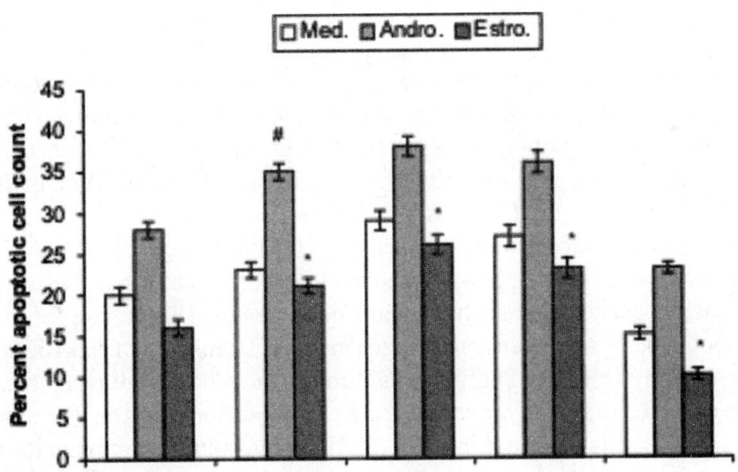

Fig. 22.10 Percentage of apoptotic DL cells treated with androgen and estrogen in the presence of antibodies. Values shown are mean ± S.D. * $p < 0.05$ vs. DL cells incubated in medium containing androgen or estrogen without antibody. # p<0.05 vs. values for DL cells incubated in medium containing androgen without antibody.

Expression of mRNA for Androgen and Estrogen Receptors in DL Cells.

DL cells obtained from male and female tumor-bearing mice on day 11 of tumor transplantation0were processed for RT-PCR of mRNA for androgen and estrogen receptors as described in the materials and methods. The results are shown in Fig 22.11. DL cells obtained from both male and female mice showed expression of mRNA for androgen and estrogen receptors.

DISCUSSION

Results of the present study demonstrate that progressive growth of a T cell lymphoma displays gender dimorphism owing to: 1) a differential rate of tumor cell death, and 2) gender dimorphism in the expression of proteins regulating tumor growth and cell death Although the precise mechanism(s) underlying the observed gender dimorphism of the differential induction of tumor cell death and growth remains unclear, some of the possibilities were considered. As sex hormones, proapoptotic cytokines and reactive nitrogen intermediates have been implicated in the induction of apoptosis in

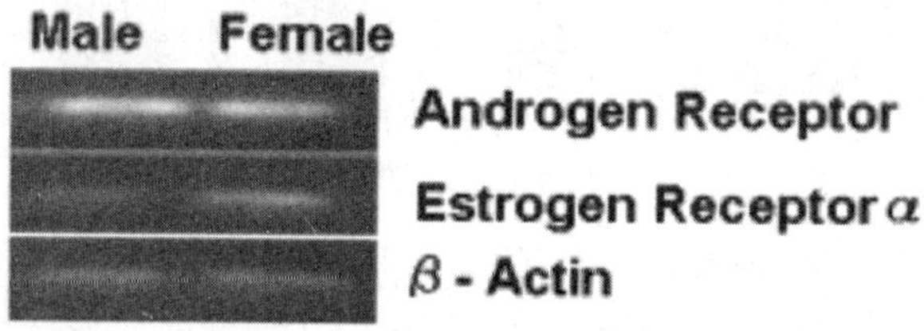

Fig. 22.11 RT-PCR for expression of Estrogen receptor (alpha) and androgen receptor in DL cells. DL cells obtained from male and female mice 11 days after tumor transplantation were processed for RT-PCR analysis for expression of mRNA for androgen and estrogen receptors. Expression of beta actin was carried out as an internal control.

a variety of target cells (5,30,39), we checked the role of such molecules in manifestation of gender dimorphism of T cell lymphoma. In vitro experiments indicated that androgen and estrogen differentially affected growth and apoptosis of tumor cells (Fig. 22.1, 22.3). The mechanism of the action of the hormones on the tumor cells could be of both direct and indirect nature. In the direct action of the hormones their effects on the DL cells could be mediated via their specific receptors on these cells (Fig 22.11). On the other hand indirect action of the hormones could be mediated through the DL and/or host derived growth regulatory molecules. Additionally the following set of indirect evidences indicate the existence of such receptors on these cells: 1. DL cell survival and death was differentially modulated by androgen and estrogen in vitro. 2. Presence of specific antagonists against androgen and estrogen, which are known to act through the blocking of receptors of the respective hormones, were observed to partially reverse the effect of these hormones on the induction of apoptosis and cell survival of DL cells in vitro (Fig. 22.1, 22.3). In vivo administration of the hormone antagonists reversed the effect of gender on tumor cell survival in vitro and the life span of the tumor-bearing male and female mice. Thus the hormone antagonists could block the action of the respective hormones by blocking the respective hormone receptors. It can be suggested that androgen and estrogen could possibly act directly through their respective receptors on tumor cells to regulate apoptosis and proliferation. Indeed a number of evidences indicate the presence of receptors for gonadal hormones on T lymphocytes (12, 29) and DL is a T cell-derived tumor.

The results of the present study also demonstrated that DL cells obtained from male mice showed a higher expression of proapoptotic proteins: CAD and P53, suggesting that induction of apoptosis in tumor cells of male mice was dependent on expression of these cell growth regulatory proteins. Moreover, these apoptotic pathways have been shown to be regulated by gender-specific hormones like testosterone, androgen, estrogen, progesterone and other proapoptotic factors like cytokine and reactive free radicals (40-44). Therefore, we also checked the involvement of other factors known to regulate cell death and proliferation through these pathways. The ascitic fluid of tumor-bearing male and female mice showed a differential level of IFN-γ, TGF-β and IL-2 cytokines (Fig.7). Nevertheless DL cells of femalc tumor-bearing mice also showed a higher level in expression of IL-2R (Fig.22.8). TGF-β, IL-2 and IL-2R have been shown to promote growth of cells of T cell lineage and antagonize induction of apoptosis (30). IFN-γ on the other hand has been demonstrated to directly regulate apoptosis in lymphoma cells (45,46). Studies also demonstrate a differential effcct of gender-specific hormones on the production of IFN-γ, IL-2, TGF-β, IL-1, IL-4, and IL-10 in various cell types (47). Two lines of experimental evidences in the present study corroborated the role of hormone-dependent cytokines in regulation of gender dimorphism of tumor cell death. Firstly that androgen treated DL cells were found to produce-enhanced amount of IFN-γ, whereas estrogen treated cells elaborated more of TGF-β, IL-2 and IL-2R (Fig.22.9). Secondly the presence of anti-bodies for the respective cytokines significantly altered the count of apoptotic tumor cells compared to that in the presence of estrogen or androgen alone in th bsence of antibodies (Fig 22.10). Thus it is suggested that the action of androgen and estrogen, in differentially regulating tumor cell apoptosis, could be direct as well as through apoptosis regulating cytokines produced by DL cells which in turn could manifest regulatory effect in an autocrine manner. The possibility of the gender-specific hormones causing a modulation of some other host-derived apoptosis regulating factors is also possible. Review of literature indicates that androgen and estrogen can modulate production of Th1 and Th2 cytokines and monokines (47), some of which could have direct and/or indirect effect on tumor cell apoptosis and growth.

The level of IFN-γ was found to increase in the ascitic fluid of DL-bearing male mice and also in the culture supernatant of DL cells treated with androgen (Fig. 22.7, 22.9). As IFN-γ has been shown to activate macrophages to tumoricidal state (48), we explored the possibility of the involve-ment of macrophages in gender-dependent differential induction of apoptosis in tumor cells. This possibility is also suggested by one of our earlier reports, where we had shown gender dimorphism in the level of monokines: IL-1 and TNF in the ascitic fluid of tumor-bearing mice (29). In a close correlation in the present study we demonstrated that the ascitic fluid of male tumor-bearing mice contained a higher level of NO. Moreover NO has been demonstrated to have a variety of effects on tumor cell growth and apoptosis (24). However, we could not detect the presence of NO in the culture supernatant of DL cells treated with androgen or estrogen (data not shown), indicating that the source of NO in the ascitic fluid could be of non-DL origin. As we had earlier reported an increase in the number of TAM along with tumor progression (21), we checked if TAM of DL-bearing mice showed gender-dependent dimorphism of NO production. Indeed TAM of male tumor-bearing mice showed a higher responsiveness to activation signals of LPS and IFNγ for production of NO compared to that of female mice (Fig. 22.5).

We also checked the expression of VEGF protein in DL cells treated with androgen or estrogen in vitro. DL cells from female tumor-bearing mice or those treated with estrogen showed an enhanced VEGF expression (Fig.22.9) compared to that of DL cells from male mice or those treated with androgen. VEGF has been demonstrated to not only augment and support angiogenesis in a progressively growing tumor but has also been assigned a number of non-angiogenic functions like antagonizing of apoptosis and regulation of cytokine production from a variety of cells types (49). The role of VEGF in antagonizing the induction of apoptosis in tumor cells treated with hormones in vitro was also confirmed by antibody-dependent blocking experiment (Fig.22.10). VEGF has been shown to down-regulate expression of bcl-2 and increase bax protein expression and thus antagonize apoptosis (50). Moreover studies have demonstrated that estrogen can up-regulate expression of VEGF in a variety of target cells promoting angiogenesis (51-52). On the other hand androgen has been shown to inhibit VEGF expression (53-54). Overall these observations indicate that VEGF could be an additional factor involved in the manifestation of gender dimorphism of tumor growth.

Further DL cells obtained from female tumor-bearing mice also showed an enhanced expression of Hsp70 and SOCS-5 proteins (Fig.22.8). Under specific conditions of tumor growth, Hsp70 over-expression has been shown to be associated with an increase in the proliferative ability of tumor cells with a concomitant ‘switching off’ of the apoptotic pathways (31). Thus it can be suggested that the gender dimorphism of Hsp70 expression in tumor cells may contribute to the differential growth rate of the tumor cells in male and female tumor-bearings host. Nevertheless role of Hsp70 in promoting tumor angiogenesis has been reported through its synergistic action with VEGF (55). Simultaneous expression of VEGF and Hsp70 has been shown to play a vital role in tumor progression (56). Moreover VEGF has also been reported to induce expression of Hsp70 (57). Our study is supported by evidences demonstrating that estrogen also increases Hsp70 expression (58). On the basis of present investigation SOCS-5 protein is indicated to play a role in gender dimorphism of T cell lymphoma. SSurveys of literature reveal that SOCS-5 has a role in anatomization of apoptosis (59). An expression of SOCS in cancer cell has been shown to be upregulated by estrogen receptor (60). Thus SOCS may play an important role in promoting tumor growth in female host.

Despite the unsolved problems regarding the mechanism(s) involved, on the basis of the afore-said observations it can be suggested that cooperation between hormones, cytokines and other apoptosis regulatory molecules underlies manifestation gender dimorphism of tumor growth.

REFERENCES

1. Hellberg D, Lindstrom AK, Stendahl U. Anticancer Research **2005,** 25, 611-616.
2. Fanale, M.A.; Uyei, A.R.; theriault, R.L.; Thompson, R.A. Clin. Breast Cancer. **2005**, 6, 354-356.
3. Sinha, P.; Clements, V.K.; Miller, S.; Ostrand-rosenberg, S. Cancer Immunol. Immunther. **2005**. 54, 1137-1142.
4. Hammacher, A.; Thompson, E.W.; Williams, E.D. Int. J. Biochem. Cell. Biol. **2005**, 37, 442-450.
5. Reiche, E.M.; Nunes, S.C.; Morimoto, H.K. Stress, depression, the immune system, and cancer. Lancet Oncol. **2004**, 5, 617-625.
6. Kousodontis, G.; Vasilaki, E.; Chou, W.C.; Papakosta, P; Kardassis, D. Biochem. J. **2005**, 389 (Pt 2): 443-55.
7. Borg, S.A.; Kerry, K.E.; Royds, J.A.; Battersby, R.D.; Jones, T.H. Eur. J. Endocrinol. **2005**, 152, 293-300.
8. Tarvainen, L.; Surronen, R.; Lindqvist, C.; Malila, NOral Dis. **2004**, 10, 167-172.
9. Nakamura, S. Gan to Kagaku ryoho. **2004**, 31, 149-157.

10. Moll, A.; Niwald, A.; Gratek, M.; Stolarska, M. Klin Oczna. **2004**, 106, 783-787.

11. Zhou, J.; Mauerer, K.; Farina, L.; Gribben, J.G. Front Biosci. **2005**,10, 1581-1596.

12. Liu, H.B.; Loo, K.K.; Palaszynski, K., Ashouri, J.; Lubahn, D.B.; Voskuhl, R.R. J. Immunol.**2003**, 171, 6936-6940.

13. Klein, G. comparative Exp. Cell Res. **1951**, 2, 518-524.

14. Goldie, H.; Felix, M.D. Cancer Res. **1951**, 11, 73-80.

15. Udaychander, M.; Menakshi, A.; Muthiah, R.; Sivanandham, R. Int. J. Radiat. Oncol. Biol. Phys.**1987**, 13, 1713-1718.

16. Khynriam, D.; Prasad, S.B. Mutat. Res. **2003**, 526, 9-18.

17. Kumar, A.; Singh, S.M.. Immunol. Invest. **1996**, 25, 413-423.

18. Kumar, A.; Singh, S.M.; Sodhi, A. Int. J. Immunopharmacol. **1997**, 19, 129-133.

19. Parajuli, P.; Singh, S.M. J. Immunopathol. Pharmacol. **1995**, 8, 103-111.

20. Parajuli, P.; Singh, S.M.,. Cancer Lett. **1996**, 107, 249-256.

21. Parajuli, P.; Singh, S.M.; Kumar, A.; Sodhi, A. Cancer J. **1997**, 10, 22-227.

22. Bharti, A.; Singh, S.M,. Immunol. Lett. **2000**, 72, 39-48.

23. Bharti, A.; Singh, S.M.,. Int. Immunopharmacol. **2001**, 1, 155-165.

24. Bharti, A.; Singh, S.M., Nitric Oxide. **2003**, 8, 75-82.

25. Singh, N.; Singh, S.M.; Srivastava, P. Immunopharmacol. Immunotoxicol. **2004**, 26, 1-18.

26. Srivastava, P,; Singh, S.M.; Singh, N.. Cancer Investigation. **2005**, 23, 316-322.

27. Shankar, A.; Singh, S.M.; Sodhi, A., Tumor Biol. **2000 a**, 21, 315-327.

28. Shankar, A,; Singh, S,M,; Sodhi, A.; Tumor Biol. **2000 b**, 21, 288-298.

29. Singh, M.P.; Rai, A.K.; Singh, S.M., J. Rep. Immunol. **2005**, 65, 17-32.

30. Singh, M.P.; Sharma, H.; Singh, S.M.,. Cancer Invest. **2006**, 24, 1-10.

31. Evan, G.I.; Vousden, K.H., Nature **2001**, 411, 342-348.

32. Hanahan, D,; Weinberg, R.A., Cell, **2000**, Vol. 100, 57-70.

33. Singh, M.P.; Singh, G.; Singh, S.M., Comp. Immunol., Micro. & Infect. Dis. **2005**, 28, 231-248.

34. Mossman, T.; J. Immunol. Methods. **1998**. 65, 53-63.

35. Sellins, K.S,; Cohen, J.J., J. Immunol. **1987**, 139, 199-206.

36. Ding, A.H.; Nathan, C.F.; Stuehr, D.J.; J. Immunol. **1988**, 141, 2407-12.

37. Shankar, A.; Singh, S.M.; Sodhi, A., FEMS Immunol Med microbiol. **2000,** 27, 247-255.

38. Hayflick, L (ed. P.K. Kruse, jr and M.K. patterson, Jr), **1973**, pp 121-31. IRL Press, Oxford.

39. Deftos, L.J.; Barken, I.; Burton, D.W.; Hoffman, R.M.; Geller, J. Biochem. Biophys. Res. Commun. **2005**, 327,. 468-472.

40. Ling, S.; Dai, A.; Williams, M.R.; Myles, K.; Dilley, R.J.; Komesaroff, P.A.; Sudhir, K. Endocrinology. **2002**, 143, 1119-25.

41. Hatzoglou, A.; Kampa, M.; Kogia, C.; Charalaampopoulos, I.; Theodoropoulos, P.A.; Anezinis, P.; Dambaki, C.; Papakonstanti, E.A.; Stathopoulos, E.N.; Stiurnaras, C.; Gravanis, A.; Castanas, E.; The J. of Clin. Endocrin. **2005**, 90, 893-903.

42. Lewis, J.S.; Meeke, K.; Osipo, C.; Ross, E.A.; Kidawi, N.; Li, T.; Bell, E,; Chandel, N.S.; Jordan, V.C.'. J. Natl. cancer Inst. **2005**, 97, 1746-1759.

43. Kirschenbaum, X_H., Liu, S., Yai, G., Narla, S.L., Freidman, J.A.. Carcinogenesis, 2006, 27, 216-224.

44. Zhang, Y., Champagne, N., Beitel, L.K>, Goodyer, G.C., Trifiro, M, Blanc A.. J. Neurosci. 2004, 5315-5321.
45. Sangfelt, O.; Einhorn, S.; bjorklund, A.C.; Wiman, K.G.; Okan, I.; Grander, D. Int. J. Cancer. **1996**, 67, 106-112.
46. Nitsu, N.; Higasshihara, M.; Honma, Y., Leuco Res. **2002**, 26, 745-755.
47. Bouman, A.; Heineman, M.J.; Fass, M.M., Human Reproduc. **2005**, 11, 411-423.
48. Mantovani, A., Sica, A. and Locati, M.. Immunity. 2005, 23, 344-346
49. Neufeld, G.; Cohen, T.; Gengrinovitch, S.; Poltorak, Z., The FASEB J. 1999, 13, 9-22.
50. Zhang H, Lu J.J, Gao QZ, Zhang J. Zhonghua Wai Kc Za Zhi. 2006, 44, 382-395.
51. Liang Y, Brekken RA, Hyder SM. Endocr Relat Cancer, 2006, 13, 905-919.
52. Hyder SM. Sex-steroids regulation of vascular endothelial growth factor in breast cancer. Endocr Relat Cancer. 2006, 13, 667-687.
53. Rinaldo F, Li J, Wang E, Muders M, Datta K.. Oncogene, **2006** Sep 11: (Epub ahead of print)
54. Boddy J.L., Fox SB, Han C, Campo L, Turkey H, Kanga S, Malone PR, Harris AL.. Clin Cancer Res. **2005**, 11, 7658-7663.
55. Bernardini C, Zannoni A, Turba ME, Fantinati P, Tamanini C, Bacci ML, Forni M. Cell Stress Chaperones. **2005**, 10, 340-348.
56. Canoz O, Gunnes T, Deniz K, akgun H, Balkanli S. APMIS. **2006**, 114, 10-24.
57. Hu, MJ.; Liu, Y.; Deng, C.G.; Chang, Y.Q.; Wang, J.N.; Dong, Y.Z., Di Yi Jun da Xue Xue Bao, **2003**, 23, 720-722.
58. Al-Khlaiwi, T.; Al-Dress, A.; Gursoy, E.; Qureshi, I.; biber, T.; Kalimi, M. J. Cardiovas. Pharmacol. **2005**, 45, 217-224.
59. Morita, Y.; Naka, T.; Kawazoe, Y.; Fujimoto, M.; Narazaki, M.; Nagagawa, R.; Fukuyama, H.; Nagata, S.; Kishimoto, T., Proc Natl Acad Sci USA, **2000**, 97, 5405-5410.
60. Matthews, J.; Almlof, T.; Kietz, S.; Leers, J.; Gustafsson, J.A.,. Biochem Biophys Res Commun, **2005**, 335, 168-74.

23
CHAPTER

Humoral Immune Response Against Sperm Associated Antigen 9 (SPAG9) in Epithelial Ovarian Cancer

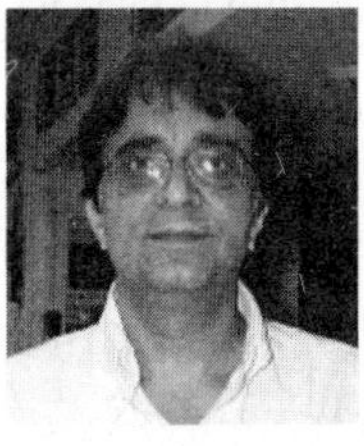

Manoj Garg[1], Deepika Kanojia[1], Namrata Dudha[1], Satish Sati[1], Sudha Salhan[2], Amar Bhatnagar[2], Sushma Suri[2], Anju Gupta[3] and Anil Suri[1]

[1]Cancer Microarray, Genes and Proteins Laboratory, National Institute of Immunology, Aruna Asaf Ali Marg, J.N.U. Campus, [2]Safdarjung Hospital and Vardhman Mahavir Medical College; and [3]Moolchand Hospital, New Delhi–110067

Ovarian cancer is the major cause of death from gynecologic malignancy. The overall mortality of ovarian cancer has remained unchanged despite new chemotherapeutic agents, which have significantly improved the 5-year survival rate [2]. The main reason is lack of success in diagnosing ovarian cancer at an early stage, and therefore, the majority of patients with ovarian cancer are diagnosed only in the advanced stages. Detecting cancers at their earliest stages, even in the premalignant state, means that current or future treatment modalities might have a higher likelihood of a true cure. The lack of preventive methods, early diagnostic methods, and effective therapies to treat recurrent ovarian tumors points toward a pressing need for identification of molecular targets for diagnosis as well as therapy.

Recently, a novel testis-specific sperm associated antigen 9 (SPAG9) gene was characterized [3], a new member of c-Jun NH_2-terminal kinase (JNK)–interacting protein family [4] involved in molecular interactions during sperm-egg fusion and mitogen- activated protein kinase signaling pathway [4, 5]. The expression pattern of SPAG9 was shown in different histotypes of epithelial ovarian cancer (EOC) tissues and ovarian cancer cell lines [1]. The presence of SPAG9 antibodies were demonstrated in the patients suffering from different ovarian malignancies. The expression of both SPAG9 mRNA and protein was detected in majority of cancer specimens. In addition, the presence of specific humoral response against SPAG9 was shown in EOC patients which further relate SPAG9 immunogenicity with early stages of EOC, suggesting its important role in early diagnostics. The present review extends the application of SPAG9, a novel member of cancer testisantigen family, as a potential target for the development of diagnostic and therapeutic methods in EOC.

CANCER TESTIS ANTIGENS

Cancer testis antigens represent a unique class of tumor antigens, which are expressed in a variety of cancerous tissues and are silent in normal tissues, except for the testis [6]. A characteristic commonly shared by cancer testis antigens is, aside from the highly tissue-restricted expression profile, their likely correlation with tumor progression and immunogenicity in cancer patients. To date, 89 individual CT antigen genes or isoforms have been described, which are organized into 44 families [6, 7]. From these, 19 families are testis-restricted and 11 show additional expression in one or two somatic tissues. Nine are expressed in 3–6 tissue types beside testis, and 5 are ubiquitously somatically expressed. Expression of CT antigens was first shown in melanoma, and all of the classic CT antigens are expressed in this type of tumor; however, since the 1980s, expression in various other tumors have also been recognized [6] but coordinated humoral and cellular immune responses have been reported for only a few cancer testis antigens, including NY-ESO-1, CAGE, and XAGE [8-10]. Because of their broad expression in cancer and restricted expression in normal tissues and high immunogenicity, cancer testis antigens are the most attractive targets for cancer immunotherapy and serum biomarker.

SPERM ASSOCIATED ANTIGEN 9 AS CANCER TESTIS ANTIGEN

A novel testis-specific sperm associated antigen 9 (SPAG9), an acrosomal molecule involved in the human sperm-egg interaction is a new member of JNK–interacting protein family. This novel testis-specific protein is exclusively expressed in testis. *In situ* hybridization of human testis section showed SPAG9 mRNA expression in round spermatids only [6]. SPAG9 is a single-copy gene mapped to human chromosome 17q21 [4], a region involved in amplification and expression of cancer related genes as well as a hotspot for chromosomal aberrations in various cancers. Serologic studies of ovarian tumor antigens showed a bias towards antigens encoded on 17q21, suggesting that elevated expression of genes encoded within this region of chromosome 17 is an important event in ovarian tumors [11]. Expression of SPAG9 gene along with other important much-studied genes has been reported in breast tumors [12], cervix carcinoma cells [13], dermatofibrosarcoma protuberans [14], and esophageal adenocarcinoma [15] by employing gene expression microarray analysis. Recently, the chromatin immunoprecipitation-paired end ditag sequencing approach was used to identify novel p53 target genes. It was demonstrated that SPAG9, along with antiapoptotic genes (BCL2A1 and TNFAIP8), is down-regulated in wild-type p53 tumors compared with the p53 mutant-type tumors [16]. Further, the higher expression of these p53- repressed genes in p53 mutant-type tumors was shown to be linked to the development of distant metastasis in more aggressive tumors. Therefore, SPAG9 expression characteristics *in vivo* can potentially be used as molecular gauges of tumor aggressiveness and clinical outcome.

EXPRESSION OF SPAG9 IN EPITHELIAL OVARIAN CANCER

SPAG9 expression was detected in ovarian cancer tissues at both mRNA and protein level. RT-PCR and *in situ* hybridization were employed to detect the expression of SPAG9 at mRNA level in EOC tissues. The PCR product was confirmed as SPAG9 by nucleotide sequencing. The relationship between SPAG9 mRNA expression and pathologic and clinical features is shown in Table 23.1. SPAG9 expression was detected in all the early-stage (I and II) and in most of the late-stage (III and IV) EOC tissues. Hence, SPAG9 expression was independent of tumor stage, indicating no correlation between tumor stages and SPAG9 expression.

Table 23.1 SPAG9 expression (RT-PCR/ immunohistochemistry), humoral response (ELISA/Western blot), and Clinicopathologic features in EOC

Pathologic and clinical features	SPAG9 expression by RT-PCR/IHC (Positive/Tested)	ELISA/Western blot (Positive/Tested)
All Tumors FIGO Stage	18/20 (90%)	20/30 (67%)
I	1/1	2/2
IB	2/2	2/3
IC	1/1	0/1
II	1/1	1/2
Subtotal of FIGO stages I and II	5/5 (100%)	5/8 (62.5%)
III	4/5	7/9
IIIA	1/1	0/1
IIIC	1/1	1/2
IV	7/8	7/10
Subtotal of FIGO stages III and IV	13/15 (87%)	15/22 (68%)
Histology		
Adenocarcinoma		
Serous	15/17 (88%)	11/19 (58%)
Clear cell	1/1 (100%)	2/2 (100%)
Mucinous	2/2 (100%)	3/3 (100%)
Unclassified		4/6 (67%)

In situ hybridization with digoxigenin-labeled riboprobes was employed to detect SPAG9 mRNA expression in different subtypes of ovarian cancer tissues. The mRNA expression was detected on the development of chocolate brown reaction product formed after the hybridization of antisense riboprobe, indicating the presence of SPAG9 mRNA in ovarian cancer tissues as shown in Fig. 23.1 (D-F). No localization of SPAG9 was detected with sense riboprobe (Fig. 23.1 G-I).

SPAG9 expression was detected at the protein level in ovarian cancer tissues by employing immunohistochemistry using anti-SPAG9 antibodies. A distinct immunoreactivity of SPAG9 protein was demonstrated in human testis by immunohistochemistry (Fig 23.2A). It was demon-

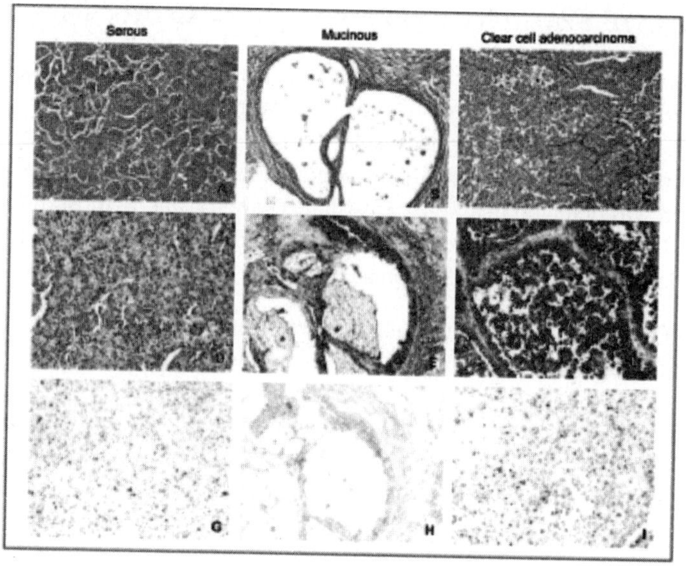

Fig. 23.1 *In situ* hybridization showing SPAG9 expression in different subtypes of EOC tissue. Representative H&E-stained sections from serous (A), mucinous (B), and clear cell adenocarcinoma (C).Tissue sections from the same specimens were hybridized with digoxigenin-labeled SPAG9 antisense (D, serous; E, mucinous; F, clear cell adenocarcinoma) and sense (G, serous; H, mucinous; I, clear cell adenocarcinoma) riboprobes. Signal was developed using alkaline phosphatase nitroblue tetrazolium/ 5-bromo-4-chloro-3-indolyl phosphate. Original magnification, x200; objective, 20x.

strated that immunolocalization of SPAG9 protein was restricted to sperm head and not in any other cell types of seminiferous tubules. Among the EOC specimens, 90% of the ovarian cancer samples showed the expression of SPAG9 protein (Table 23.1). SPAG9 expression was detected in both the epithelial and stromal components of mucinous carcinoma tissues (Fig. 23.2B). In serous carcinoma, most of the samples displayed immunoreactivity throughout the tumor tissue section (Fig. 23.2C) and in some samples heterogeneous staining was detected for SPAG9 with areas corresponding to invasive foci and regions with poor histological differentiation displayed a stronger staining. Strong SPAG9 immunoreactivity was detected in ovarian tissue section diagnosed with clear cell carcinoma.

SPAG9 expression was also detected in ovarian cancer cell lines by employing indirect immunofluorescence using the anti-SPAG9 antibodies. Strong SPAG9 immunoreactivity was demonstrated in the ovarian cancer cells. Predominantly cytoplasmic expression of SPAG9 was detected in fixed and permeabilized ovarian cancer cells whereas surface localization of SPAG9 was detected in live cells (Fig. 23.3 B). Surface localization of SPAG9 in ovarian cancer cells was also demonstrated by Flow cytometry (Fig. 23.3 C). No or very low surface distribution (0.23% fluorescence intensity) was detected in the control cells, whereas 40.70% fluorescence intensity or displacement of fluorescence on X axis was detected in cells probed with anti-SPAG9 antibody, indicating surface localization of SPAG9 protein.

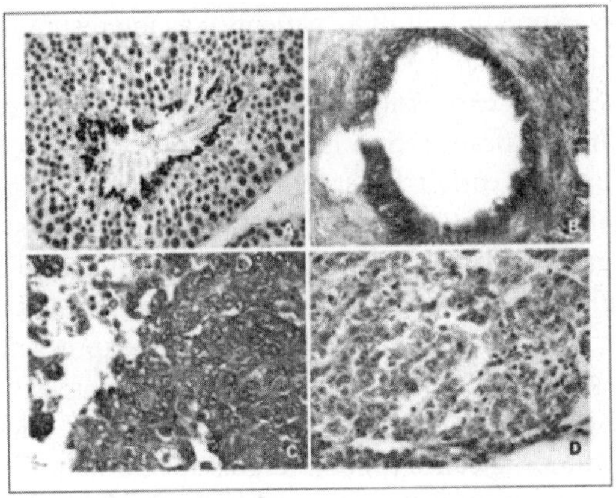

Fig. 23.2 Analysis of SPAG9 expression in EOC tissues. A, immunohistochemical staining of normal testis. SPAG9 protein was detected in the sperm head and not in any other cell type. B to D, cytoplasmic localization of SPAG9 protein was observed in mucinous (B), serous (C), and clear cell carcinoma (D). Original magnification, x400; objective, 40x.

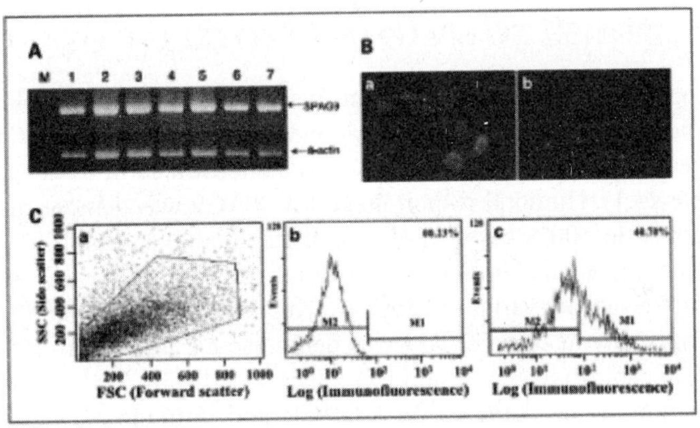

Fig. 23.3 A, RT-PCR analysis for SPAG9 mRNA expression yielded 1.2 kb product. mRNA from serous (lane1), mucinous (lane 2), and clear cell carcinoma (lane 3) tissues; from three ovarian cancer cell lines, A-10 (lane 4), SKOV-6 (lane 5), and Caov-2 (lane 6); and from testis (lane 7). b-actin gene expression was used as an internal control. B, evaluation of SPAG9 protein expression in ovarian cancer cells by indirect immunofluorescence microscopy. a, SKOV-6 cells revealed predominant cytoplasmic SPAG9 expression in fixed and permeabilized cell stained with anti-SPAG9 antibodies; b, surface localization of SPAG9 was observed in live SKOV-6 cells. Cells were stained with 4',6-diamidino-2-phenylindole to show the nucleus. The fluorescence images were merged using Image-Pro Plus version 5.1. Original magnification, x400; objective, 40x. C, fluorescence-activated cell sorting analysis of SPAG9 expression in SKOV-6 cells. a, side scatter (SSC) versus forward scatter (FSC) gate analysis; b, percentile fluorescence (displacement of fluorescence on X axis) of control cells stained with secondary antibody only; c, percentile fluorescence of SPAG9-expressing cells probed with anti-SPAG9 antibodies (M1).M1, gating of fluorescence-positive cells; M2, gating of fluorescence-negative cells.

The predominant SPAG9 expression in EOC patients was interesting when compared with other known potential cancer testis antigens. Sperm protein 17 mRNA has been reported to be expressed in 68% of ovarian tumors. SPAG9 expression was detected in both the epithelial and stromal components of mucinous carcinoma tissues. Similar finding of stromal cell staining in few ovarian cancer samples was also reported earlier for sperm protein 17 expression [17]. Another study on testis-specific synaptonemal complex protein-1 reported mRNA expression in only 15% of ovarian cancer specimens. However, immunohistochemical studies showed no detectable protein expression in synaptonemal complex protein-1 mRNA-positive ovarian tumor samples [18]. A well-characterized cancer testis antigen NYESO-1 mRNA and protein expression was reported in 43% of EOC specimens [19]. In contrast, SPAG9 mRNA and protein expression was detected in 90% of EOC tissues analyzed irrespective of disease stage and histotypes. This is one of the important criteria toward identifying tumor-specific protein targets for immunotherapy and development of cancer biomarker. Moreover, tumor stages have no effect on the frequency of SPAG9 expression in different malignant histotypes of epithelial ovarian tissues. The presence of SPAG9 expression in early-stage EOC tissues thereby ensures its important role as potential biomarker for early diagnosis of ovarian malignancies. Hence, SPAG9 is an important candidate molecule, which shows a considerable merit over other cancer testis antigens.

HUMORAL RESPONSE TO SPAG9 IN EPITHELIAL OVARIAN CANCER

Humoral response against SPAG9 in EOC patients was demonstrated by employing ELISA. High-titer IgG antibodies directed at SPAG9 protein were detected by ELISA in EOC patients irrespective of disease stages. SPAG9 immunoreactivity was demonstrated in 67% patients with different disease stages (Table 23.1). Humoral response against SPAG9 was demonstrated in 58% cases of serous adenocarcinoma, in 100% cases of clear cell carcinoma, and in 100% cases of mucinous adenocarcinoma. It is interesting to note that humoral response against SPAG9 was detected in 62.5% of patients suffering from various histotypes with early stages of ovarian cancer (stages I and II). *In vivo* immunogenicity against SPAG9 was demonstrated in 68% of patients suffering from later stages of ovarian cancer (stages III and IV). More specifically 72% of the EOC patients with SPAG9-expressing tumors, as detected by RT-PCR and immunohistochemistry, showed the presence of SPAG9 antibody suggesting that SPAG9 antibody was most likely generated as a consequence of SPAG9 expression.

The presence of SPAG9 antibody in the patient's serum was also detected by employing western blotting. Specific SPAG9 antibodies were detected in sera of 67% of ovarian cancer patients irrespective of malignant histotypes. However, no specific SPAG9 antibodies were detected in sera from healthy individuals. Further, the specificity of SPAG9 antibody from patient's sera was also demonstrated by neutralization of SPAG9 antibodies in patient's serum with recombinant SPAG9. Incubation of the patient's serum with recombinant SPAG9 showed loss in the immunoreactivity of SPAG9 protein (Fig. 23.4B). It was demonstrated on the basis of available tumor stage information for EOC patients that the occurrence of antibodies against SPAG9 in EOC patients was not a feature of advanced-stage disease.

It is interesting to note that NY-ESO-1, the most immunogenic cancer testis antigen with well-documented spontaneous and vaccine-induced immunity [20], showed antibodies to NY-ESO-1 in only 12.5% of ovarian cancer patients [21]. In another study, antibody response against synovial sarcoma on X chromosome 4 was demonstrated in only 1 of 44 ovarian cancer patients [22]. Similarly, no antibody response was detected in synaptonemal complex protein-1–expressing ovarian cancer patients [18]. However, the SPAG9 antibody response was demonstrated in 67% of serum samples, indicating strong immunogenicity of SPAG9 protein in ovarian cancer patients. Furthermore, the expression of antibodies to NY-ESO-1, p53, HER2/neu, HOXB7, and MAGE family gene products is reported in late-stage ovarian cancer patients, and possible existence of these responses in a significant proportion of early-stage ovarian cancer patients remains unknown [6]. Significant proportion of immune response against SPAG9 was demonstrated in 62.5% of early-stage (I and II) and 68% of late-stage (III and IV) ovarian cancer patients. This is an important finding where significant number (62.5%) of early-stage EOC patients showed strong humoral response against SPAG9 expression, supporting its potential role as a serum biomarker.

CONCLUSION

In conclusion, SPAG9 is expressed at both mRNA and protein level in majority of epithelial ovarian cancers. SPAG9-specific humoral response is demonstrated in various histotypes with different stages of ovarian cancer, indicating that SPAG9 is a promising candidate biomarker for early diagnostics, prognosis, and tumor aggressiveness. This review extends the application of SPAG9 for its potential use as a prognostic marker in tissue biopsies.

REFERENCES

1. Garg M, Chaurasiya D, Rana R, Jagadish N, Kanojia D, Dudha N, Kamran N, Salhan S, Bhatnagar A, Suri S, Gupta A, Suri A. Sperm-associated antigen 9, a novel cancer testis antigen, is a potential target for immunotherapy in epithelial ovarian cancer. Clin Cancer Res. 2007; 13(5):1421-8.
2. Jemal A, Tiwari RC, Murray T, et al. Cancer statistics, 2004. CA Cancer J Clin 2004; 54:8-29.
3. Shankar S, Mohapatra B, Suri A. Cloning of a novel human testis mRNA specifically expressed in testicular haploid germ cells, having unique palindromic sequences and encoding a leucine zipper dimerization motif. Biochem Biophys Res Commun 1998; 243: 561-5.
4. Jagadish N, Rana R, Selvi R, et al. Characterization of a novel human sperm-associated antigen 9 (SPAG9) having structural homology with c-Jun N-terminal kinase-interacting protein. Biochem J 2005; 389:73-82.
5. Jagadish N, Rana R, Mishra D, Kumar M, Suri A. Sperm associated antigen 9 (SPAG9): a new member of c-Jun NH_2-terminal kinase (JNK) interacting protein exclusively expressed in testis. Keio J Med 2005; 54:66-71.
6. Suri A. Cancer testis antigens - their importance in immunotherapy and in the early detection of cancer. Expert Opin Biol Ther 2006; 6:379 -89.
7. Scanlan MJ, Simpson AJ, Old LJ. The cancer/testis genes: review, standardization, and commentary. Cancer Immun 2004; 4:1.
8. Tureci O, Mack U, Luxemburger U, et al. Humoral immune responses of lung cancer patients against tumor antigen NY-ESO-1.Cancer Lett 2006; 236:64-71.
9. Nakagawa K, Noguchi Y, Uenaka A, et al. XAGE-1 expression in non-small cell lung cancer and antibody response in patients. Clin Cancer Res 2005; 11: 5496-503.

10. Iwata T, Fujita T, Hirao N, et al. Frequent immune responses to a cancer/testis antigen, CAGE, in patients with microsatellite instability-positive endometrial cancer. Clin Cancer Res 2005; 11:39 49-57.
11. Stone B, Schummer M, Paley PJ, et al. Serologic analysis of ovarian tumor antigens reveals a bias toward antigens encoded on 17q. Int. J Cancer 2003; 104:73 - 84.
12. Willis S, Hutchins AM, Hammet F, et al. Detailed gene copy number and RNA expression analysis of the 17q12-23 region in primary breast cancers. Genes Chromosomes Cancer 2003; 36:382-92.
13. Kitahara O, Katagiri T, Tsunoda T, et al. Classification of sensitivity or resistance of cervical cancers to ionizing radiation according to expression profiles of 62 genes selected by cDNA microarray analysis. Neoplasia 2002; 4:295-303.
14. Linn SC, West RB , Pollack JR, et al. Gene expression patterns and gene copy number changes in dermatofibrosarcoma protuberans. Am J Pathol 2003; 163: 2383-95.
15. Helm J, Enkemann SA, Coppola D, et al. Dedifferentiation precedes invasion in the progression from Barrett's metaplasia to esophageal adenocarcinoma. Clin Cancer Res 2005; 11:2478-85.
16. Wei CL, Wu Q, Vega VB, et al. A global map of p53 transcription-factor binding sites in the human genome. Cell 2006; 124:207-19.
17. Straughn JM, Jr., Shaw DR, Guerrero A, et al. Expression of sperm protein 17 (Sp17) in ovarian cancer. Int J Cancer 2004; 108:805-11.
18. Tammela J, Jungbluth AA, Qian F, et al. SCP-1cancer/ testis antigen is a prognostic indicator and a candidate target for immunotherapy in epithelial ovarian cancer. Cancer Immun 2004; 4:10-6.
19. Odunsi K, Jungbluth AA, Stockert E, et al. NY-ESO-1and LAGE-1cancer-testis antigens are potential targets for immunotherapy in epithelial ovarian cancer. Cancer Res 2003; 63:6076-83.
20. Jager D, Stockert E, Karbach J, et al. Urine antibody against human cancer antigen NY-ESO-1. Cancer Immun 2002; 2:10 - 8.
21. Stockert E, Jager E, Chen YT, et al. A survey of the humoral immune response of cancer patients to a panel of human tumor antigens. JExpMed1998; 187: 1349-54.
22. Hasegawa K, Koizumi F, Noguchi Y, et al. SSX expression in gynecological cancers and antibody response in patients. Cancer Immun 2004; 4:16.

24
CHAPTER

Molecular Staging of Glial Tumors

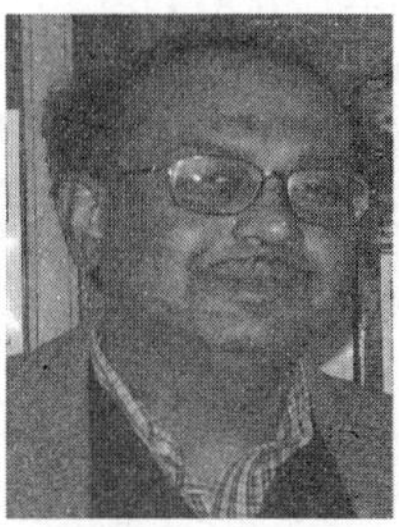

Tapasya Srivastava[1], Kunzang Chosdol[1], Anjan Misra[1,4], Parthaprasad Chattopadhyay[1], Chitra Sarkar[2], Ashok K. Mahapatra[3,5] and Subrata Sinha[1]

Department of Biochemistry[1], Pathology[2] and Neurosurgery[3], All India Institute of Medical Sciences, New Delhi.
[4]Present address: Barrow Neurological Institute, St. Joseph's Hospital and Medical Center, Phoenix, AZ, USA.
[5]Present address: Sanjay Gandhi Post Graduate Institute of Medical Sciences (SGPGI), Raebareli Road, Lucknow

Glial cells are the supporting cells of the central nervous system (CNS) and important for nurturing and sustaining the neurons. They are the most abundant cell type in CNS and are present in the vicinity of the neurons. They are also known to play a role in signaling in response to stimuli and are the mediators of cross-talk between neurons and endothelial cells. Glial cells are of three sub-types, astrocytes, oligodendrocytes and microglia.

GLIAL TUMORS

Prevalence

Glial tumors may arise from the astrocytes (astrocytomas), oligodendrocytes (oligodendrogliomas) or ependymal (ependydomas) of the brain. This heterogenous group of tumors are the most frequent neoplasms of the central nervous system. In adults, gliomas account for about 2% of the primary malignant tumors and are the second most common tumors to affect the age of 35 years, next to hematological malignancies. Age and performance status of the patient, together with tumor type and grade are the determining prognostic factors of the gliomas. However, the survival time of a particular tumor grade shows variation amongst individuals.

In our lab, we have mostly worked on tumors arising from cells of the astrocytic lineage i.e. the astrocytic tumors.

WHO Classification and Presentation

WHO grading of tumors arising from astrocytes is according to their degree of malignancy assessed by histopathological analysis based on the presence or absence ofnuclear atypia, mitosis, microvascular proliferation, and necrosis. By and large, the survival time is inversely proportionate to the degree of malignancy. Histologic features of the tumor and the patient's age and performance status are major prognostic factors and have more influence than any specific therapy on the outcome.

WHO Grade I or Pilocytic astrocytomas are benign tumors which typically are not a part of the progressive astrocytomas and mostly occur in children.

WHO Grade II or Diffuse Astrocytomas (DA) are the least malignant of the gliomas and occur in late middle age. Their pathology shows a poor definition, few proliferating and more differentiated cells. These tumors on resection have a great chance of recurrence and present with a pathology more malignant than the original tumor.

WHO Grade III or Anaplastic Astrocytomas (AA) are tumors with increased hyper cellularity, pleomorphic cells and hyperchromatism. AA show increased malignancy as compared to DA.

WHO Grade IV or Glioblastoma multiforme (GBM) are the most malignant of all astrocytic tumors. These tumors have very poor prognosis and their pathology shows increased necrosis and cysts. The DA and AA may progress to GBM with time.

Behavior and Outcome

The outcome of glial tumors has not really changed with time inspite of development of state-of-the-art non-invasive detection and current treatment modalities. The mean survival time of DA is six years, surgery being the preferred corrective treatment. However, the chances of recurrence are high and invariably the recurrent tumor presents with increased malignancy and stage. The range of survival of these young patients is broad and unpredictable. The survival rate of patients with AA is considerably less as compared to DA. The mean time is only about two years. AA responds well to chemotherapy and radiotherapy, and again, there is no consistency amongst individuals. GBM, being the most malignant tumor, has very poor prognosis and the survival time is only about one year. The astrocytic tumors are difficult to treat and quite drug resistant, combination therapy has shown better results than stand-alone treatment. To improve the prognosis and outcome of the patient, the primary focus of current laboratory and clinical research is to better understand unique challenges such as the heterogeneity of individual tumors, the delivery of drugs or other agents into the central nervous system, and the neurotoxic effects of therapy.

MOLECULAR STAGING: TUMORIGENESIS AND PROGRESSION

Oncogenesis is a complex process and no individual gene/protein has overall control on either initiation or progression of the oncogenic process. Development of astrocytic tumors, like many other tumors, is a multistep process which involves occurrence of many genetic events which compel a normal cell towards tumor phenotype. Amplification of oncogenes, suppression of tumor suppressor genes (TSGs) and altered expression of growth factors, which are specific for different stages of tumor progression are some of the common factors studied to understand the process of tumorigenesis and also further progression of malignancy. Specific factors have been consistently shown to be associated with various stages of the tumor and also with the transition of tumor phenotypes.

The characterization of the heterogeneity of tumor type in glial tumors in terms of its molecular profile is necessary to not only understand the tumor evolution but also to design therapeutic modalities which provide the best efficacy and survival. Molecular staging has vast implications in treatment of recurrent gliomas. At the molecular level there are many reports in literature which specifically show the involvement of various (including chromosomal locations of putative) tumor suppressor and oncogene in the development and progression of the astrocytic tumor. A summary of various factors contributing to glial tumorigenesis and progression reported in literature is given in Table1{modified from [1]} .

Tumorigenesis; Diffuse Astrocytoma (DA)

The low grade, DA are associated with alterations such as those of p53, activation of tumor growth factors such as PDGF (platelet derived growth factor), Fibroblast growth factor (FGF) and loss of chromosome 22q in 20-30% DA [2]. p53 alteration are known to occur in all stages of astrocytic tumors. Our lab has also reported that about 7/19 (37%) DA and 11/23 (48%) AA+GBM show loss of heterozygosity (LOH) at p53 indicating that p53 mutations are involved in glial tumorigenensis without any predilection to a particular phenotype [3]. In particular 3' rearrangements of c-myc oncogene were observed to be associated with dysregulation (increase) of c-myc protein in low grade, DA [4]. We have also reported the significant association of LOH at mismatch repair gene hMLH1 gene to be associated with DA [5]. LOH was also observed at the putative tumor suppressor hFAT locus, (q34-35) in DA (unpublished data).

Progression to Anaplastic Astrocytoma (AA)

Various reports indicate DA to AA transition to be associated with loss of chromosome13q13 which houses the Rb (retinoblastoma) gene. Rb gene, when hyperphosphorylated or absent results in dysregulaton of the cell cycle and continuous progression through G1/S phase. Rathore et al have also shown an aberrant phosphoRb expression to be increasing associated with high grade tumors and in their report [6] showed a heterogenous and aberrant pRb expression detected by histochemistry in 2/16 DA, 4/19 AA and 7/22 GBM. The same report also confirms our LOH findings on association of p53 mutations with all grades of astrocytic tumors and an increased expression by histochemical analysis (indicative of a mutant p53) was observed in 10/16 DA, 15/19 AA and 20/22 GBM. The loss of p16 or p15 genes on chromosome 9p21 is also known to occur commonly in higher grade of tumor [7]. Gene amplification of cdk4 or cyclin D1 is also observed in high grade gliomas [8]. The MDM2 gene as well as GLI gene on chromosome 12q are known to amplify at later stages of tumor progression [9].

Glioblastoma Multiforme (GBM)

The majority of cases (>90%) are primary glioblastomas that develop rapidly *de novo*, without clinical or histological evidence of a less malignant precursor lesion. They affect mainly the elderly and are associated with dysregulation of EGFR/PTEN/Akt/mTOR pathway and is genetically characterized by LOH at 10q, EGFR amplification, p16^{INK4a} deletion, and PTEN mutations. Secondary glioblastomas develop through progression from low-grade diffuse astrocytoma or anaplastic astrocytoma and manifest in younger patients. the TP53/MDM2/p14^{ARF} pathway is dysregulated in the pathway to secondary glioblastoma [10]. TP53 mutations are the most frequent and earliest detectable genetic alteration, already present in 60% of precursor low-grade astrocytomas. LOH at 10q is associated with both types of GBM and it is associated with overall reduction in survival time of patient [11]. The gene DCC, deleted-in-colon carcinoma (18q21) is also known to be deleted in 53% GBM as compared to 7% DA suggesting a role in genesis of GBM [12]. LOH at 22q is significantly more frequent in secondary glioblastomas (82%) than in primary glioblastomas (41%)[13]. We have also reported a region on chromosome 17p13.3 whose LOH is associated with high grade tumors, AA and GBM [3]. What is of special interest is that one AA tumor which on microdissection showed explicit demarcation of a region with low and high malignancy tumor regions. The heterozygosity status at 17p13.3 region on DNA extracted from these two regions showed LOH only in the more malignant area while no LOH was seen at p53 locus in either areas. This led us to speculate that a tumor suppressor gene is located in this region of the chromosome 17 (17p13.3) which is independent of p53 (17p13.1). This is an interesting example of molecular heterogeneity within a particular histological grade translating into phenotypic characteristic. We have also observed that LOH at 17p13.3 is associated with increased proliferation in astrocytic tumors [14] indicating that alterations at one or more putative tumor suppressor genes present at this locus results in higher rate of proliferation within a histological grade. We have also report aberrantly higher expression of hMSH2 protein in GBM as compared to DA by immunohistochemistry [15]. LOH at this region, however, did not show a significant difference between DA and GBM indicating that the higher protein expression detected may be under control of other cellular factors.

GENOMIC AND PROTEOMIC APPROACHES

A global analysis of genes with the help of microarray provide an excellent platform for further analysis of specific genes. Characterization and cataloging of the genetic alterations and molecular markers that correlate with the clinical behavior of gliomas are needed to establish the comprehensive molecular fingerprint of these tumors. A high-throughput technology, such as microarray, may facilitate the molecular profiling of human tumors considerably. Thousands of genes can now be analyzed in a simple microarray hybridization. The expression profile from a single tumor reflects the state of events of an individual malignancy at a certain time point. To generalize the findings and provide conclusive evidence for the involvement of a molecular alteration, it is often necessary to analyze a large number of tumors at a time. DNA microarrays such as cDNA and oligo array as well as tissue array are currently in use for characterizing tumors. Glioma profiling has also been done using this powerful technology and has given insight into novel genes involved in specific stages of glial tumorigenesis and progression.

Rickman et al [16] used DNA microarrays to identify gene expression differences between high-grade and low-grade glial tumors. They compared the transcriptional profile of 45 astrocytic tumors including 21 GBMs and 19 pilocytic astrocytomas using oligonucleotide-based microarrays. Of the ~ 6800 genes that were analyzed, a set of 360 genes provided a molecular signature that distinguished between GBMs and pilocytic astrocytomas. Overexpression of the EGFR, MDM2, CDK4, CD44, and IGFBP2 genes is well described in gliomas and the results validated the available

Table 24.1 Genetic alterations in different grades of glioma Chosdol et al (1)

Alteration	Astrocytoma	Anaplastic astrocytoma	Glioblastoma multiforme	
			Progressive	Primary
Deletion/mutation of tumor suppressor gene				
P53 gene (17p13)	L	L	L	-
Rb gene (13q13)	L	LL	LL	-
PTEN gene (10q24)	-	-	-	LL
Chromosome 9p21 (CDKN2A/Band p14 gene)	-	L	L	L
Chromosome 22q	L	L	L	-
Chromosome 19q	L	L	L	-
Chromosome 6q	-	L	L	-
Chromosome 17p13.3	-	L	L	?
hMLH1 gene (3p22)	LL	-	L	?
hMSH2 gene (2p21)	L	-	L	?
hFAT gene (4q34-35)	L	-	L	?
Amplification/overexpression of oncogene/growth factors				
PDGF/PDGFR	G	G	G	-
FGF2	G	GG	GG	-
CNGF	G	G	G	-
Chromosome 12q (CDK4, MDM2, GLI)	-	G	GG	-
EGFR (7p12)	-	-	G	G
IL13R	-	-	G	G
c-*myc*	G	G	G	G
hMSH2	G	-	GG	-
hMLH1	G	-	G	-

literature. They were also able to identify new genes with distinct patterns in low and high grade tumors such as FOXG1B (also known as Brain factor-1 is a putative oncogene) and FOXM1 which encode for the proteins fork head box G1B and fork head box M1, respectively. These were observed to be greatly increased in GBM. Sallinen et al [17] also used a cDNA microarray to identify more than 200 gene expression alterations from glioblastomas, whereas relatively few changes were reported by them in grade II and grade III tumors. The most distinct progression-related expression change was the up-regulation of the insulin-like growth factor binding protein 2 (IGFBP2) gene and also of vimentin. They also conducted a high-density tissue microarray of 418 brain tumors constructed for clinical validation of gene expression changes. Godard et al [18] performed cDNA-array analysis of 53 patient biopsies, comprising low-grade astrocytoma, secondary glioblastoma (respective recurrent high-grade tumors), and newly diagnosed primary glioblastoma. They observed that low-grade astrocytoma have the most specific and similar expression profiles, whereas primary glioblastoma exhibit much larger variation between tumors. Secondary glioblastoma display features of both other groups. They have tried to comprehensively sort their data into those that: (a) can be associated with specific biological functions; and (b) can effectively differentiate tumor class. One prominent gene cluster discriminating primary versus non-primary glioblastoma comprises mostly genes involved in angiogenesis, including VEGF fms-related tyrosine kinase1 but also IGFBP2, that has not yet been directly linked to angiogenesis. As a verification, they used in situ hybridization demonstrating coexpression of IGFBP2 and VEGF in pseudopalisading cells surrounding tumor necrosis as evidence for a possible involvement of IGFBP2 in angiogenesis. Raza et al [19] used a cDNA microarray to analyze mRNA expression of 588 universal cellular genes in 15 surgically resected human GBM samples with varying degrees of necrosis. Gene expression was correlated with the degree of necrosis using rank correlation coefficients. They also compared the expression of identified genes with their expression in tissue samples from 5 anaplastic astrocytomas (AAs). Their results showed Ras, Akt, TNF-α, NF-αB, apoptosis, procoagulation, and hypoxia may be important to necrogenesis because all of the 26 differentially expressed genes identified had functions associated with these factors. Of the 26 genes that may play a role in necrogenesis, only the ephrin type A receptor 1, prostaglandin E_2 receptor EP4, interleukin 7 receptor subunit, G_1-S-specific cyclin E, and thrombomodulin gene products showed a significant correlation with the process.

Oligonucleotide based array was used by Maher et al [20] to identify some notable genes in GBM, these include EPS15 (1p32), WNT7A (3p26.3-3p24.3), and RASSF3, a RAS association family member (12q14.2), and in loss/deletion MCRs IRF2BP2, an IFN regulatory factor 2 repressor (1q42.2) and MKK4/JNKK1 (6q26). Some notable candidates not previously ascribed to glioblastoma include extracellular signal–regulated kinase (ERK)-8 (8q23-24 amplicon), a novel member of the RAS-mitogen-activated protein kinase family that is activated by a SRC-independent mechanism, and TMPO/LAP2 (12q22 deletion), a protein that anchors Rb in the nucleoskeleton and regulates Rb function.

One of the outputs of Human Genome Project is the beginning of the proteomics era. Identification of sequences has translated into studying global protein patterns of tumors sub-types. Protein signatures provide tremendous potential in early disease detection and also may act as a predictor of drug sensitivity. Proteomic pattern analysis has been greatly facilitated by advances in 2 D electrophoresis analysis, high-throughput mass spectrometry, a recent addition being surface-enhanced laser desorption ionization time-of-flight (SELDI-TOF) analysis. Banerjee et al [21] have used protein chip SELDI-TOF to identify several potential biomarkers in astrocytomas as compared to normal astrocytes. Jiang et al [22] constructed a glioma protein lysate array from 82 different primary glioma tissues, and surveyed the expression and phosphorylation of 46 different proteins involved in signaling pathways of cell proliferation, cell survival, apoptosis, angiogenesis, and cell invasion. They could identify 12 proteins as powerful discriminators between high and low grade gliomas: IBalpha, EGFRpTyr845, AKTpThr308, phosphatidylinositol 3-kinase (PI3K), BadpSer136, insulin-like growth factor binding protein (IGFBP) 2, IGFBP5, matrix metalloproteinase 9 (MMP9), vascular endothelial growth factor (VEGF), phosphorylated retinoblastoma protein (pRB), Bcl-2, and c-Abl. Protein microarray technology thus has the potential to monitor complex intracellular protein expression and to simultaneously study the interaction between proteins and a large number of potential interaction partners.

Global views of cellular function with the help of genomic and proteomic technologies have tremendous potential in quality care and personalization of diagnosis and treatment of patients.

CURENTLY USED MOLECULAR MARKERS IN GLIOMA MANAGEMENT

There are two clear molecular indicators which have been accepted in practice of gliomas management. These are a) LOH at 1p and 19q as a diagnostic and chemosensitivity marker for oligodendrogliomas [23] b) Hypermethylation of MGMT liocus as a predictor of Temozolomide sensitivity/ resistance [24]. However, these cover only a limited subset of tumors and further improvement in molecular sub-classification of gliomas would translate into benefits to the patients.

GENOMIC INSTABILITY IN GLIAL TUMORS

We needed to study a bigger part of the tumor genome and be able to assess the overall genomic instability in comparison to its normal counterpart. A comprehensive estimate of genome wide changes occurring in a tumor cell would provide us an insight into larger fragments which may be deleted or amplified or rearranged in a tumor genome. A more intensive examination of such an analysis wll provides a molecular fingerprint that will distinguish individual cancer through the stages of occurrence, and this is of tremendous significance in heterogenous tumors like gliomas. To address this issue, we have successfully used the robust and reproducible technique of RAPD-PCR to initially assess the changes present in the tumor genome simultaneously at multiple loci.

RAPD Analysis of Tumor Stage: More Clonal Mutations and Extensive Intra-tumor Heterogeneity in DA

Locus non-specific random decamer generates a fingerprinting profile of patient tumor DNA as well as leucocyte DNA. RAPD analyses is done simply on an agarose gel and the technique is quite robust and reproducible. The 10mer RAPD primers are not biased for a locus, and bind randomly throughout the genome. This locus non-specific binding gives a good estimate of overall genome change. A number of such primers (about 15) were used amplification for each tumor DNA and its leucocyte control DNA. The snap frozen tumor was microdissected and every 15th section was histopathologically checked for % tumor cells. Only those microdissected slides with 70% or more of tumor tissue were used for DNA extraction. In our study on of RAPD profiling with 18 primers of 24 gliomas, a number of primers generated a polymorphic profile [25]. We also microdissected chunks of tumor and pooled slides for DNA extraction every 15th section to look for intra-tumor heterogeneity. Our results showed extensive mutations within a tumor with their RAPD profile, more so in low grade DA than in GBM [26]. One of our broad aims was to make a comprehensive quantitative estimation of these changes. This was done in 17 low grade (Grade II, Diffuse Astrocytoma) and 16 high grade (Grade IV, GBM) studied with 15 RAPD primers by two methods of analyses. With both estimations, we observed a significantly greater number of alterations in low grade DA than in the high grade GBM [27].

Higher LOH at Mismatch Repair Gene Locus In Da; Evidence For Accumulation of Mutations

The RAPD data on overall changes being more in DA is strengthened by studies on the heterozygosity status of two common constitutive mismatch repair genes, hMLH1 and hMSH2 in 22 low grade, DA and 21 high grade, GBM. We mostly chose markers which were close to the gene of concern (within 5cM) as well as those further away. One of the hMLH1 markers was intra-genic. Markers in close proximity to these genes would give more information than an overall microsatellite instability study (with markers spread across the genome) which tends to be a consequence of mutations in the genes involved in repair including hMLH1 and hMSH2. Our results showed a significantly higher LOH of hMLH1 gene in DA than in GBM indicating that alterations in hMLH1 may be key to accumulation of mutations in low grade tumors as is proposed by the mutator hypothesis [5].

Validity of Mutator Hypothesis in Glial Tumors

The presence of more mutations in low grade DA is suggestive of the mutator hypothesis given by Loeb [28] which proposes that accumulations of mutations in tumors early on in the stage of progression would prove to be beneficial for tumor growth and accumulation of such 'clonal' mutations does not influence the phenotype of a cell. At a later stage, such mutations would prove to be detrimental to the tumor and so during the course of progression, the tumor might select out certain cells which favor its survival and these would outgrow and in the process select against the pre-existing mutations. Primary human glial tumors hence provide an *in vivo* model for demonstrating the applicability of the mutator hypothesis [5, 26, 27]

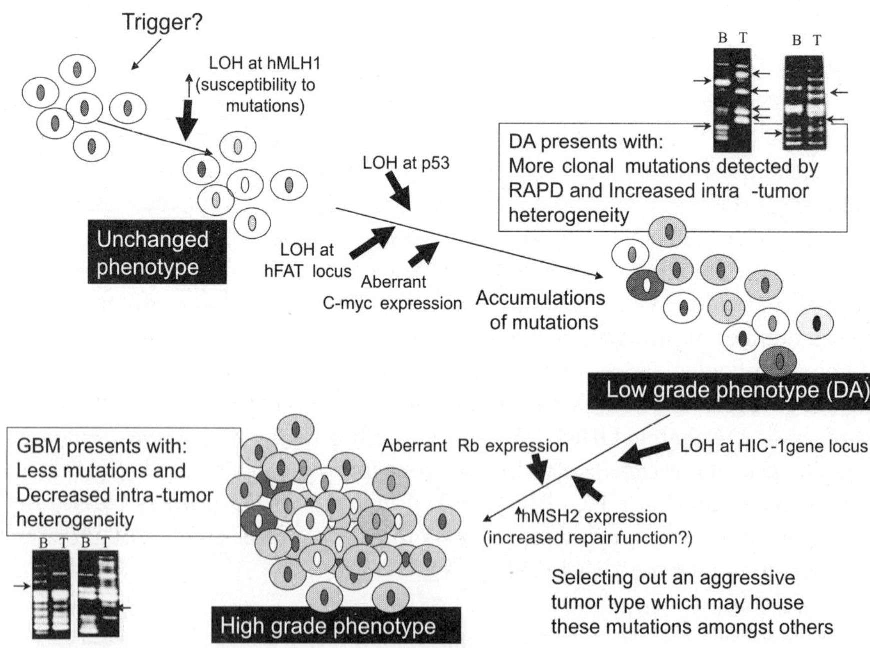

Fig. 24.1

Molecular Perspective of Tumor Classification

Histopathologic evaluations are an indispensable tool in the clinician's armamentarium, but variations of tumor behaviour within a hstological grade not uncommon. These may not take into account some of the unique molecular attributes that determine biological behavior and treatment responsiveness in individual glioma patients. In order to improve glioma classification, recent efforts have been directed to supplementing histopathologic diagnosis with molecular characterization of mutational damage. We have tried to use a two-pronged approach for attempting to elucidate the glial tumorigenic and progression pathway by (1) defining a small number of specific glioma-associated gene alterations and (2) studying the overall changes in tumor DNA. Simultaneous analysis of morphologic features and molecular attributes offers more potential towards significant improvement in glioma diagnosis, prognostication, classification and treatment.

REFERENCES

1. Chosdol K, Chattopadhyay P and Sinha S Molecular pathways of glial tumorigenesis, Curr Sci, 2002, 82 (6); 648-654.
2. Holland, E. C., Gliomagenesis: genetic alterations and mouse models. Nat. Rev. Genet., 2001, **2**, 120-9.
3. Chattopadhyay P, Rathore A, Mathur M, Sarkar C, Mahapatra AK, Sinha S. Loss of heterozygosity of a locus on 17p13.3, independent of p53, is associated with higher grades of astrocytic tumours. Oncogene. 1997 Aug 14;15(7):871-4.
4. Chattopadhyay P, Banerjee M, Sarkar C, Mathur M, Mohapatra AK, Sinha S. Infrequent alteration of the c-myc gene in human glial tumours associated with increased numbers of c-myc positive cells. Oncogene. 1995 Dec 21;11(12):2711-4.
5. Srivastava T, Chosdol K, Chattopadhyay P, Mahapatra AK, Sarkar C, Sinha S. Frequent loss of heterozygosity encompassing the hMLH1 locus in low grade astrocytic tumors. J Neurooncol. 2007 Feb;81(3):249-55.
6. Rathore A Kamarajan P, Mathur M, Sinha S and Sarkar C. Simultaneous alterations of Retinoblastoma and p53 protein expression in astrocytic tumors. Pathol Oncol Res 1999, 5(1): 21-27.
7. Schmidt, E. E., Ichimura, K., Messerle, K. R., Goike, H. M. and Collins, V. P., Infrequent methylation of CDKN2A(MTS1/p16) and rare mutation of both CDKN2A and CDKN2B(MTS2/p15) in primary astrocytic tumours. Br. J. Cancer, 1997, **75**, 2-8.
8. Reifenberger, G., Reifenberger, J., Ichimura, K., Meltzer, P. S., Collins, V. P., Amplification of multiple genes from chromosomal region 12q13-14 in human malignant gliomas: preliminary mapping of the amplicons shows preferential involvement of CDK4, SAS, and MDM2. Cancer Res., 1994, **54**, 4299-303.
9. Forus A, Myklebost O, A physical map of a 1.3-Mb region on the long arm of chromosome 12, spanning the GLI and LRP loci. Genomics, 1992, **14**, 117-20.
10. Ohgaki H, Kleihues P: Genetic Pathways to Primary and Secondary Glioblastoma. *Am J Path.* 2007;170:1445-1453.
11. Fujisawa H, Kurrer M, Reis RM, Yonekawa Y, Kleihues P, Ohgaki H: Acquisition of the glioblastoma phenotype during astrocytoma progression is associated with loss of heterozygosity on 10q 25-qter. Am J Pathol 1999, 155:387-394.

12. Reyes-Mugica, M., Rieger-Christ, K., Ohgaki, H., Ekstrand, B. C., Helie, M., Kleinman, G., Yahanda, A., Fearon, E. R., Kleihues, P., Reale, M. A., Loss of DCC expression and glioma progression. Cancer Res., 1997, **57**, 382-6.

13. Nakamura M, Ishida E, Shimada K, Kishi M, Nakase H, Sakaki T, Konishi N: Frequent LOH on 22q12.3 and TIMP-3 inactivation occur in the progression to secondary glioblastomas. Lab Invest 2005, 85:165-175.

14. Sarkar C, Chattopadhyay P, Ralte AM, Mahapatra AK, Sinha S. Loss of heterozygosity of a locus in chromosomal region 17p13.3 is associated with increased cell proliferation in astrocytic tumors. Cancer genet Cytogenet 144(2): 156-164.

15. Srivastava T, Chattopadhyay P, Mahapatra AK, Sarkar C and Sinha S. Increased hMSH2 Protein Expression in Glioblastoma Multiforme. J Neuro-oncol 2004 Jan 66 (1-2): 51-57.

16. Rickman DS, Bobek MP, Misek DE, Kuick R, Blaivas M, Kurnit DM, Taylor J, Hanash SM. Distinctive Molecular Profiles of High-Grade and Low-Grade Gliomas Based on Oligonucleotide Microarray Analysis. 2001 Cancer Res 61, 6885-6891.

17. Sallinen S, Sallinen PK, Haapasalo HK, Helin HJ, Helén PT, Schraml P, Kallioniemi O, Kononen J. Identification of Differentially Expressed Genes in Human Gliomas by DNA Microarray and Tissue Chip Techniques. 2000. Cancer Res 60, 6617-6622.

18. Godard S, Getz G, Delorenzi M, Farmer P, Kobayashi H, Desbaillets I, Nozaki M, Diserens A, Hamou M, Dietrich P, Regli L, Janzer RC, Bucher P, Stupp R, de Tribolet N, Domany E, Hegi ME. Classification of Human Astrocytic Gliomas on the Basis of Gene Expression: A Correlated Group of Genes with Angiogenic Activity Emerges As a Strong Predictor of Subtypes. Cancer Res 63, 6613-6625.

19. Raza SM, Fuller GN, Rhee CH, Huang S, Hess K, Zhang W, Sawaya R.Identification of Necrosis-Associated Genes in Glioblastoma by cDNA Microarray Analysis. 2004 Clinical Cancer Research Vol. 10, 212-221.

20. Maher EA, Brennan C, Wen PY, Durso L, Ligon KL, Richardson A, Khatry D, Feng B, Sinha R, Louis DN, Quackenbush J, Black P, Chin L, DePinho RA. Marked Genomic Differences Characterize Primary and Secondary Glioblastoma Subtypes and Identify Two Distinct Molecular and Clinical Secondary Glioblastoma Entities. 2006 *Cancer Res* 66, 11502-11513.

21. Banerjee H, Hawkins Z, Williams J, Blackshear M, Sawyer C, Cezares L, Pramanik SK, Williams A. Search for a novel biomarker for the brain cancer astrocytoma by using surface enhanced laser desorption/ionisation (SELDI) technique. 2004 Cell Mol Biol (Noisy-le-grand). Sep;50(6):733-6.

22. Jiang R, Mircean C, Shmulevich I, Cogdell D, Jia Y, Tabus I, Aldape K, Sawaya R, Bruner JM, Fuller GN, Zhang W. Pathway alterations during glioma progression revealed by reverse phase protein lysate arrays. 2006 Proteomics. May;6(10):2964-71.

23. van den Bent M, Chinot OL, Cairncross JG. Recent developments in the molecular characterization and treatment of oligodendroglial tumors. Neuro Oncol. 2003; 5(2):128-38.

24. Hegi ME, Diserens AC, Gorlia T, Hamou MF, de Tribolet N, Weller M, Kros JM, Hainfellner JA, Mason W, Mariani L, Bromberg JE, Hau P, Mirimanoff RO, Cairncross JG, Janzer RC, Stupp R.MGMT gene silencing and benefit from temozolomide in glioblastoma. 2005 N Engl J Med. Mar 10;352(10):997-1003.

25. Dil-Afroze, Misra, A., Sulaiman, I. M., Sinha, S., Sarkar, C., Mahapatra, A. K., Hasnain, S. E., Genetic alterations in brain tumors identified by RAPD analysis. Gene, 1998, 206, 45-8.

26. Misra, A., Chattopadhyay, P., Dinda, A. K., Sarkar, C., Mahapatra, A. K., Hasnain, S. E., Sinha, S., Extensive intra-tumor heterogeneity in primary human glial tumors as a result of locus non-specific genomic alterations. J. Neurooncol., 2000, 48, 1-12.

27. Misra A, Chattopadhyay P, Chosdol K, Sarkar C, Mahapatra AK and Sinha S.Clonal mutations in primary human glial tumors: evidence in support of the mutator hypothesis. BMC Cancer.

28. Loeb, L. A., Many Mutations in Cancers, in Tooze, J., Franks, L. M., Sinclair, C. E., Lindahl, T., eds., Cancer Surveys, Genetic Instability in Cancer, Volume 28, Cold Spring Harbor Laboratory press, 1996, pp. 329-42.

25
CHAPTER

Tumour Microenvironment and Inflammation: Role in Glioblastoma Progression

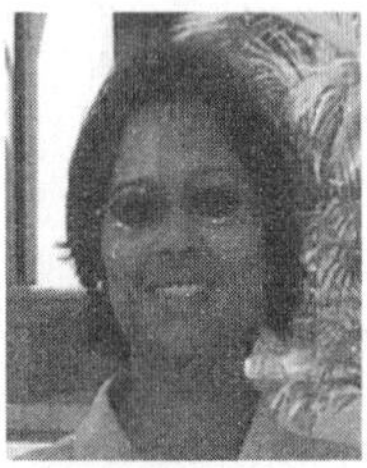

Vivek Sharma and Ellora Sen*

National Brain Research Centre, Manesar, Haryana 122 050

ABSTRACT

Gliomas of astrocytic, oligodendroglial and ependymal origin are the most common type of primary central nervous system (CNS) neoplasm accounting for more than 70% of all brain tumors. Among the gliomas, astrocytoma is the most common type of brain cancer constituting more than half of all brain tumors. Glioblastoma multiformes (GBM) represents the most common and malignant astrocytoma characterized by intense proliferation and widespread invasion of poorly differentiated cells. Primarily because of its diffuse nature, there is no effective treatment for GBM and despite current advances in therapy, the morbidity and mortality of GBM remain very high (1).

Emerging evidences indicate that inflammation contributes to initiation and/or propagation of a wide range of cancers (2, 3). The increased presence of pro-inflammatory mediators in the tumor microenvironment plays a major factor in inducing malignancy (4). Chronic inflammation results in up-regulation of various cytokines, including interleukin-1 (IL-1α/ß), interferon (IFN-α), and tumor necrosis factor (TNF-) in inflammatory cells. These nonspecific pro-inflammatory cytokines induce expression of pro-inflammatory mediators, including cyclooxygenase-2 (COX-2) (5). In addition, pro-inflammatory cytokines acts as a tumour promoter by regulating cascade of cytokines, chemokines, adhesions, matrix metalloproteinases (MMPs) and pro-angiogenic activities (7). A complex network of chemokines and their receptors also influences the development of primary tumors and metastases (6). MMPs promote tumour progression, activate angiogenesis and mediate many of the actions of inflammatory cells in neoplasms (8, 9). Perhaps the best evidence for the significance of inflammation during neoplastic progression comes from study that nonsteroidal anti-inflammatory drugs (NSAIDs) inhibit COX; involved in inducing inflammatory reactions in damaged tissues, which underlies one of their mechanism of chemoprevention (3).

Chronic inflammatory processes produce an excess of reactive oxygen species (ROS) and DNA-reactive aldehydes from lipid peroxidation, which can modify cellular macromolecules and drive to malignancy. Most cancer cells are under oxidative stress associated with increased metabolic activity and production of ROS (7) which has been shown to induce oxidative damage to DNA directly are capable of damaging proteins involved in DNA repair (8). A possible role for pro-inflammatory cytokines in DNA damage and regulation of stability of chromosomes has also been reported (9). In addition, inflammation affects the activity of drug transporters responsible for the systemic disposition of lipophilic and amphipathic drugs, thereby potentially altering the pharmacokinetics of drugs that are substrates of drug transporters (14). Therefore, it is clearly evident that inflammation is a critical component in tumor progression.

Increased expression of pro-inflammatory mediators has been implicated as a possible prognostic indicator in GBM and to play a role in tissue edema and angiogenesis in GBM (10). Hypoxia-inducible factor-1 (HIF-1?) involved in controlling the expression of several genes implicated in angiogenesis, metabolism and cell survival is over expressed in GBM, and HIF-1.? expression level correlates with the highest grade of malignancy. As both HIF-1? and inflammation play critical role in GBM progression, the effect of pro-inflammatory cytokines on the expression of HIF-1?? and its target genes such as vascular endothelial growth factor (VEGF), inducible nitric oxide synthetase (iNOS), and COX-2, in GBM is being investigation. It is increasingly becoming clear that anti-inflammatory therapy is efficacious towards neoplastic progression and malignant conversion. GBM remains one of the most challenging solid cancers to treat due to its highly proliferative, angiogenic and invasive nature. As the causal relationship between inflammation and cancer is widely accepted, our studies aim to provide insight into how GBM aggressiveness is regulated by inflammation and to evaluate the potential of novel therapeutics as anti-inflammatory therapeutic approaches to glioblastoma treatment.

REFERENCES

1. Surawicz TS, Davis F, Freels S, Laws ER, Jr., Menck HR. Brain tumor survival: results from the National Cancer Data Base. J Neurooncol 1998;40(2):151-60.
2. Beachy PA, Karhadkar SS, Berman DM. Tissue repair and stem cell renewal in carcinogenesis. Nature 2004;432(7015):324-31.
3. Pikarsky E, Porat RM, Stein I, *et al.* NF-kappaB functions as a tumour promoter in inflammation-associated cancer. Nature 2004;431(7007):461-6.
4. Coussens LM, Werb Z. Inflammation and cancer. Nature 2002;420(6917):860-7.
5. Dubois RN, Abramson SB, Crofford L, *et al.* Cyclooxygenase in biology and disease. Faseb J 1998;12(12):1063-73.

6. Balkwill F. Cancer and the chemokine network. Nature reviews 2004;4(7):540-50.
7. Szatrowski TP, Nathan CF. Production of large amounts of hydrogen peroxide by human tumor cells. Cancer research 1991;51(3):794-8.
8. Jaiswal M, LaRusso NF, Burgart LJ, Gores GJ. Inflammatory cytokines induce DNA damage and inhibit DNA repair in cholangiocarcinoma cells by a nitric oxide-dependent mechanism. Cancer research 2000;60(1):184-90.
9. Higashimoto T, Panopoulos A, Hsieh CL, Zandi E. TNFalpha induces chromosomal abnormalities independent of ROS through IKK, JNK, p38 and caspase pathways. Cytokine 2006;34(1-2):39-50.
10. Chang CY, Li MC, Liao SL, Huang YL, Shen CC, Pan HC. Prognostic and clinical implication of IL-6 expression in glioblastoma multiforme. J Clin Neurosci 2005;12(8):930-3.

26

CHAPTER

Seeding the Discovery and Development of New Drugs for Advanced-Stage Cancers

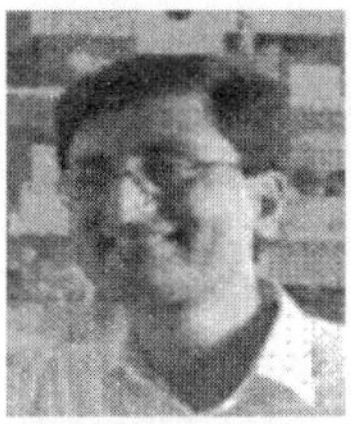

Ashok R. Venkitaraman

University of Cambridge School of Clinical Medicine,
The Cambridge Molecular Therapeutics Programme and
The Medical Research Council Cancer Cell Unit, Hutchison/
MRC Research Centre, Hills Road, Cambridge CB2 0XZ, UK.

ABSTRACT

The discovery, and early clinical development, of new drugs for advanced stage malignancies is widely acknowledged to be a major priority, but the process is beset with challenges that make it difficult, expensive and protracted. One key challenge is the limited repertoire of molecular targets that have successfully been 'drugged', including enzymes like protein kinases or G-protein-coupled receptors. When compared with the large number of molecular targets that have been implicated in cancer, it has been estimated that over 95% of new drugs are being made against less than 5% of the potential targets.

Most clinically validated opportunities for the treatment of cancer involve molecules classed as novel or difficult targets for small molecule therapeutics. These include atypical enzymes, protein–protein interactions that form macromolecular complexes, or tertiary nucleic acid structures. These targets are generally inaccessible to conventional methods for lead identification based on combinatorial chemistry and high-throughput screening using assays of target activity. Although targets involved in macromolecular interactions may appear intractable, recent work highlights many examples containing well-defined structural features that are attractive candidates for modulation by specific, potent drugs. However, robust approaches to lead discovery for these difficult targets remain to be developed.

The Cambridge Molecular Therapeutics Programme (CMTP) is a recently established multi-disciplinary initiative at the University of Cambridge, one of whose key aims is to pioneer new methods for the discovery of small-molecule leads against novel or difficult targets, through the development of inventive enabling technologies, including fragment-based screening, chemical genetics and biophysical assays. In fragment-based screening, small fragments (rather than complete drug molecules) are soaked into crystals of the target protein to identify the site and nature of the binding interaction, and this information is used in the design and synthesis of the next generation of inhibitors. This approach provides a wealth of information about protein–ligand interactions. Structural determination of the macromolecular target also allows *in silico* screening of libraries of chemical fragments by computational modelling, as well as their design and elaboration by diversity-oriented chemical synthesis.

A second key challenge is the high attrition rate of investigational new drugs in Phase II trials of efficacy, even after the successful completion of Phase I trials of safety. This arises largely from the difficulty in selecting the appropriate combination in which to trial investigational agents, and from the difficulty in selecting the clinical (or genetic) features of patients who are most likely to benefit.

Work in the CMTP seeks to meet this challenge through the development of innovative mechanisms to guide the better design of clinical trials to test new drugs in patients, and to identify 'biomarkers' which help to distinguish patients most likely to benefit from the new treatments.

A clear example of this approach is emerging from our recent work. Taxanes, including paclitaxel and docetaxel, are amongst the most successful agents currently used for the treatment of advanced-stage cancers. They act as anti-mitotics by inhibiting the dynamic instability of the microtubules of the mitotic spindle, which is essential for the segregation of chromosomes to daughter cells during mitotic cell division. The resistance of many cancers to taxane therapy represents an important clinical challenge.

We reasoned that genetic alterations in cancer cells might contribute to taxane resistance. One of the most common genetic alterations found in epithelial malignancies of tissues like the breast, ovary, pancreas, colon or prostate involves the over-expression of the protein Aurora-A. Aurora-A is a protein serine-threonine kinase, whose activity in normal cells is restricted to mitosis, and is essential for progression through mitotic cell division. Aurora-A over-expression at the protein level has been documented in as many as 10-60% of common epithelial cancers.

We have used retrovirus-mediated gene transfer to recapitulate in vitro the over-expression of Aurora-A at levels found in cancer cells. Over-expression leads, as previously reported by us and others, to the formation of abnormal numbers of centrosomes, and the seeding from them of multi-polar or otherwise structurally aberrant mitotic spindle microtubules.

We have found using deconvolution confocal microscopy that Aurora-A over-expression leads to the frequent failure of microtubule attachment to the kinetochores of condensed chromosomes during the metaphase of mitotic division. Normally, failure of kinetochore-microtubule attachments activates the mitotic checkpoint for spindle assembly, which triggers an arrest in progression at the metaphase-anaphase transition.

Remarkably, we find that Aurora-A overexpression over-rides the mitotic spindle assembly checkpoint, and cells continue to progress into anaphase despite the failure of kinetochore-microtubule attachments. We reasoned that this characteristic elicited by Aurora-A overexpression might lead to taxane resistance, since taxanes induce their cytotoxic effects on cancer cells by activating the mitotic spindle assembly checkpoint. Consistent with our proposal, Aurora-A overexpressing cells demonstrate resistance to apoptosis induced by paclitaxel at therapeutically relevant concentrations.

These data suggest first that Aurora-A overexpression in cancers is a biomarker for resistance to taxanes and other anti-mitotic drugs, and second, that investigational new drugs which inhibit Aurora kinase activity might enter clinical trials of efficacy in combination with taxanes. These principles, now tested in preliminary studies on human patients, are now being used to formulate a new type of 'proof-of-concept' clinical trial design in which to test the efficacy of an investigational small-molecule inhibitor of Aurora kinase activity in combination with paclitaxel for the treatment of advanced-stage cancers.

Index